Mycotoxins in Feed and Food Chain

Mycotoxins in Feed and Food Chain

Present Status and Future Concerns

Editor

Filippo Rossi

MDPI • Basel • Beijing • Wuhan • Barcelona • Belgrade • Manchester • Tokyo • Cluj • Tianjin

Editor
Filippo Rossi
Catholic University
Italy

Editorial Office
MDPI
St. Alban-Anlage 66
4052 Basel, Switzerland

This is a reprint of articles from the Special Issue published online in the open access journal *Toxins* (ISSN 2072-6651) (available at: https://www.mdpi.com/journal/toxins/special_issues/mycotoxins_feed_food_chain).

For citation purposes, cite each article independently as indicated on the article page online and as indicated below:

LastName, A.A.; LastName, B.B.; LastName, C.C. Article Title. *Journal Name* **Year**, *Article Number*, Page Range.

ISBN 978-3-03936-874-7 (Hbk)
ISBN 978-3-03936-875-4 (PDF)

Contents

About the Editor vii

Filippo Rossi
A Long Road to Safer Food
Reprinted from: *Toxins* **2020**, *12*, 453, doi:10.3390/toxins12070453 1

Patricia A. Quevedo-Garza, Genaro G. Amador-Espejo, Rogelio Salas-García, Esteban G. Ramos-Peña and Antonio-José Trujillo
Aflatoxin M_1 Determination in Infant Formulae Distributed in Monterrey, Mexico
Reprinted from: *Toxins* **2020**, *12*, 100, doi:10.3390/toxins12020100 3

Andrea Zentai, Mária Szeitzné-Szabó, Gábor Mihucz, Nóra Szeli, András Szabó and Melinda Kovács
Occurrence and Risk Assessment of Fumonisin B_1 and B_2 Mycotoxins in Maize-Based Food Products in Hungary
Reprinted from: *Toxins* **2019**, *11*, 709, doi:10.3390/toxins11120709 11

Jianhua Wang, Shuangxia Wang, Zhiyong Zhao, Shanhai Lin, François Van Hove and Aibo Wu
Species Composition and Toxigenic Potential of *Fusarium* Isolates Causing Fruit Rot of Sweet Pepper in China
Reprinted from: *Toxins* **2019**, *11*, 690, doi:10.3390/toxins11120690 25

Hamed K. Abbas, Nacer Bellaloui, Cesare Accinelli, James R. Smith and W. Thomas Shier
Toxin Production in Soybean (*Glycine max* L.) Plants with Charcoal Rot Disease and by *Macrophomina phaseolina*, the Fungus that Causes the Disease
Reprinted from: *Toxins* **2019**, *11*, 645, doi:10.3390/toxins11110645 39

Hamed K. Abbas, Nacer Bellaloui, Alemah M. Butler, Justin L. Nelson, Mohamed Abou-Karam and W. Thomas Shier
Phytotoxic Responses of Soybean (*Glycine max* L.) to Botryodiplodin, a Toxin Produced by the Charcoal Rot Disease Fungus, *Macrophomina phaseolina*
Reprinted from: *Toxins* **2020**, *12*, 25, doi:10.3390/toxins12010025 53

Miroslav Flieger, Eva Stodůlková, Stephen A. Wyka, Jan Černý, Valéria Grobárová, Kamila Píchová, Petr Novák, Petr Man, Marek Kuzma, Ladislav Cvak, Kirk D. Broders and Miroslav Kolařík
Ergochromes: Heretofore Neglected Side of Ergot Toxicity
Reprinted from: *Toxins* **2019**, *11*, 439, doi:10.3390/toxins11080439 69

Nathan Meijer, Geert Stoopen, H.J. van der Fels-Klerx, Joop J.A. van Loon, John Carney and Guido Bosch
Aflatoxin B_1 Conversion by Black Soldier Fly (*Hermetia illucens*) Larval Enzyme Extracts
Reprinted from: *Toxins* **2019**, *11*, 532, doi:10.3390/toxins11090532 85

Paola Giorni, Umberto Rolla, Marco Romani, Annalisa Mulazzi and Terenzio Bertuzzi
Efficacy of Azoxystrobin on Mycotoxins and Related Fungi in Italian Paddy Rice
Reprinted from: *Toxins* **2019**, *11*, 310, doi:10.3390/toxins11060310 97

Guro Brodal, Heidi Udnes Aamot, Marit Almvik and Ingerd Skow Hofgaard
Removal of Small Kernels Reduces the Content of *Fusarium* Mycotoxins in Oat Grain
Reprinted from: *Toxins* **2020**, *12*, 346, doi:10.3390/toxins12050346 107

Amritha Johny, Christiane Kruse Fæste, André S. Bogevik, Gerd Marit Berge, Jorge M.O. Fernandes and Lada Ivanova
Development and Validation of a Liquid Chromatography High-Resolution Mass Spectrometry Method for the Simultaneous Determination of Mycotoxins and Phytoestrogens in Plant-Based Fish Feed and Exposed Fish
Reprinted from: *Toxins* **2019**, *11*, 222, doi:10.3390/toxins11040222 . . . . **127**

Sara Ahlberg, Delia Randolph, Sheila Okoth and Johanna Lindahl
Aflatoxin Binders in Foods for Human Consumption—Can This be Promoted Safely and Ethically?
Reprinted from: *Toxins* **2019**, *11*, 410, doi:10.3390/toxins11070410 . . . . **149**

Madhu Kamle, Dipendra K. Mahato, Sheetal Devi, Kyung Eun Lee, Sang G. Kang and Pradeep Kumar
Fumonisins: Impact on Agriculture, Food, and Human Health and their Management Strategies
Reprinted from: *Toxins* **2019**, *11*, 328, doi:10.3390/toxins11060328 . . . . **161**

Francesco Crudo, Elisabeth Varga, Georg Aichinger, Gianni Galaverna, Doris Marko, Chiara Dall'Asta and Luca Dellafiora
Co-Occurrence and Combinatory Effects of *Alternaria* Mycotoxins and Other Xenobiotics of Food Origin: Current Scenario and Future Perspectives
Reprinted from: *Toxins* **2019**, *11*, 640, doi:10.3390/toxins11110640 . . . . **185**

About the Editor

Filippo Rossi was born in Piacenza (1963) and graduated in Agricultural Sciences in 1989 (Catholic University, of Piacenza, Italy). In 1992, the Italian Ministry of Research awarded him with a Ph.D. in Molecular Biotechnology. Since 1993, he has been working at the Department of Food Science and Nutrition of the Faculty of Agricultural Sciences in Piacenza, where he is in charge of the Human Nutrition course in the Food Science and Technology degree. His research interests cover the role of food in the prevention of noncommunicable disease, particularly Mediterranean Diet and breast cancer, mycotoxins and liver cancer, dairy foods and hypertension, and starch digestion and obesity. Since 2004 (EU fundend project "Safe Food"), he has been involved in research regarding the prevention of mycotoxins contamination in the feed and food chain.

toxins

MDPI

Editorial

A Long Road to Safer Food

Filippo Rossi

Section of Food Science and Nutrition, Department of Animal Sciences, Food and Nutrition, Faculty of Agricultural, Food and Environmental Sciences, Catholic University of Sacred Heart, Via Emilia Parmense 84, 29122 Piacenza, Italy; filippo.rossi@unicatt.it

Received: 17 June 2020; Accepted: 10 July 2020; Published: 14 July 2020

As a side effect of food production, mycotoxins have always accompanied humanity, even if the danger posed by these molecules has only recently been understood and new research has begun to identify and study ways to reduce their presence in food.

This Special Issue of *Toxins* includes papers on new findings concerning well-known mycotoxins, results of studies regarding emerging mycotoxins, such as alternaria and botryodiplodin, and new techniques to reduce mycotoxin contamination in processed cereals.

Reliable data on the presence of mycotoxins in food is very important in the toxicological evaluation of the risk associated with these toxic fungal compounds. Two papers cover this subject: Quevedo-Garza et al. [1] analyze Mexican infant formula food for aflatoxin M1 and Zentai et al. [2] determine the fumonisins in Hungarian maize-based food.

Fusarium spp., together with *Aspergillus* spp., are the most relevant fungi genus responsible for mycotoxin production. Researchers have focused their attention on cereals, while neglecting other crops. A paper from a Chinese group reports on the identification of the *Fusarium* species causing sweet pepper fruit rot and on the kinds of mycotoxins produced by these microorganisms [3].

A new toxic molecule produced by a fungal parasite of soybean is the focus of two papers from Abbas et al. who investigate the production of botryodiplodin [4] and its toxicity [5], while another contribution [6] considers secalonic acids, which are the main ergot ergochromes in overall ergot toxicity.

We have observed not only the appearance of new or emerging mycotoxins, but also of new foods, such as insects, that can also be contaminated by mycotoxins. On this topic, a paper in this Special Issue studies the metabolism of aflatoxin B1 in the larvae of the black soldier fly (*Hermetia illucens*) [7].

The reduction of mycotoxin contamination can be obtained by intervening during the cultivation or storage of products. Research carried out by Giorni et al. [8] tested the efficacy of the fungicide azoxystrobin on fungal parasites of rice and obtained a strong reduction (−67%) of sterigmatocystin while deoxynivalenol remained unaffected.

A clear reduction in *Fusarium*-produced toxins can be observed in the paper of Brodal et al. [9], by sieving oat grains and removing broken kernels, which are more contaminated than intact ones.

The last research article of the Special Issue describes an analytical method for the detection of 19 mycotoxins and three phytoestrogens in fish feed and fish meat [10]. The reduction of the risk posed to human health by mycotoxins requires the development and validation of reliable methods to monitor mycotoxins in feed and food.

The three reviews included in the Special Issue cover as many topics. Issues related to the use of lactic acid bacteria as aflatoxin binders in developing countries are discussed in the review of Ahlberg et al [11]. Kamle et al. [12] summarize the effect of fumonisin on human health and the strategies to reduce the level of this toxin in food. A group of emerging mycotoxins, those produced by *Alternaria*, is the focus of Crudo et al [13], who analyze "the most relevant data concerning the occurrence and toxicity of mycotoxins produced by *Alternaria* spp., (....) alone or in combination with other mycotoxins and bioactive food constituents".

In conclusion, all the contributions to this Special Issue expand our current knowledge and, as Guest Editor, I am happy and proud to present this issue to the community of scientists involved in research on mycotoxins.

All research and review articles proposing novelties and overviews, respectively, were successfully and carefully selected for this Special Issue after rigorous revision by the expert peer reviewers. As the Guest Editor, I would like to express my deep appreciation to all the selfless and fair reviewers.

Acknowledgments: The editor would like to thank all the authors who contributed to this Special Issue and the reviewers for their evaluation work. The editor is also grateful to the MDPI management team for their valuable support.

Conflicts of Interest: The author declares no conflict of interest.

References

1. Quevedo-Garza, P.A.; Amador-Espejo, G.G.; Salas-García, R.; Ramos-Peña, E.G.; Trujillo, A.-J. Aflatoxin M_1 Determination in Infant Formulae Distributed in Monterrey, Mexico. *Toxins* **2020**, *12*, 100. [CrossRef] [PubMed]
2. Zentai, A.; Szeitzné-Szabó, M.; Mihucz, G.; Szeli, N.; Szabó, A.; Kovács, M. Occurrence and Risk Assessment of Fumonisin B_1 and B_2 Mycotoxins in Maize-Based Food Products in Hungary. *Toxins* **2019**, *11*, 709. [CrossRef] [PubMed]
3. Wang, J.; Wang, S.; Zhao, Z.; Lin, S.; Van Hove, F.; Wu, A. Species Composition and Toxigenic Potential of *Fusarium* Isolates Causing Fruit Rot of Sweet Pepper in China. *Toxins* **2019**, *11*, 690. [CrossRef] [PubMed]
4. Abbas, H.K.; Bellaloui, N.; Accinelli, C.; Smith, J.R.; Shier, W.T. Toxin Production in Soybean (*Glycine max* L.) Plants with Charcoal Rot Disease and by *Macrophomina phaseolina*, the Fungus that Causes the Disease. *Toxins* **2019**, *11*, 645. [CrossRef] [PubMed]
5. Abbas, H.K.; Bellaloui, N.; Butler, A.M.; Nelson, J.L.; Abou-Karam, M.; Shier, W.T. Phytotoxic Responses of Soybean (*Glycine max* L.) to Botryodiplodin, a Toxin Produced by the Charcoal Rot Disease Fungus, *Macrophomina phaseolina*. *Toxins* **2020**, *12*, 25. [CrossRef] [PubMed]
6. Flieger, M.; Stodůlková, E.; Wyka, S.A.; Černý, J.; Grobárová, V.; Píchová, K.; Novák, P.; Man, P.; Kuzma, M.; Cvak, L.; et al. Ergochromes: Heretofore Neglected Side of Ergot Toxicity. *Toxins* **2019**, *11*, 439. [CrossRef] [PubMed]
7. Meijer, N.; Stoopen, G.; van der Fels-Klerx, H.; van Loon, J.J.; Carney, J.; Bosch, G. Aflatoxin B_1 Conversion by Black Soldier Fly (*Hermetia illucens*) Larval Enzyme Extracts. *Toxins* **2019**, *11*, 532. [CrossRef] [PubMed]
8. Giorni, P.; Rolla, U.; Romani, M.; Mulazzi, A.; Bertuzzi, T. Efficacy of Azoxystrobin on Mycotoxins and Related Fungi in Italian Paddy Rice. *Toxins* **2019**, *11*, 310. [CrossRef] [PubMed]
9. Brodal, G.; Aamot, H.U.; Almvik, M.; Hofgaard, I.S. Removal of Small Kernels Reduces the Content of *Fusarium* Mycotoxins in Oat Grain. *Toxins* **2020**, *12*, 346. [CrossRef] [PubMed]
10. Johny, A.; Fæste, C.K.; Bogevik, A.S.; Berge, G.M.; Fernandes, J.M.; Ivanova, L. Development and Validation of a Liquid Chromatography High-Resolution Mass Spectrometry Method for the Simultaneous Determination of Mycotoxins and Phytoestrogens in Plant-Based Fish Feed and Exposed Fish. *Toxins* **2019**, *11*, 222. [CrossRef] [PubMed]
11. Ahlberg, S.; Randolph, D.; Okoth, S.; Lindahl, J. Aflatoxin Binders in Foods for Human Consumption—Can This be Promoted Safely and Ethically? *Toxins* **2019**, *11*, 410. [CrossRef] [PubMed]
12. Kamle, M.; Mahato, D.K.; Devi, S.; Lee, K.E.; Kang, S.G.; Kumar, P. Fumonisins: Impact on Agriculture, Food, and Human Health and their Management Strategies. *Toxins* **2019**, *11*, 328. [CrossRef] [PubMed]
13. Crudo, F.; Varga, E.; Aichinger, G.; Galaverna, G.; Marko, D.; Dall'Asta, C.; Dellafiora, L. Co-Occurrence and Combinatory Effects of *Alternaria* Mycotoxins and Other Xenobiotics of Food Origin: Current Scenario and Future Perspectives. *Toxins* **2019**, *11*, 640. [CrossRef] [PubMed]

toxins

MDPI

Article

Aflatoxin M_1 Determination in Infant Formulae Distributed in Monterrey, Mexico

Patricia A. Quevedo-Garza [1], Genaro G. Amador-Espejo [2], Rogelio Salas-García [1], Esteban G. Ramos-Peña [1] and Antonio-José Trujillo [3,*]

1 Facultad de Salud Pública y Nutrición, Universidad Autónoma de Nuevo León, Monterrey 64460, N.L.; Mexico; patricia.quevedog@uanl.mx (P.A.Q.-G.); rogelio.salasg@uanl.mx (R.S.-G.); esteban.ramosp@uanl.mx (E.G.R.-P.)

2 CONACYT–Centro de Investigación en Biotecnología Aplicada-IPN, Ex-Hacienda San Juan Molino Carretera Estatal Tecuexcomac, Tlaxcala 90700, Mexico; genaroamador2014@gmail.com

3 Centre d'Innovació, Recerca i Transferència en Tecnologia dels Aliments (CIRTTA), TECNIO-UAB, MALTA-Consolider Team, Departament de Ciència Animal i dels Aliments, Facultat de Veterinària, Universitat Autònoma de Barcelona, 08193 Bellaterra, Spain

* Correspondence: toni.trujillo@uab.es

Received: 27 December 2019; Accepted: 31 January 2020; Published: 4 February 2020

Abstract: The occurrence of aflatoxin M_1 (AFM_1) in infant formulae commercialized in the metropolitan area of Monterrey (Nuevo León, Mexico) was determined by using immunoaffinity column clean-up followed by HPLC determination with fluorimetric detection. For this, 55 infant formula powders were classified in two groups, starter (49 samples) and follow-on (6 samples) formulae. Eleven of the evaluated samples (20%) presented values above the permissible limit set by the European Union for infant formulae (25 ng/L), ranging from 40 to 450 ng/L. The estimated daily intake (EDI) for AFM_1 was determined employing the average body weight (bw) of the groups of age in the ranges of 0–6 and 6–12 months, and 1–2 years. The results evidenced high intake values, ranging from 1.56 to 14 ng/kg bw/day, depending on the group. Finally, with the EDI value, the carcinogenic risk index was determined, presenting a high risk for all the evaluated groups. Based on these results, it is a necessary extra effort by the regulatory agencies to reduce the AFM_1 presence in infant formulae consumed in Mexico.

Keywords: AMF_1; infant formulae; estimated daily intake; carcinogenic risk index; Monterrey (Mexico)

Key Contribution: Aflatoxin B_1 can be metabolized by mammals to aflatoxin M_1 (AFM_1), a form that retains potent carcinogenicity and which can be excreted into milk. There is scarce information on the occurrence of AFM_1 in milk and dairy products, and no data are available in Mexico concerning infant formulae contamination by this mycotoxin. The results of the present study further demonstrate the potential risk for the infant population associated with the AFM_1 presence in the infant formulae marketed in Monterrey (Mexico).

1. Introduction

Aflatoxins' presence in food products is one of the major health concerns of the regulatory agencies around the world. These toxins include around 20 metabolites produced by molds such as *Aspergillus flavus* and *A. parasiticus*, which is the most important of the aflatoxin B_1 (AFB_1) and is normally found in foods, especially those having high carbohydrate and/or fat contents [1]. Its occurrence has been reported in numerous food and feedstuff, including cereals and cereal-derived products [2].

Cattle feed with contaminated crops of AFB_1 may lead to the formation of a hydroxylated metabolite named aflatoxin M_1 (AFM_1), which is excreted in the milk of lactating animals and whose name is due to the source detected [3]. Numerous researchers have reported a linear relationship of about 0.3–6.2% between the amount of AFM_1 detected in milk and AFB_1 in feed consumed by the animals [4]. Nevertheless, the percent of AFM_1 excreted depends on various factors, including concentration of AFB_1 in feed, milk yield, stage of lactation and breed [5].

Even though AFM_1, the main monohydroxylated derivate of AFB_1, presents less carcinogenic and mutagenic activity than AFB_1, it exhibits a high level of genotoxic activity and certainly represents a health risk because of its elevated possibility of accumulation and binding to DNA [6]. Based on this, different health agencies such as the World Health Organization and the International Agency for Research on Cancer (IARC) have published articles in which AFM_1 is a strong genotoxic and hepatotoxic agent [7]. Therefore, AFM_1 has been evaluated as a possible human carcinogen agent, and although until 2002 it was classified in the 2B Group, with a tolerable daily intake (TDI) of 2 ng/kg bw [8], based on numerous scientific evidence that demonstrated carcinogenic and other (teratogenic, genotoxic and immunosuppressive) effects, it was reclassified into the first group [7].

Hence, the elimination of risk sources represents a major assignment for government agencies and food processors, not only for the contaminated products directly consumed by humans but also in feeding cattle that consume contaminated crops, whose products can reach the human being. Government regulations around the world concerning AFM_1 limits differ from one other. The lowest AFM_1 concentration was approved by the European Union (EU) and the Codex Alimentarius, fixing a maximum admissible level of 50 ng/L in fluid milk and dried or processed milk products [9,10]. On the contrary, higher AFM_1 concentrations (500 ng/L) are permitted in the United States of America (USA) and some Latin American countries (such as Mexico and the MERCOSUR agreement), and China allows a maximum limit of 62.5 ng/L [11–14]. However, because of the higher susceptibility of infants to AFM_1, the EU and the Codex Alimentarius fixed the maximum admissible level of 25 ng/L for infant formulae, follow-on formulae and dietary foods for medical purposes intended specifically for infants [9].

Another major problem concerning the presence of AFM_1 in milk is the different dairy products it's included in (e.g., liquid milk, yogurt, cheese, milk powder, ice cream, regular cream, among others) and the fact that the aflatoxin cannot be eliminated by regular heat treatments such as pasteurization or ultra-high temperature processing [15]. Besides, one of the most important products manufactured from milk are the infant formulae, in which there is significant risk of AFM_1 intoxication because small amounts of this toxin in the product may represent an important portion of aflatoxin intake [16].

Despite the danger associated to the AFM_1 presence in milk, only a few articles are available regarding the presence of this toxin in milk and dairy products in Mexico [17,18], and no studies have been published regarding its presence in infant formulae or intake assessment for AFM_1 in the country. Based on this, the aim of this study was to evaluate the AFM_1 occurrence in infant formulae and to estimate the exposure of infant milk consumers to AFM_1 by means of a sampling of the infant formulae brands distributed in Monterrey (Nuevo León, Mexico).

2. Results and Discussion

2.1. Occurrence of AFM_1 in Infant Formulae

Table 1 shows the results obtained from the analyzed samples, with 20% of them being positive for the toxin in a range of 40 to 450 ng/L, and an average AFM_1 concentration of 40 ± 99 ng/L for all analyzed samples, which is higher than the limit established for AFM_1 in infant formulae by the Codex Alimentarius (25 ng/L) [11]. Nevertheless, when the infant formulae were evaluated separately (starter and follow-on groups), it can be observed that the AFM_1 values increased from one group to another. In the starter formulae, the percentage of samples exceeding the AFM_1 limit was 14%, remarkably lower than the percentage of samples above the limit in the follow-on formulae (67%). Furthermore, the media in the starter formulae (20 ± 67 ng/L) was below the EU or Codex Alimentarius AFM_1 limit (25 ng/L), compared to the follow-on formulae, with an average (180 ± 185 ng/L) exceeding the AFM_1 limit. Although the AFM_1 levels in starter formulae were significantly ($p < 0.05$) lower than those in follow-on formulae, it is important to notice the small number of samples evaluated in the follow-on formulae, compared to the infant formula evaluated in the starter group.

Table 1. Aflatoxin M_1 presence in infant formulae.

Infant Formulae	*N*	Positive Samples	AFM_1 (ng/L)	
			Range	Mean ± SD
Total of samples	55	11 (20%) *	0.00–450	40 ± 99
Starter formula	49	7 (14%)	0.00–420	20 ± 67 [b]
Follow-on formula	6	4 (67%)	0.00–450	180 ± 185 [a]

* Value in parentheses indicates the samples percentage above the limit set by the Codex Alimentarius (25 ng/L) with respect to the total. [a,b] Different online letters indicate significant mean differences among the different types of infant formulae ($p < 0.05$).

Regarding legislation about AFM_1 limits in infant formulae, most of the countries do not have an established limit, which is the case of most of the Latin-American countries (including Mexico), which tends to apply the limit established by the Codex Alimentarius or the EU regulation (25 ng/mL) [11,19].

The occurrence of AFM_1 in infant formulae varies in different countries. Gomez-Arranz and Navarro-Blasco [20] evaluated the presence of AFM_1 in infant formulae in Spain, testing 69 samples and detecting the presence of AFM_1 in 26% of them. In this case, all the detected samples were below the EU established limit. More recently, Akhtar et al. [21] determined the AFM_1 presence in infant formulae in Pakistan, evaluating 13 samples, in which 53.84% of the samples were positive to the toxin presence and 30.76% exceeded the EU limit. Kanungo and Bhand [22] evaluated the AFM_1 presence in infant formulae in India, determining that in 72 evaluated samples, all of them were above the EU permitted limit (25 ng/kg) and 75% of the samples exceeded the USA and Indian Food regulation limit (500 ng/kg). Er et al. [4] published a study evaluating the AFM_1 presence in infant formula in Turkey, evaluating 84 samples with only one sample positive for the toxin. In this sense, Li et al. [14] detected the presence of AFM_1 in powder base for infant formulae in China, evaluating a total of 1207 samples, with 56 samples being positive for the toxin without passing the Chinese limit (62.5 ng/kg). Awaisheh et al. [23] determined the AFM_1 content in infant formulae (120 samples; 48 starter and 72 follow-on formulae) distributed in Jordan, with 58 positive samples for the toxin presence, with a media of 69 and 84 ng/kg for the starter and follow-on formulae, respectively.

2.2. *Infant Formulae Daily Intake by Age Group*

The present study is the first evaluation of the daily intake by Mexican minors, based on average consumption and body weight (Table 2). The Mexican Standard NOM-031-SSA2-1999 [24] classifies infants in two groups of infant formulae consumption: i) minor lactating (0–12 months), and ii) major lactating (one to two years). The consumption in these groups is starter and follow-on formulae for the first and the second year, respectively.

Based on the occurrence of AFM_1 in infant formulae and the body weight of infants, the estimated daily intake (EDI) for AFM_1 was in a range of 1.56 to 14 ng/kg bw per day, which represents the values estimated for one year-old infants when they are fed with starter or with follow-on formulae, respectively. However, when major lactating groups gain weight and reduce the follow-on formula intake (i.e., two years old), the EDI is reduced up to 4.28 ng/kg bw/day. Awaisheh et al. [23] have evaluated the infant formulae consumed in Jordan, presenting an EDI of 1.57 and 1.55 ng/kg bw/day for infants aged six and 12 months, respectively. On the other hand, Ismail et al. [25] reported an EDI value of 4.1 ng/kg bw/day for children aged one to three years in Pakistan. It is considerable the work developed by the food agencies seeking to reduce the presence of AFM_1 in milk and infant formulae. In this sense, Oliveira et al. [26] published an article evaluating the presence of AFM_1 in infant formulae in Brazil with a daily intake of 22 ng/kg bw/day. In contrast, almost 20 years later, Ishikawa et al. [27] determined the AFM_1 presence in infant formulae in the same country, presenting an important reduction in EDI values (0.078–0.306 ng/kg bw/day). Likewise, lower EDI values than the present study were detected in infant formulae consumed in Spain (n = 69) (0.02–0.13 ng/kg bw/day) [4]. Further, Ruangwises et al. [28] evaluated AFM_1 presence in milk powder distributed in Thailand (90 samples) showing EDI values of 0.16 ng/kg bw/day in milk consumed by infants up to three years.

Table 2. Estimated aflatoxin M_1 daily intake by average body weight and carcinogenic risk index (CRI) in children population based on the ENSANUT (2012).

Age (years)	Average Body Weight (bw) (kg)	Intake Type	Average Consumption		* CRI (2 ng/kg bw/day)
			Infant Formula Intake Range (L/day)	AFM_1 Intake (ng/kg bw/day)	
0–0.5	3.55–7.3	Starter infant formula	0.78–0.93	4.39–2.55	Risk
0.5–1	7.3–10.8	Starter infant formula	0.93–0.84	2.55–1.56	Risk
1–2	10.8–13.03	Follow-on infant formula	0.84–0.31	14–4.28	Risk

* According to the Kuiper-Goodman equation [8].

Comparing the results of AFM_1 occurrence in infant formulae and in breast milk in Mexico, the results are quite similar. Thereby, Cantú-Cornelio et al. [29] evaluated the presence of AFM_1 in breast milk of nursing mothers in central Mexico (112 samples), with an EDI value of 2.35 ng/kg bw/day, comparable results to the values obtained in the present study. These results show the importance of evaluating the presence of AFB_1 in different products consumed by nursing mothers in order to reduce the toxin that may be transformed into AFM_1 and reach infants by breast milk.

Table 2 also presents the result of the carcinogenic risk index (CRI) for the evaluated population. At this day, up to our knowledge, no CRI study evaluating the infant population of Mexico has been published. The AFM_1 ingestion obtained in this study was greater than the TDI value (2 ng/kg bw/day) calculated by Kuiper-Goodman [8] dividing the TD50 by the safety factor 5000, indicating that there is a potential high risk for liver cancer due to the consumption of infant formulae in Mexican consumers groups studied.

3. Conclusions

The results of the current study have shown a high presence of AFM_1 in infant formulae distributed in the Monterrey (Mexico) metropolitan area. From fifty-five samples evaluated, 20% exhibited a toxin content above the EU and Codex Alimentarius limit (25 ng/L), presenting a range of 40–450 ng/L. Further, in classifying the samples by the type of infant formulae and infant age for consumption (starter formula for minor infants up to one year, and follow-on formula for major infants between one and two years), different levels of AFM_1 were obtained (20 ng/L for starter and 180 ng/L for follow-on formulae). Besides, based on the average body weight of the evaluated groups, the EDI value was calculated, with values in the range of 1.56–14 ng/kg bw/day. Finally, with the EDI data, the CRI was determined, obtaining a result of risk in all the evaluated groups. Based on these results, an important effort should be carried out by the regulatory agencies and milk producers in order to reduce AFM_1 levels in milk in general, and, in particular, in batches that will be employed for infant formulae elaboration because of the high cancer risk associated with AFM_1 presence and the infant consumers' vulnerability.

4. Materials and Methods

4.1. Sample Collection

Fifty-five infant formula samples from drug stores and supermarkets sold in Monterrey (Nuevo León, Mexico) were obtained. From these, 49 were starter formulae (0–12 months) and 6 were follow-on formulae (1–2 years). Among the starter formulae, 6 were pre-term formulae (formulated for prematurely born, regurgitation episodes by immature esophageal sphincter, or low birth weight infants), 11 were hypoallergenic formulae (specialized formula based on casein, whey or soy protein hydrolysates) and 9 were lactose free formulae (designed for lactose intolerant infants based on lactose hydrolysis by β-galactosidase or formulated from soy protein isolates).

All formulae were supplied as powder milks. Infant formula containers (cans or bags) were stored in dark at room temperature until analyses were performed.

4.2. Sample Preparation

Powder-based formula samples were suspended in deionized warm water according to the manufacturer instructions. The method used for sample preparation and AFM_1 determination was that specified by the method ISO 14,501 [30]. Suspended infant formula samples were centrifuged at 4200 × *g* for 15 min to separate and remove the milk fat. Aliquots of skimmed milk (50 mL) were filtered (Whatman no. 4 filter paper) and slowly passed (1–2 drops/s) through an immunoaffinity column (AflaM1 HPLC, VICAM, Milford, MA, USA) fitted on a vacuum manifold, and washed twice with 10 mL of distilled water. Thereafter, the AFM_1 was eluted with 4 mL of acetonitrile, allowing a time contact of at least 60 s. The eluate was collected in amber vials, the solvent was evaporated in a water bath at 40 °C with nitrogen, and the residue reconstituted in water:acetonitrile (67:33) and filtered by Millipore filters (0.45 µm) in amber vials.

4.3. HPLC Analysis

The HPLC analysis was carried out in a Varian HPLC model 9012 (Agilent Technologies, Santa Clara, CA, USA) connected with a fluorescence detector Varian ProStar (Agilent Technologies Santa, Clara, CA, USA). The separation column was a Phenomenex C18 with 4.5 × 250 mm and 5 µm of particle size (Phenomenex, Torrance, CA, USA). Water and acetonitrile mixture were used as a mobile phase in a proportion of 67:33 (v/v), at a flow rate of 1 mL/min, and an injection volume of 100 µL. Fluorometric detection was achieved at 360 nm excitation and 440 nm emission wavelength.

To assess the performance of the analytical method, linearity, limits of detection (LOD) and quantification (LOQ), recovery and precision (repeatability) were studied. Linearity was evaluated using standard calibration curves that were constructed by plotting the peak area versus the analyte concentration. The calibration curves were established using eight levels of concentrations from LOQ to 100 times LOQ. The regression curve obtained was $y = 287.78\,x + 75.10$ giving appropriate value for the linearity ($R^2 = 0.998$). LOD (2 ng/L) and LOQ (5 ng/L) were calculated as the sample blank value plus 3 and 10 times its standard deviation, respectively. In order to determine the recovery, reconstituted milk was added with 3 levels of AFM_1 concentrations (50, 100 and 200 ng/L). The obtained values of recovery were between 83% and 104%. The precision (15.18%) was calculated as repeatability by means of triplicates in each of the levels analyzed in the recovery assay.

4.4. Determination of AFM_1 Exposure in the Population

The determination of the exposure level or estimated daily intake (EDI) in the population of Monterrey to the AFM_1 due to the consumption of infant formulae was carried out by combining data on the average daily consumption of milk by groups of age, with the average concentration of AFM_1 found in this work, as well as the average body weight (bw) of the population by age groups. For this, Equation (1) was applied:

$$\text{Estimated AFM1 daily intake}\left(\frac{\text{ng}}{\text{kg bw}}/\text{day}\right) = \frac{\text{Milk intake (L)} \times \text{AFM1}\left(\frac{\text{ng}}{\text{L}}\right)}{\text{Body weight (kg)}} \quad (1)$$

where: Milk intake is the average amount of milk that the infant population ingests daily, expressed in liters. AFM_1 is the average concentration of AFM_1 contained in the analyzed samples, expressed in ng/L. Body weight is the bw average in the population by age groups in kilograms.

The data corresponding to the daily milk consumption by age groups was obtained from the National Survey of Health and Nutrition of Mexico (ENSANUT) [31], in the section corresponding to Nuevo León State.

In order to obtain the daily intake of AFM_1 in the infant population, it was necessary to separate the population, as indicated by Mexican Standard NOM-031-SSA2-1999 [24] in: (1) minor lactating (newborn up to 6 months), at this stage of the infant's life, their diet is only based on breast milk or infant formulae for initiation; (2) minor lactating (from 6 to 12 months), at this stage, ablactation occurs, and the starter infant formulae and dairy infant formulae containing cereals and honey are taken as the infant diet at this stage of life; (3) major lactating (from 12 to 24 months), at this stage the dairy intake is determined by the follow-on formulae and those containing cereals and honey. From the ENSANUT [31] survey, the average weights of the infant population (minor and major lactating) were obtained.

Likewise, the CRI was estimated based on the proposal of Kuiper-Goodman [8], which estimates the TDI of AFM_1 by dividing the TD50 (threshold dose by body weight; 10,380 ng/kg bw per day for AFM_1) by the safety factor 5000, to give an estimated value of 2 ng/kg bw per day. A CRI of AFM_1 higher than 2 ng/kg bw indicates liver cancer risk to consumers [8,32].

4.5. Statistical Analysis

All infant formulae were analyzed in duplicates. Collected data were statistically evaluated using the nonparametric Wilcoxon rank sum test with continuity correction of R Core Team (Vienna, Austria) [33]. AFM_1 concentrations were expressed as mean ± standard deviation in order to show the occurrence of the toxin in infant formulae.

Author Contributions: Research concept, design and supervision: P.A.Q.-G. and A.-J.T.; HPLC method validation: P.A.Q.-G. and R.S.-G.; AFM_1 analysis in infant formulae: P.A.Q.-G. and E.G.R.-P.; writing and correcting of the manuscript: P.A.Q.-G.; A.-J.T.; R.S.-G.; E.G.R.-P.; G.G.A.-E. All authors have read and agreed to the published version of the manuscript.

Funding: The authors appreciate the funding provided by the Universidad Autónoma de Nuevo León, Monterrey, México, through the PAICYT – UANL program, and by the CIRTTA of Universitat Autònoma de Barcelona, Bellaterra, Spain, for this study.

Acknowledgments: The authors are very grateful to Jesús Piedrafita (UAB, Spain) for his support in statistical analysis.

Conflicts of Interest: The authors declare no conflict of interest.

Abbreviations

AFB_1	Aflatoxin B_1
AFM_1	Aflatoxin M_1
bw	Body weight
CRI	Carcinogenic risk index
EDI	Estimated daily intake
EU	European Union
HPLC	High Performance Liquid Chromatography
TDI	Tolerable daily intake
USA	United States of America

References

1. Prandini, A.; Tansini, G.; Sigolo, S.; Filippi, L.; Laporta, M.; Piva, G. On the occurrence of aflatoxin M1 in milk and dairy products. *Food Chem. Toxicol.* **2009**, *47*, 984–991. [CrossRef] [PubMed]

2. European Food Safety Authority. Aflatoxins (sum of B_1, B_2, G_1 and G_2) in cereals and cereal-derived food products [Internet]. *Supporting Publication, EN–406.* Available online: http://www.efsa.europa.eu/en/supporting/pub/406e.htm. (accessed on 15 January 2015).
3. Torović, L. Aflatoxin M1 in processed milk and infant formulae and corresponding exposure of adult population in Serbia in 2013–2014. *Food Addit. Contam. Part B* **2015**, *8*, 235–244.
4. Er, B.; Demirhan, B.; Yentür, G. Investigation of aflatoxin M1 levels in infant follow-on milks and infant formulas sold in the markets of Ankara, Turkey. *J. Dairy Sci.* **2014**, *97*, 3328–3331. [CrossRef] [PubMed]
5. Bakirci, I. A study on the occurrence of aflatoxin M1 in milk and milk products produced in Van province of Turkey. *Food Control* **2001**, *12*, 47–51. [CrossRef]
6. Kocasari, F.S. Occurrence of aflatoxin M 1 in UHT milk and infant formula samples consumed in Burdur, Turkey. *Environ. Monit. Assess.* **2014**, *186*(10), 6363–6368. [CrossRef] [PubMed]
7. Inetrnational Agency for Research on Cancer. *Monographs on the Evaluation of Carcinogenic Risks on Humans;* World health organization: Lyon, France, 2002; pp. 225–248.
8. Kuiper Goodman, T. Prevention of human mycotoxicoses trough risk assesment and risk management. In *Mycotoxins in Grain, Compounds Other Than Aflatoxin;* Miller, J.D., Trenholm, H.L., Eds.; Eagan Press: St. Paul, MN, USA, 1994; pp. 439–469.
9. European Commission. Commission Regulation (EU) No 165/2010 of 26 February 2010 amending Regulation (EC) No 1881/2006 setting maximum levels for certain contaminants in foodstuffs as regards aflatoxins. *Off. J. Eur. Comm.* **2010**, *50*, 8–12.
10. Codex Alimentarius Comission. *Commission submitted on the draft maximum level for aflatoxin M1 in milk Codex Committee on Food Additives and Contamination 33rd Session;* FAO: Hague, The Netherlands, 2001.
11. Food and Drug Administration (FDA). *CPG Sec. 527.400 Whole Milk, Low Fat Milk, Skim Milk–Aflatoxin M1;* Silver Spring: Rockville, MD, USA, 2005.
12. MERCOSUR/GMC/Res. No 25/02. Regulamento Técnico Mercosul Sobre límites Máximos de Aflatoxinas Admissíveis no leite, no Amendoim, no Milho. 2002. Available online: http://gd.mercosur.int/SAM/GestDoc/PubWeb.nsf/Normativa?ReadForm&lang=ESP&id=208FC19902A9C152032576340064C15D. (accessed on 17 November 2016).
13. Salud, S.d. NORMA Oficial Mexicana NOM-184-SSA1–2002, Productos y servicios. Leche, fórmula láctea y producto lácteo Combinado. *Especificaciones sanitarias. Mexico.* 2002. Available online: http://www.salud.gob.mx/unidades/cdi/nom/184ssa12.html. (accessed on 22 February 2017).
14. Li, S.; Min, L.; Wang, G.; Li, D.; Zheng, N.; Wang, J. Occurrence of Aflatoxin M1 in Raw Milk from Manufacturers of Infant Milk Powder in China. *Int. J. Environ. Res. Public Health* **2018**, *15*, 879. [CrossRef]
15. Joint FAO/WHO Expert Committee on Food Additives. Evaluation of certain mycotoxins in food. *Fifty sixth report of the Joint FAO/WHO expert committee on food additives;* World Health Organization: Geneva, Switzerland, 2001. Available online: https://apps.who.int/iris/bitstream/handle/10665/42448/WHO_TRS_906.pdf (accessed on 3 May 2018).
16. Zinedine, A.; González-Osnaya, L.; Soriano, J.M.; Moltó, J.C.; Idrissi, L.; Manes, J. Presence of aflatoxin M1 in pasteurized milk from Morocco. *Int. J. Food Microb.* **2007**, *114*, 25–29. [CrossRef]
17. Quevedo-Garza, P.A.; Amador-Espejo, G.G.; Cantú-Martínez, P.C.; Trujillo-Mesa, J.A. Aflatoxin M1 occurrence in fluid milk commercialized in Monterrey, Mexico. *J. Food Saf.* **2018**, *38*, e12507.
18. Ortiz-Martinez, R.; De Luna-Lopez, M.C.; Valdivia-Flores, A.; Quezada-Tristan, T. Aflatoxins: Occurrence in animal feeds and milk from dairy farms in Aguascalientes, Mexico. *Toxicol. Let.* **2014**, S224–S225.
19. European Comission. Commission Regulation 1881/2006 of 19 December setting maximum levels for certain contaminants in foodstuffs. *Off. J. Eur. Union* **2006**, *364*, 5–24.
20. Gomez-Arranz, E.; Navarro-Blasco, I. Aflatoxin M1 in Spanish infant formulae: Occurrence and dietary intake regarding type, protein-base and physical state. *Food Addit. Contam.* **2010**, *3*, 193–199. [CrossRef] [PubMed]
21. Akhtar, S.; Shahzad, M.A.; Yoo, S.; Yoo, S.; Aneela, I.A. Determination of Aflatoxin M1 and Heavy Metals in Infant Formula Milk Brands Available in Pakistani Markets. *Kor. J. Food Sci. An.* **2017**, *37*, 79–86. [CrossRef] [PubMed]
22. Kanungo, L.; Bhand, S. A survey of Aflatoxin M1 in some commercial milk samples and infant formula milk samples in Goa, India. *Food Agr Immunol.* **2014**, *25*, 467–476. [CrossRef]

23. Awaisheh, S.S.; Rahahleh, R.J.; Algroom, R.M.; Al-Bakheit, A.A.A.; Al-Khaza'leh, J.F.M. Al-Dababseh, B.A. Contamination level and exposure assessment to Aflatoxin M1 in Jordanian infant milk formulas. *Ital. J. Food Saf.* **2019**, *8*, 8263.
24. Norma Oficial Mexicana NOM-031-SSA2-1999, Norma para la Atención a la Salud del niño. Available online: http://www.salud.gob.mx/unidades/cdi/nom/031ssa29.html. (accessed on 15 January 2015).
25. Ismail, A.; Riaz, M.; Levin, R.E.; Akhtar, S.; Hameed, A. Seasonal prevalence level of aflatoxin M1 and its estimated daily intake in Pakistan. *Food Cont.* **2016**, *60*, 461–465. [CrossRef]
26. Oliveira, C.A.; Germano, P.M.; Bird, C.; Pinto, C.A. Immunochemical assessment of aflatoxin M1 in milk powder consumed by infants in São Paulo, Brazil. *Food Addit. Contam.* **1997**, *14*, 7–10.
27. Ishikawa, A.; Takabayashi-Yamashita, C.; Ono, E.; Bagatin, A.; Rigobello, F.; Kawamura, O.; Itano, E. Exposure assessment of infants to aflatoxin M1 through consumption of breast milk and infant powdered milk in Brazil. *Toxins* **2016**, *8*, 246. [CrossRef] [PubMed]
28. Ruangwises, N.; Saipan, P.; Ruangwises, S. Estimated daily intake of aflatoxin M1 in Thailand. In *Aflatoxins—Biochemistry and Molecular Biology*; Guevara-Gonzalez, R.G., Ed.; InTech: Rijeka, Croatia, 2011; Volume 21, pp. 439–446.
29. Cantú-Cornelio, F.; Aguilar-Toalá, J.E.; de León-Rodríguez, C.I.; Esparza-Romero, J.; Vallejo-Cordoba, B.; González-Córdova, A.F. Hernández-Mendoza, A. Occurrence and factors associated with the presence of aflatoxin M1 in breast milk samples of nursing mothers in central Mexico. *Food Cont.* **2016**, *62*, 16–22. [CrossRef]
30. International Organization for Standardization. *ISO 14501: 2007-Milk and milk powder- determination of aflatoxin M1 content- clean up by immunoaffinity chromatography and determination by high-performance liquid chromatography*; ISO: Geneva, Switzerland, 2007.
31. ENSANUT. Secretaria de Salud. Encuesta Nacional de Salud y Nutrición. Mexico. 2012. Available online: https://ensanut.insp.mx/. (accessed on 18 June 2016).
32. Shundo, L.; Navas, S.; Lamardo, L.; Ruvieri, V.; Sabino, M. Estimate of aflatoxin M_1 exposure in milk and occurrence in Brazil. *Food Cont.* **2009**, *20*, 655–657. [CrossRef]
33. R Core Team. R: A language and environment for statistical computing. R Foundation for Statistical Computing, Vienna, Austria. 2018. Available online: http://www.R-project.org/. (accessed on 20 January 2020).

toxins

MDPI

Article

Occurrence and Risk Assessment of Fumonisin B_1 and B_2 Mycotoxins in Maize-Based Food Products in Hungary

Andrea Zentai [1], Mária Szeitzné-Szabó [2], Gábor Mihucz [2], Nóra Szeli [2], András Szabó [2,3,*] and Melinda Kovács [2,3]

1. System Management and Supervision Directorate, National Food Chain Safety Office, 1024 Budapest, Hungary; zentaia@nebih.gov.hu
2. Faculty of Agricultural and Environmental Sciences, University of Kaposvár, Guba S. u. 40., 7400 Kaposvár, Hungary; dr.szabomaria@gmail.com (M.S.-S.); mihucz.gabor@ke.hu (G.M.); szeli.nora@ke.hu (N.S.); kovacs.melinda@ke.hu (M.K.)
3. MTA-KE-SZIE Mycotoxins in the Food Chain Research Group, Kaposvár University, Guba S. u. 40., 7400 Kaposvár, Hungary

* Correspondence: szan1125@freemail.hu

Received: 24 October 2019; Accepted: 3 December 2019; Published: 5 December 2019

Abstract: Fumonisins are toxic secondary metabolites produced mainly by *Fusarium verticillioides* and *Fusarium proliferatum*. Their toxicity was evaluated, and health-based guidance values established on the basis of both Joint FAO/WHO Expert Committee on Food Additives (JECFA) and European Food Safety Authority (EFSA) recommendations. This study presents the results of fumonisin analyses in different maize- and rice-based food products in Hungary and the potential health risk arising from their dietary intake. In total, 326 samples were measured in 2017 and 2018 to determine fumonisins B_1 and B_2 levels. Three-day dietary record data were collected from 4992 consumers, in 2009. For each food category, the average concentration values were multiplied by the relevant individual consumption data, and the results were compared to the reference values. With respect to the maximum limits, one maize flour, two maize grits, and two samples of other maize-based, snack-like products had total fumonisin content minimally exceeding the EU regulatory limit. The mean daily intake for all maize-product consumers was 0.045–0.120 μg/kg bw/day. The high intake (95 percentile) ranged between 0.182 and 0.396 μg/kg bw/day, well below the 1 μg/kg bw/day tolerable daily intake (TDI) established by EFSA. While the intake calculations resulted in comforting results, maize-based products may indeed be contaminated by fumonisins. Therefore, frequent monitoring of fumonisins' levels and evaluation of their intakes using the best available data are recommended.

Keywords: fumonisin; human exposure; maize products

Key Contribution: Fumonisin intake of Hungarian consumers from maize-based products is below the health-based guidance values. Maize-based products may be contaminated by fumonisins

1. Introduction

Fumonisins are secondary metabolites produced mainly by *Fusarium verticillioides* and *Fusarium proliferatum* [1]. Maize and maize-based products are most commonly contaminated by fumonisins, but fumonisins can be detected in several other cereal grains, such as rice, wheat, barley, rye, and oat [2,3]. More than 15 fumonisin homologues have been described, including fumonisin A, B, C, and P, and, among them, fumonisin B_1 (FB_1), FB_2, and FB_3 are the most frequent naturally occurring fumonisins [1,4]. FB_1 typically accounts for 70%–80% of the total fumonisin produced, while FB_2 usually makes up 15%–25% and FB_3 3%–8% when cultured on maize, rice, or in liquid medium [1].

Among fumonisins, FB_1 is the most toxic compound and has been shown to promote tumour growth in rats as well as equine leukoencephalomalacia [5] and porcine pulmonary oedema [6]. It was classified by the International Agency for Research on Cancer (IARC) in Group 2B (possibly carcinogenic in humans) [7]. FB_1 also causes chronic liver and kidney toxicity when administered in repeated doses to rodents.

Fumonisin B toxins, as structural analogues of sphingoid bases, inhibit ceramide synthases, causing the disruption of the sphingolipid metabolism and leading to sphinganine (and sphingosine) accumulation in cells and tissues [8]. Toxicity studies have mainly focused on the effects of FB_1, but $FB_{2\text{–}4}$ appear to have similar toxicological profiles. Acute toxicity is not relevant for fumonisins.

The Scientific Committee on Food (SCF) as well as the European Food Safety Authority (EFSA) in Europe and the Joint FAO/WHO Expert Committee on Food Additives (JECFA) evaluated the dietary risk of fumonisin intakes [9–15].

The SCF established a tolerable daily intake (TDI) of 2 μg/kg bw/day for FB_1 in 2000, based on an overall level of no observed adverse effect (NOAEL) of 0.2 mg/kg bw for liver and kidney in rodents [9]. This TDI was expanded into group TDI in relation to the total amounts of fumonisin B_1, B_2, and B_3, alone or in combination [10]. JECFA published a risk assessment on FB_1, FB_2, FB_3 in 2001 [11]. The assessment was essentially based on FB_1 data, and the other toxins were considered as having similar toxicological profiles. A group provisional maximum tolerable daily intake (PMTDI) of 2 μg/kg bw/day per day was allocated based on a NOAEL of 0.2 mg FB_1/kg bw per day for renal toxicity in a subchronic and a chronic rat study [11]. The PMTDI established by JECFA was retained in 2011 and in 2016 as well [12,13].

EFSA discussed food safety issues of mycotoxins, including fumonisins, in several documents. The chemical structure of mycotoxins can be altered by the defense reaction of plants, rendering them extractable conjugated and/or non-extractable bound mycotoxins or mycotoxin metabolites. Since these modified toxins are usually not detected during the analysis of mycotoxins, they are commonly termed "masked" or "bound". EFSA issued a scientific opinion in 2014 regarding certain modified mycotoxins in food and feed [14].

More recently, EFSA published a scientific opinion on the appropriateness to set a group health-based guidance value for fumonisins and their modified forms in 2018 [15]. For the establishment of the TDI, the benchmark dose lower confidence limit (BMDL10) of 0.1 mg/kg bw per day for induction of megalocytic hepatocytes in mice was used. Taking into account an uncertainty factor (UF) of 100 for intra- and interspecies variability, the TDI was established at 1.0 μg FB_1/kg bw per day. FB_2, FB_3, and FB_4 were included in the TDI, based on structural similarity and the limited available data indicating similar mode of action (MoA) and toxic potencies.

In Europe, Commission Regulation (EC) No 1881/2006, setting the maximum levels for certain contaminants in foodstuffs, established the maximum limits for fumonisins (sum of B_1 and B_2) in different commodities, including unprocessed maize, maize intended for direct human consumption, maize-based foods for direct human consumption, maize-based breakfast cereals, maize-based snacks, processed maize-based foods and baby foods for infants and young children, different milling fractions of maize, and other maize milling products not used for direct human consumption. Table 1 presents the specified maximum limits by commodities.

This article presents the results of fumonisin analyses in different maize- and rice-based food products in Hungary and, consequently, the potential health risk arising from their dietary intake.

Table 1. Maximum limits (μg/kg) for fumonisins established by Commission Regulation (EC) No 1881/2006.

2.6	Fumonisins	Sum of B_1 and B_2
2.6.1	Unprocessed maize, with the exception of unprocessed maize intended to be processed by wet-milling	4000
2.6.2	Maize intended for direct human consumption, maize-based foods for direct human consumption, with the exception of foodstuffs listed in 2.6.3 and 2.6.4	1000
2.6.3	Maize-based breakfast cereals and maize-based snacks	800
2.6.4	Processed maize-based foods and baby foods for infants and young children	200
2.6.5	Milling fractions of maize with particle size >500 μm, falling within CN code 1103 13 or 1103 20 40, and other maize milling products with particle size >500 μm not used for direct human consumption, falling within CN code 1904 10 10	1400
2.6.6	Milling fractions of maize with particle size ≤500 μm, falling within CN code 1102 20, and other maize milling products with particle size ≤500 μm not used for direct human consumption, falling within CN code 1904 10 10	2000

2. Results and Discussion

2.1. An Overview of the Measured Fumonisin Content

Altogether, 326 samples were measured for fumonisins B_1 and B_2 mycotoxins levels. The types of samples were from the food categories of maize flour, maize grits, corn flakes, canned maize, other maize-based, snack-like products, white and brown rice, and other rice-based products. The limit of detection (LOD) and the limit of quantification (LOQ) for FB_1 were 0.031 and 0.093 mg/kg, while those for FB_2 were 0.051 and 0.154 mg/kg.

In total, 70 and 256 samples were analyzed in 2017 and 2018, respectively, and were considered together in our assessment.

We measured 64 maize flour samples, of which 33 (51.6%) had detectable FB_1 content, and 6 (9.4%) had detectable FB_2 content. The highest FB_1 value was 1.46 mg/kg. The average FB_1 and FB_2 concentrations were 0.17–0.20 mg/kg for FB_1 and 0.05–0.10 mg/kg for FB_2. In no instance was FB_2 detected if FB_1 was undetected. Only in six cases, both FB_1 and FB_2 were detected at a measurable level (above LOQ), while FB_2 was never detected alone.

Then, 62 maize grits were analyzed; 26 samples (41.9%) presented detectable FB_1, and 4 (6.5%) detectable FB_2. The highest concentrations found were 1.96 mg/kg for FB_1 and 0.58 mg/kg for FB_2. The average FB_1 content was 0.13–0.16 mg/kg, while the average FB_2 content was 0.03–0.08 mg/kg. Four samples contained both FB_1 and FB_2 above the LOQ.

Altogether, 8 of the 64 corn flakes samples (12.5%) had measurable FB_1 content, whereas FB_2 was not detectable in any of them. The average fumonisin B_1 content ranged between 0.03 and 0.07 mg/kg, and the highest measured value was 0.46 mg/kg.

Only one of the 18 canned maize samples contained measurable FB_1, but none of them contained FB_2. The relevant FB_1 concentration was 0.20 mg/kg.

Fumonisin B_1 was measured in 20% of the other maize-based, snack-like products (17 of the 85 samples), and FB_2 in only 2 samples. The average FB_1 content ranged between 0.07 and 0.10 mg/kg, with a maximum content of 1.1 mg/kg.

Regarding white rice and brown rice samples and other rice-based products, FB_1 and FB_2 contents were in all cases below the LOQ. These commodities were therefore not included in our further risk assessment. The most important parameters of the analysis results for each food categories are summarized in Tables 2 and 3.

Table 2. Classification of the samples analyzed in this study in relation to fumonisins' limit of detection (LOD), limit of quantification (LOQ) *, and the regulatory limit.

		Fumonisin B_1			Fumonisin B_2			
Commodity Category	**Nr**	**<LOD**	**LOD-LOQ**	**>LOQ**	**<LOD**	**LOD-LOQ**	**>LOQ**	**Samples Over the Regulatory Limit (Regarding FB_1 + FB_2 Content)**
Maize flour	64	12	19	33	48	10	6	1 (1.6%)
Maize grits	62	18	18	26	51	7	4	2 (3.2%)
Corn flakes	64	37	19	8	63	1	0	0
Canned maize	18	17	0	1	17	1	0	0
Maize-based, snack-like products	85	48	20	17	78	5	2	2 (2.4%)
Brown rice	10	9	1	0	10	0	0	0
White rice	16	14	2	0	16	0	0	0
Rice-based products	7	7	0	0	7	0	0	0

* LOD and LOQ for FB_1: 0.031 and 0.093 mg/kg, LOD and LOQ for FB_2: 0.051 and 0.154 mg/kg. Nr: number of samples.

Table 3. Descriptive statistics of the results obtained for in the different maize-based food categories.

		Fumonisin B_1 (mg/kg)				Fumonisin B_2 (mg/kg)			
Commodity Category	**Nr**	**Mean (LB)***	**Mean (UB)***	**P95 (LB)**	**Max**	**Mean (LB)**	**Mean (UB)**	**P95 (LB)**	**Max**
Maize flour	64	0.17	0.20	0.66	1.46	0.05	0.10	0.32	0.73
Maize grits	62	0.13	0.16	0.50	1.96	0.03	0.08	0.12	0.58
Corn flakes	64	0.03	0.07	0.12	0.46	na	na	Na	na
Canned maize	18	0.01	0.04	0.03	0.20	na	na	Na	na
Maize-based, snack-like products	85	0.07	0.10	0.36	1.10	0.01 **	0.06 **	0.05 **	0.17 **
All maize samples analyzed	293	0.09	0.12	0.46	1.96	0.02	0.07	0.05	0.73

* Method of mean calculation: Results below the LOD and between LOD and LOQ were taken into account in two ways. In the lower-bound (LB) scenario, 0 and LOD were inserted for values below LOD and between LOD and LOQ, respectively. In the upper-bound (UB) scenario, LOD and LOQ were inserted for values below LOD and between LOD and LOQ, respectively. ** There were only two measured values for the concerned food category and mycotoxin; na: not applicable. Nr: number of samples.

Considering these results in light of the current maximum limits, one maize flour, two maize grits, and two samples of the other maize-based, snack-like products (mexicorn and a maize wafer) had total fumonisin contents minimally exceeding the regulatory limit (the sum was calculated according to the upper-bound (UB) scenario in case of a non-detectable value of FB_2).

Our results were also compared with fumonisin contents measured and published in the previous decades in Hungary. Fazekas et al. [16] measured considerably high fumonisin concentrations in maize collected during storage and harvesting in 1993 and 1994. Of the moldy maize samples collected in the period of storage, 70.8% contained fumonisin B_1 (0.05–19.8 mg/kg; average concentration: 2.6 mg/kg). Fumonisin B_1 content measured in maize ears more or less affected by molds (affected sample), collected in the period of harvesting, ranged between 0.095 and 52.4 mg/kg, with an average content of 6.64 mg/kg in 70% of the samples. Of the "average samples", 30% were contaminated with fumonisin B_1 (0.06–5.1 mg/kg; average: 1.52 mg/kg). Fumonisin concentrations were determined by high-performance liquid chromatography methods.

Tóth et al. [17] investigated *Aspergillus* and *Penicillium* species and their mycotoxins in maize in Hungary in two consecutive years after harvest. Mycotoxin concentrations were measured with HPLC–MS technique. Fumonisins (B_1 + B_2) were observed in quantities exceeding the EU limit in some samples collected in different regions (4.66 mg/kg; 10.15 mg/kg; 5.13 mg/kg; 7.55 mg/kg) in 2010.

The IARC report cites contamination data in maize for Europe, including Hungary. Fumonisin B_1 was detected in 248 out of 714 maize samples, at a concentration range of 0.007–250 mg/kg [7]. Similarly, the WHO series of Environmental Health Criteria dealt with fumonisin B_1 in 2000 [18]. The report specifically cites the results of the Hungarian authors Fazekas et al. [19], measuring 0.05–75.10 mg/kg fumonisin B_1 in 56 out of 92 maize samples.

Comparing our results with those of the above reports, fumonisin contamination in Hungary in recent years seems to be lower than that measured in previous decades. However, our measurements focused on processed food products (targeting the end consumer), which obviously have lower fumonisin contents than unprocessed maize samples.

2.2. Correlation between FB_1 and FB_2 Levels

FB_2 content was always lower than FB_1 content in our samples and was detected only in those samples also containing FB_1. The relationship between fumonisin B_1 and B_2 contents was further analyzed, to understand whether a possible correlation coefficient could be set up.

The commodity groups of at least one sample containing measurable quantities of FB_1 and FB_2 together were maize flour (six samples), maize grits (four samples), and the other maize-based snacks (two samples). The correlation coefficient calculated for the maize flour commodity group based on the numerical concentrations was 0.95, indicating a strong correlation.

Taking into account all 35 samples where, beside FB_1, FB_2 was also detected but not measurable (i.e., between LOD and LOQ), the correlation coefficients were 0.79 and 0.77 in the lower-bound (LB) and UB scenarios, respectively. Considering only the pooled maize flour and maize grits samples (26 samples), the correlation coefficient values were 0.86 and 0.82 in the LB and UB scenarios, respectively.

These results suggest a possible correlation between the levels of fumonisins B_1 and B_2; however, a higher number of samples with measured fumonisin B_1 and B_2 concentrations would be necessary to draw further conclusions.

2.3. Risk Assessment

The resulting intake values—both mean and high percentile—were well below the reference values established by EFSA and JECFA. Table 4 presents the calculated population mean and 95 percentile intakes for the five commodity groups (maize flour, maize grits, corn flakes, canned maize, and other maize-based, snack-like products) concerned.

Table 4. Calculated mean and 95 percentile (P) for fumonisin intakes (μg/kg bw/day). The percentage of European Food Safety Authority (EFSA) tolerable daily intake (TDI) is included in brackets.

Intake Level	All Consumers (LB Scenario)	All Consumers (UB Scenario)	Children (LB Scenario)	Children (UB Scenario)
Mean intake	0.045 (4.5%)	0.120 (12.0%)	0.056 (5.6%)	0.167 (16.7%)
95P intake	0.182 (18.2%)	0.396 (39.6%)	0.244 (24.4%)	0.537 (53.7%)

The mean daily intake for all maize-product consumers based on the LB and UB scenarios was 0.045–0.120 μg/kg bw/day. In addition, the high intake (95 percentile) ranged between 0.182 and 0.396 μg/kg bw/day, well below 1 μg/kg bw/day.

Regarding children (aged 0–18 years), the mean intake was 0.056–0.167 μg/kg bw/day, and the high intake (95 percentile) was 0.244–0.537 μg/kg bw/day.

Figure 1 presents the relative and cumulative frequencies of the resulting distributions of total fumonisin intakes for both total consumer population and children. The figure shows that most intakes cumulated below 0.5 μg/kg bw/day.

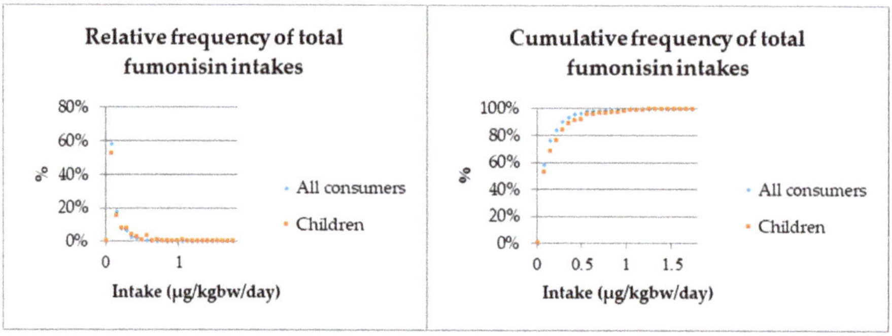

Figure 1. Relative and cumulative frequencies of total fumonisin intakes derived from maize-based products.

The results were compared to those of the exposure assessment conducted by EFSA in 2014 on the occasion of a derogation request for the maximum levels of several mycotoxins, including fumonisins [20]. On the basis of French contamination data of 2013, the mean exposure levels in children groups ranged between 0.17 and 1.52 μg/kg bw/day in the LB scenario and between 0.47 and 2.11 μg/kg bw/day in the UB scenario. The high (95 percentile) exposure levels ranged between 0.54 and 3.44 μg/kg bw/day and between 1.09 and 4.39 μg/kg bw/day in the LB and UB scenarios, respectively. In adult groups, the mean exposure levels were between 0.03 and 0.81 μg/kg bw/day in the LB scenario and between 0.15 and 1.19 μg/kg bw/day in the UB scenario. The 95th percentile, however, ranged between 0.08 and 1.76 μg/kg bw/day in the LB scenario and between 0.31 and 2.30 μg/kg bw/day in the UB scenario.

Our present results are in the same range or—especially in the case of children—considerably lower than reported results (Table 5).

Although the estimated mean and high intakes remained below both the JECFA and the EFSA reference values in all scenarios, it is worth noting that the maximum and some high values (over the 95 percentile) exceeded the 1 μg/kg bw TDI set by EFSA in 2018. In the case of all consumers, these high values amounted to 0.97% of the population, whereas in the case of children, they amounted to 2.36%. The maximum estimated intake value was 1.81 μg/kg bw. These specific high values were predominantly children's intake values, derived mainly from the consumption of canned and sweet maize and other maize-based snack-like products.

Considering that these intake results are based on the actually registered consumptions, representing only 4.8% of the total population and 7.6% of children consumers, the consequent health risk is probably negligible.

Table 5. Summary of estimated intakes (μg/kg bw/day) in comparison with EFSA estimations and health-based guidance values.

Comparison with EFSA Results and Reference Intakes	Children's Mean Exposure		Children's High Exposure		Adults' Mean Exposure *		Adults' High Exposure *	
	LB Scenario	UB Scenario	LB Scenario	UB Scenario	LB Scenario	UB Scenario	LB Scenario	UB Scenario
Our results	0.056	0.167	0.244	0.537	0.045	0.120	0.182	0.396
EFSA 2014	0.17–1.52	0.47–2.11	0.54–3.44	1.09–4.39	0.03–0.81	0.15–1.19	0.08–1.76	0.31–2.30
% of JECFA PMTDI	2.8	8.4	12.2	26.9	2.2	6.0	9.1	19.8
% of EFSA TDI	5.6	16.7	24.4	53.7	4.5	12.0	18.2	39.6

* All (adult + children) consumers included in our calculations. JECFA: Joint FAO/WHO Expert Committee on Food Additives, PMTDI: provisional maximum tolerable daily intake.

2.4. *Commodity Contributions*

The contributions of different commodities to the summed intake estimated from all maize-based foods are presented in Table 6.

Table 6. Contribution of different commodities to total fumonisin intake from maize-based products.

Scenario	Average Intake and % Contribution	Maize Flour	Maize Grits *	Corn Flakes	Canned Maize	Maize-Based, Snack-Like Products	All Maize-Based Products
Total population (LB scenario)	average intake of FB (μg/kg bw/day)	0.013	0.001	0.007	0.005	0.019	0.045
	% contribution	29.1%	2.1%	15.1%	10.4%	43.3%	100%
Total population (UB scenario)	average intake of FB (μg/kg bw/day)	0.018	0.001	0.027	0.033	0.041	0.120
	% contribution	14.8%	1.2%	22.3%	27.4%	34.3%	100%
Children (LB scenario)	average intake of FB (μg/kg bw/day)	0.005	0	0.011	0.006	0.034	0.056
	% contribution	8.2%	0.0%	20.2%	11.2%	60.4%	100%
Children (UB scenario)	average intake of FB (μg/kg bw/day)	0.006	0	0.045	0.044	0.072	0.167
	% contribution	3.7%	0.0%	26.8%	26.5%	43.0%	100%

* Data are shown, but conclusions cannot be made due to extremely low registered consumption.

Considering the LB scenarios, maize-based, snack-like products contributed the most to the fumonisin intake of the total (all consumers) population (43.3%), followed by maize flour (29.1%) and corn flakes (15.1%). In the case of children, the main contributors in the LB scenario were, similarly, maize-based, snack-like products (60.4%), corn flakes (20.2%), and canned maize (11.2%) (see Figure 2).

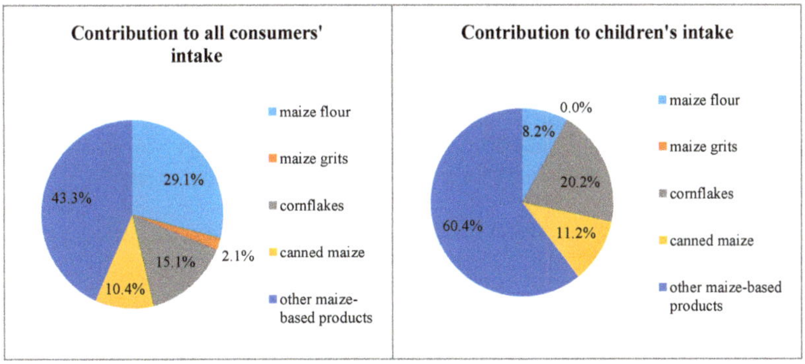

Figure 2. Contribution of food commodities to total fumonisin intake from maize-based products.

2.5. Uncertainty Considerations

It should be mentioned that this assessment focused only on the intake of fumonisins B_1 and B_2 from five different maize-based commodity types. Other types and the modified or masked forms of fumonisins were not analyzed. Total fumonisin intake of the population could be somewhat higher, if all relevant (including also non-maize-based) commodity types were considered. However, given that maize is the focal commodity in relation to fumonisin contamination, the contribution of other food products to total fumonisin intake is considered low.

The effect of household food processing on fumonisin content (relevant only for maize flour and grit) was not taken into account in our calculations. While the change of fumonisin content as a result of processing operations was studied by several authors [21–25], and heating was reported to lead to some losses of the toxin, the results from different studies are variable [13]. Our approach might have led to a slight overestimation of exposure, taking into account that the effect of heating would lower the calculated intakes; however, this would not change our conclusions, considering that our results do not indicate serious health concern.

The fact that we took into account only those consumption days for which actual consumptions were registered also adds uncertainty. Given that maize-based commodities are non-staple commodities in Hungary, consumed only occasionally by the majority of the population, averaging the occasionally registered consumption values would be misleading. Similarly, including the zero-consumptions in our assessment would "dilute" the results.

However, it needs to be mentioned that current trends indicate an increase in gluten-free foods consumption, which is not strictly linked to the number of consumers intolerant to gluten. Regular consumers striving for healthy diets may as well choose maize-based foods. These facts highlight the importance of focusing more attention on these kinds of food products, considering that they also tend to be the focal commodities most highly contaminated with fumonisins.

As the consumption data were collected in 2009, certain changes might have occurred since then. In the case newer/more recent consumption data are published, repeating these evaluations would be of great value. In this regard, the consumption of different maize-based products could be studied in more detail. In our calculations, we linked the concentration data of an aggregated "maize-based, snack-like products" group to the consumption of an aggregated maize-based products group, including popped maize or extruded corn flakes. These calculations, however, could be refined by separately studying the consumptions of these specific products. Our measurement results indicate a relatively high contamination rate in this kind of commodity category.

3. Conclusions

Our calculations based on recent fumonisin analyses in maize-based foods and consumption data from a Hungarian survey produced comforting results. The calculated fumonisin intakes of the total population and of children consumers were well below the reference values established by JECFA and EFSA. The values were also in the same range or lower than the European exposure rates estimated by EFSA in 2014.

However, the recent trend of increasing the consumption of alternative, "healthy" foods, including maize-based commodities, needs to be monitored. Our results suggest that maize-based products may indeed be contaminated by fumonisins. Therefore, monitoring of fumonisins' levels and the frequent re-evaluation of their dietary intakes with the best available data are recommended.

4. Materials and Methods

4.1. Sampling

Maize-based products were purchased from the Hungarian market in three metropolitan regions, i.e., Kaposvár (n = 276), Budapest (n = 29), and other cities, e.g., Debrecen, Keszthely, Székesfehérvár (n = 21). Commercial products were collected from supermarkets, retail shops, and pharmacies. A total amount of 326 samples purchased in 15 months (from August 2017 to November 2018) included maize flour (64), maize grits (62), corn flakes (64), canned maize (18), and other maize-based, snack-like products (85, extruded corn bread, tortilla chips, popcorn, nacho, maize chips, etc.). Beside these, 16 white and 10 brown rice and 7 rice-based products were also sampled. All information about the samples (i.e., producer, distributor, country of origin) was obtained from the products' labels and recorded. Samples were randomly selected, collecting as many as possible leader and minor brands available on the market.

4.2. Laboratory Analysis

4.2.1. Chemicals

Fumonisin B_1 (FB_1) and B_2 (FB_2) were purchased from Merck-Sigma Aldrich (St. Louis, LO, USA). HPLC–MS-grade acetonitrile and water were purchased from Carl Roth GmbH (Karlsruhe, Germany), HPLC–MS-grade acetic acid was purchased from Merck (Darmstadt, Germany).

4.2.2. Sample Preparation

Dry solid samples were ground using an ETA® Vital Blend II blender (ETA a.s., Praha, Czech Republic). Then, 5 g of sample was vortexed for 1 min with 20 mL of acetonitrile/water (50:50) on a VELP ZX-3 desktop vortex (Velp, Usmate, Italy) and 0.1% acetic acid and extracted for 60 min at 420 rotations/min speed on a horizontal desktop shaker (Edmund Bühler SM30A model, Bodelshausen, Germany). The supernatant of the extracted sample was centrifuged for 10 min at 14,000 rpm, and 4 °C. Aliquots of 10 μL internal standard solutions (^{13}C-FB_1, 6 μg/mL) were added to 970 μL aliquots of the supernatant of the centrifuged sample. The mixture was analyzed with LC–MS.

4.2.3. High-Performance Liquid Chromatography

Liquid chromatography and mass spectrometry (LC–MS) analysis were performed with a Shimadzu Prominence UFLC separation system equipped with an LC–MS-2020 single quadrupole (ultra-fast) liquid chromatographer–mass spectrometer (Shimadzu, Kyoto, Japan) with electrospray source. Optimized mass spectra were obtained with an interface voltage of 4.5 kV and a detector voltage of 1.05 kV in negative mode and 1.25 kV in positive mode. Samples were analyzed on a Phenomenex Kinetex 2.6 μm XB-C18 100 Å column (100 mm × 2.1 mm, Phenomenex, Torrance, CA, USA). The column temperature was set to 40 °C; the flow rate was 0.3 mL/minute. Gradient elution was performed using LC–MS-grade water (Carl Roth GmbH, Karlsruhe, Germany) (eluent A) and acetonitrile (Carl Roth GmbH, Karlsruhe, Germany) (eluent B), both acidified with 0.1% acetic acid (Merck, Darmstadt, Germany). Then, 5 μL of each samples were analyzed with the gradient: (0 min) 5% B, (3 min) 60% B, (8 min) 95% B, followed by a holding time of 3 min at 95% eluent B and 2.5 min column re-equilibration with eluent 5% B. FB_1 (diluted from 10 mg/L) standard solutions were used as references. MS parameters: source block temperature 90 °C; desolvation temperature 250 °C; heat block temperature 200 °C; drying gas flow 15.0 L/minute. Detection was performed using selected ion-monitoring (SIM) mode.

Detection (LOD) and quantification (LOQ) limits were 31 and 93 μg/kg for FB_1 and 51 and 154 μg/kg for FB_2.

For the calculation of LOD and LOQ, nine calibration points (0.1 μg/kg; 0.5 μg/kg; 1 μg/kg; 5 μg/kg; 10 μg/kg; 50 μg/kg; 100 μg/kg; 500 μg/kg; 1000 μg/kg) were measured, and the LOD and LOQ were calculated using the STHIBAYX function in Microsoft® Excel (Version 2013, Microsoft Corporation, Redmond, WA, USA). The slope of the calibration curve was determined using the nine calibration points.

$$LOD = (\text{Peak area 1, Peak area 2, ...; Concentration 1, Concentration 2,....}) \cdot \frac{3{,}3333}{\text{Slope of calibration curve}}$$

$$LOQ = (\text{Peak area 1, Peak area 2, \ldots; Concentration 1, Concentration 2,} \ldots) \cdot \frac{10}{\text{Slope of calibration curve}}$$

Ms Excel 2010 was used for the evaluation of the results.

4.3. Analysis of the Measurements and Correlation between FB_1 and FB_2 Concentrations

Main descriptive statistics (mean, maximum, 95th percentile) of the measured fumonisin contamination of the analyzed commodities were used. The measurement results were also characterized regarding the number of non-detected/not measurable values and the samples with fumonisin content exceeding the regulatory limit.

To take into account the uncertainty derived from the non-detected (<LOD) and detected but not measurable values (<LOQ), two scenarios were considered. First, to account for the worst-case option, assuming the highest possible concentration of these non-numerical values, LOD was inserted for values <LOD, and LOQ was inserted for values <LOQ, for both fumonisin B_1 and B_2 results. This was termed the upper-bound scenario. To illustrate with numbers, 0.031 mg/kg and 0.051 mg/kg were substituted for values of FB_1 and FB_2 <LOD, respectively, and 0.093 mg/kg and 0.154 mg/kg were substituted for values of FB_1 and FB_2 <LOQ, respectively.

To account for an optimistic scenario, assuming the lowest possible concentration, values <LOD were replaced with 0, and values <LOQ were replaced with the relevant LOD. This scenario was termed the lower-bound scenario. To illustrate with numbers, 0 was inserted for values of both fumonisins <LOD, and 0.031 mg/kg and 0.051 mg/kg were inserted for values of FB_1 and FB_2 <LOQ, respectively. Obviously, in the case of values >LOQ, the measured numerical values were used directly in all scenarios.

The possible correlation between fumonisin B_1 and B_2 contents in the samples was also analyzed, calculating the correlation coefficients. Besides considering only the corresponding numerical values of FB_1 and FB_2, we also analyzed a larger sample set, including those samples for which a numerical FB_1 value was accompanied by a detected but not measurable (i.e., between LOD and LOQ) FB_2 result. Lower- and upper-bound scenarios were calculated for these sample results as well.

4.4. Food Consumption Data

Consumption data were obtained from a survey carried out jointly by the Hungarian Food Safety Office (HFSO) and the Hungarian Central Statistical Office in 2009. Three-day dietary record data were collected from 4992 consumers, providing overall 14,976 daily food consumption data, including those of 934 children (aged below 18).

Relevant consumptions of maize products were recorded specifically for maize flour, maize grits, corn flakes, sweet maize, canned maize, frozen maize, extruded corn flakes, popped maize (with and without oil), and cheese-flavored popped maize. These products, and consequently their consumptions, were linked to the analyzed products, in order to perform intake calculations based on the concentration and consumption data of these specific commodities. Table 7 presents the commodities analyzed in relation to those consumed.

Table 7. Linking of analyzed values to consumed maize commodity categories by commodity name.

Commodities with Analyzed Fumonisin Content	Commodities Present in the Food Consumption Database	Number of Consumption Days (Out of 14,976 Data)	Number of Consumption Days, Children (Out of 2802 Data)
Maize flour	maize flour	54	5
Maize grits	maize grits	4	0
Corn flakes	corn flakes	399	137
Canned maize	canned maize, sweet maize, frozen maize	176	45
Maize-based, snack-like products	maize popped, extruded corn flakes, cheese flavored popped maize	102	34

The maize-based, snack-like products measured mainly consisted of different types of snacks produced from maize, including nacho, tacoshells, corn flips, tortilla chips, extruded maize snack, etc. Although they had different compositions, they were dealt with in one aggregated commodity group called maize-based, snack-like products, as their compositions were not specified in the consumption data.

The effect of processing was not taken into account for two reasons. First, the effect of milling was not relevant, as the analytical measurements and consumptions were both recorded for milled maize products, enabling a direct linkage between them. On the other hand, the effect of heating was relevant for maize flour and maize grits; however, further studies would be necessary to conclude on the quantitative effect of heating, based on the literature.

We considered only the consumption days for which consumption of the selected foods was reported. Given that maize-based products are not consumed daily, including those individuals who did not report any consumption of these foods would unrealistically dilute our data. The main statistical parameters of the consumption data are summarized in Table 8.

4.5. Risk Assessment Approach

Risk assessment was performed by semi-probabilistic means, by considering the consumption values as a distribution, since there were exact individual food consumption data available. The concentration values of FB_1 and FB_2 were summed in each sample and considered accordingly in further calculations.

For each food commodity category, the average concentration was calculated for both the LB and the UB scenarios. These values were then multiplied by the relevant individual consumption data one-by-one, resulting in the relevant calculated fumonisin intake values for each individual consumption of each commodity.

The daily individual intakes calculated from each commodity category were then summed for each individual, resulting in the summed individual daily fumonisin intake from all the selected foods. The resulting distribution of individual total daily fumonisin intakes could then be further studied on a population level. Average and high (95 percentile) values were calculated to determine the fumonisin intake of average and high consumers. These calculations were also applied for the children population of consumers. Finally, the resulting values were compared to the reference values established by JECFA [11] and EFSA [15].

To estimate the commodity contributions to the summed intake estimated from the analyzed commodities, the population average intake from each commodity was calculated separately and then compared to the average summed intake, resulting in the proportion of contribution of each commodity.

Table 8. Main statistical parameters of the consumption data.

Population	Parameter	g/Capita/Day Consumptions					g/kg bw/Day Consumptions				
		Maize Flour	**Maize Grits**	**Cornflakes**	**Canned Maize**	**Maize-Based, Snack-Like Products**	**Maize Flour**	**Maize Grits**	**Cornflakes**	**Canned Maize**	**Maize-Based, Snack-Like Products**
All consumers' data	count	54	4	399	176	102	54	4	399	176	102
	mean	47.8	70.0	16.9	73.9	83.7	0.75	1.04	0.35	1.36	1.78
	P95	96.0	111.0	50.0	200.0	200.0	1.52	1.64	0.98	3.72	4.54
	maximum	220	120	100	330	400	3.67	1.76	4.55	11.54	11.11
Children's data	count	5	0	137	45	34	5	0	137	45	34
	mean	38.4	na	20.4	61.0	74.6	0.89	na	0.57	2.12	2.69
	P95	53.2	na	60.0	150.0	150.0	1.33	na	1.96	5.52	6.75
	maximum	54	na	100	200	250	1.42	na	4.55	11.54	11.11

Na.: not applicable.

Author Contributions: Study design, M.S.-S., M.K. and A.Z.; Methodology, A.Z. and M.S.-S.; Analytics, G.M., N.S. and A.S.; Formal Analysis, A.Z.; Resources, M.K.; Original Draft Manuscript Preparation, A.Z.; Review & Editing, A.Z., M.S.-S. and A.S.; Supervision, M.K. and M.S.-S.

Funding: This research was funded by the project GINOP-2.3.2.-15-2016-00046 and the EFOP-3.6.3.-VEKOP-16-2017-00005 programs.

Conflicts of Interest: The authors declare no conflict of interest. The funders had no role in the design of the study; in the collection, analyses, or interpretation of data; in the writing of the manuscript, or in the decision to publish the results.

References

1. Rheeder, J.P.; Marasas, W.F.O.; Vismer, H.F. Production of Fumonisin Analogs by Fusarium Species. *Appl. Environ. Microbiol.* **2002**, *68*, 2101–2105. [CrossRef] [PubMed]
2. Dall'Asta, C.; Battilani, P. Fumonisins and Their Modified Forms, a Matter of Concern in Future Scenario? *World Mycotoxin J.* **2016**, *9*, 727–739. [CrossRef]
3. Cendoya, E.; Chiotta, M.L.; Zachetti, V.; Chulze, S.N.; Ramirez, M.L. Fumonisins and Fumonisin-Producing Fusarium Occurrence in Wheat and Wheat by Products: A Review. *J. Cereal Sci.* **2018**, *80*, 158–166. [CrossRef]
4. Sewram, V.; Mshicileli, N.; Shephard, G.S.; Vismer, H.F.; Rheeder, J.P.; Lee, Y.-W.; Leslie, J.F.; Marasas, W.F.O. Production of Fumonisin B and C Analogues by Several Fusarium Species. *J. Agric. Food Chem.* **2005**, *53*, 4861–4866. [CrossRef] [PubMed]
5. Marasas, W.F.; Kellerman, T.S.; Gelderblom, W.C.; Coetzer, J.A.; Thiel, P.G.; van der Lugt, J.J. Leukoencephalomalacia in a Horse Induced by Fumonisin B_1 Isolated from Fusarium Moniliforme. *Onderstepoor. Vet. Res.* **1988**, *55*, 197–203.
6. Haschek, W.M.; Gumprecht, L.A.; Smith, G.; Tumbleson, M.E.; Constable, P.D. Fumonisin Toxicosis in Swine: An Overview of Porcine Pulmonary Edema and Current Perspectives. *Environ. Health Perspect.* **2001**, *109* (Suppl. 2), 251–257.
7. IARC Working Group on the Evaluation of Carcinogenic Risks to Humans. Some Traditional Herbal Medicines, Some Mycotoxins, Naphthalene and Styrene. *IARC Monogr. Eval Carcinog. Risks Hum.* **2002**, *82*, 1–556.
8. Stockmann-Juvala, H.; Savolainen, K. A Review of the Toxic Effects and Mechanisms of Action of Fumonisin B1. *Hum. Exp. Toxicol.* **2008**, *27*, 799–809. [CrossRef] [PubMed]
9. Scientific Committee on Food. Opinion of the Scientific Committee on Food on Fusarium Toxins. Part 3: Fumonisin B_1 (FB_1). Available online: https://ec.europa.eu/food/sites/food/files/safety/docs/cs_contaminants_catalogue_out73_en.pdf (accessed on 17 October 2000).
10. Scientific Committee on Food. Updated Opinion of the Scientific Committee on Food on Fumonisin B1, B2 and B3. Available online: https://ec.europa.eu/food/sites/food/files/safety/docs/sci-com_scf_out185_en.pdf (accessed on 4 April 2003).
11. Joint FAO/WHO Expert Committee on Food Additives. Evaluation of Certain Mycotoxins in Food: Fifty-Sixth Report of the Joint FAO/WHO Expert Committee on Food Additives. Available online: https://apps.who.int/iris/handle/10665/42448?show=full (accessed on 11 September 2019).
12. Joint FAO/WHO Expert Committee on Food Additives. *Evaluation of Certain Food Additives and Contaminants: Seventy-Fourth [74th] Report of the Joint FAO/WHO Expert Committee on Food Additives*; Meeting (74th: 2011: Rome, Italy); World Health Organization: Geneva, Switzerland, 2011.
13. Joint FAO/WHO Expert Committee on Food Additives. *Evaluation of Certain Contaminants in Food: Eighty-Third Report of the Joint FAO/WHO Expert Committee on Food Additives*; (83rd); World Health Organization: Geneva, Switzerland, 2017.
14. European Food Safety Authority. Scientific Opinion on the Risks for Human and Animal Health Related to the Presence of Modified Forms of Certain Mycotoxins in Food and Feed. *EFSA J.* **2014**, *12*, 3916. [CrossRef]
15. Knutsen, H.-K.; Barregård, L.; Bignami, M.; Brüschweiler, B.; Ceccatelli, S.; Cottrill, B.; Dinovi, M.; Edler, L.; Grasl-Kraupp, B.; Hogstrand, C.; et al. Appropriateness to Set a Group Health-Based Guidance Value for Fumonisins and Their Modified Forms. *EFSA J.* **2018**, *16*, e05172. [CrossRef]
16. Fazekas, B.; Kis, M.; Hajdu, E.T. Data on the Contamination of Maize with Fumonisin B1 and Other Fusariotoxins in Hungary. *Acta Vet. Hung.* **1996**, *44*, 25–37. [PubMed]

17. Tóth, B.; Török, O.; Kótai, É.; Varga, M.; Toldiné Tóth, É.; Pálfi, X.; Háfra, E.; Varga, J.; Téren, J.; Mesterházy, Á. Role of Aspergilli and Penicillia in mycotoxin contamination of maize in Hungary. *Acta Agron. Hung.* **2012**, *60*, 143–149. [CrossRef]
18. United Nations Environment Programme; International Labour Organisation; World Health Organisation. *Environmental Health Criteria 219. Fumonisin B_1*; International Programme on Chemical Safety; World Health Organisation: Geneva, Switzerland, 2000; Available online: http://www.inchem.org/documents/ehc/ehc/ehc219.htm (accessed on 22 November 2019).
19. Fazekas, B.; Bajmócy, E.; Glávits, R.; Fenyvesi, A.; Tanyi, J. Fumonisin B1 Contamination of Maize and Experimental Acute Fumonisin Toxicosis in Pigs. *Zentralblatt Veterinarmedizin Reihe B* **1998**, *45*, 171–181. [CrossRef] [PubMed]
20. European Food Safety Authority. Evaluation of the Increase of Risk for Public Health Related to a Possible Temporary Derogation from the Maximum Level of Deoxynivalenol, Zearalenone and Fumonisins for Maize and Maize Products. *EFSA J.* **2014**, *12*, 3699. [CrossRef]
21. Saunders, D.S.; Meredith, F.I.; Voss, K.A. Control of Fumonisin: Effects of Processing. *Environ. Health Perspect.* **2001**, *109* (Suppl. 2), 333–336. [CrossRef]
22. Brera, C.; Debegnach, F.; Grossi, S.; Miraglia, M. Effect of Industrial Processing on the Distribution of Fumonisin B1 in Dry Milling Corn Fractions. *J. Food Prot.* **2004**, *67*, 1261–1266. [CrossRef] [PubMed]
23. Bryła, M.; Waśkiewicz, A.; Szymczyk, K.; Jędrzejczak, R. Effects of PH and Temperature on the Stability of Fumonisins in Maize Products. *Toxins (Basel)* **2017**, *9*, 88. [CrossRef] [PubMed]
24. Kamle, M.; Mahato, D.K.; Devi, S.; Lee, K.E.; Kang, S.G.; Kumar, P. Fumonisins: Impact on Agriculture, Food, and Human Health and Their Management Strategies. *Toxins (Basel)* **2019**, *11*, 328. [CrossRef] [PubMed]
25. Bullerman, L.B.; Ryu, D.; Jackson, L.S. Stability of Fumonisins in Food Processing. *Adv. Exp. Med. Biol.* **2002**, *504*, 195–204. [CrossRef] [PubMed]

toxins

MDPI

Article

Species Composition and Toxigenic Potential of *Fusarium* Isolates Causing Fruit Rot of Sweet Pepper in China

Jianhua Wang [1], Shuangxia Wang [2], Zhiyong Zhao [1], Shanhai Lin [1,3], François Van Hove [4] and Aibo Wu [2,*]

1 Institute for Agri-food Standards and Testing Technology, Shanghai Academy of Agricultural Sciences, 1000 Jinqi Road, Shanghai 201403, China; wangjianhua@saas.sh.cn (J.W.); zhaozhiyong@saas.sh.cn (Z.Z.); linshanhai@gxaas.net (S.L.)

2 SIBS-UGENT-SJTU Joint Laboratory of Mycotoxin Research, CAS Key Laboratory of Nutrition, Metabolism and Food Safety, Shanghai Institute of Nutrition and Health, Shanghai Institutes for Biological Sciences, Chinese Academy of Sciences, University of Chinese Academy of Sciences, Shanghai 200000, China; shuangxiawang@163.com

3 Sugarcane Research Institute, Guangxi Academy of Agricultural Sciences, Nanning 530007, China

4 Mycothèque de l'UCL catholique de Louvain (BCCMTM/MUCL), Applied Microbiology (ELIM), Earth and Life Institute (ELI), Université catholique de Louvain (UCL), B-1348 Louvain-la-Neuve, Belgium; francois.vanhove@uclouvain.be

* Correspondence: abwu@sibs.ac.cn; Tel.: +86-21-5492-0926

Received: 28 October 2019; Accepted: 21 November 2019; Published: 24 November 2019

Abstract: Apart from causing serious yield losses, various kinds of mycotoxins may be accumulated in plant tissues infected by *Fusarium* strains. Fusarium mycotoxin contamination is one of the most important concerns in the food safety field nowadays. However, limited information on the causal agents, etiology, and mycotoxin production of this disease is available on pepper in China. This research was conducted to identify the *Fusarium* species causing pepper fruit rot and analyze their toxigenic potential in China. Forty-two *Fusarium* strains obtained from diseased pepper from six provinces were identified as *F. equiseti* (27 strains), *F. solani* (10 strains), *F. fujikuroi* (five strains). This is the first report of *F. equiseti*, *F. solani* and *F. fujikuroi* associated with pepper fruit rot in China, which revealed that the population structure of *Fusarium* species in this study was quite different from those surveyed in other countries, such as Canada and Belgium. The mycotoxin production capabilities were assessed using a well-established liquid chromatography mass spectrometry method. Out of the thirty-six target mycotoxins, fumonisins B_1 and B_2, fusaric acid, beauvericin, moniliformin, and nivalenol were detected in pepper tissues. Furthermore, some mycotoxins were found in non-colonized parts of sweet pepper fruit, implying migration from colonized to non-colonized parts of pepper tissues, which implied the risk of mycotoxin contamination in non-infected parts of food products.

Keywords: *Fusarium* species; mycotoxin; toxigenic profile; mycotoxin migration; sweet pepper; fungal disease

Key Contribution: *Fusarium* species on sweet pepper in China is different from those in Canada and Belgium, and *F. equiseti*, *F. solani*, and *F. fujikuroi* were first reported causing pepper fruit rot in China. Toxigenic potential of *Fusairum* strains were analyzed in inoculated pepper fruit and diffusions of FA (fusaric acid), FB_1 (fumonisin B_1), FB_2 (fumonisin B_2), and MON (moniliformin) from lesions into the surrounding sound tissues were observed. This is the first report about the migration of FA and MON in sweet peppers.

1. Introduction

Sweet pepper or bell pepper (*Capsicum annuum* L.) is highly appreciated in the fresh vegetable markets worldwide due to its unique taste, aromas, and the multiple culinary uses. It represents one of the most important vegetables for the high content of phytochemicals, such as ascorbic acid and soluble phenols [1,2], having potential positive effects on human health. For example, ascorbic acid is an essential dietary nutrient in the human body with its vital biological function as an antioxidant. Sweet pepper is an economically important vegetable crop and widely used for direct consumption and manufacturing of sauce worldwide, where the global production reached 34.6 million tons of fresh fruit and 3.5 million tons of dried pods [3]. China is the largest producer and exporter of sweet pepper in the world, with a total fresh pepper production per year of almost 23 million tons. Sweet pepper is often grown in commercial greenhouses, which is favorable for the growth and survival of phytopathogenic fungi and the infection of pepper plants [4]. Thus, the disease poses a serious limitation to pepper cultivation, resulting in yield reduction or complete crop loss, as reported previously in the literature [4–6].

Several fungal diseases have caused economic losses in sweet pepper production in Canada, United Kingdom, and Belgium [4,7,8]. *Fusarium* infection on the stem- and blossom-end of pepper fruit caused by *F. solani* was first reported in Ontario and British Columbia in 1991 and caused approximately 5% fruit-yield loss [8–10]. Since the 1990s, this rot disease has been an increasing problem in pepper production in both Europe and North America [7,11,12]. More seriously, a severe outbreak of this disease resulting in a 50% yield loss in a greenhouse was reported in 1990 in Ontario [13].

In addition to external fruit rot, internal rot of sweet pepper fruit is also a big problem in pepper production [14]. In contrast to the external pepper fruit rot, the fruit is infected internally by a fungus. Unless severely infected and rotten, most infected fruits are difficult to cull before delivery to the market as the symptoms are not readily visible [4,8,10]. A comprehensive histopathology analysis performed by Yang et al. [10] indicated that internal fruit rot of greenhouse sweet pepper caused by *F. lactis* was initiated through the infection of the stigma and style during anthesis. Symptomless seed infection may contribute to disease spread, and air and insects also play an important role as intermediates in fungal spores spreading [15]. Based on the surveys to date, *F. lactis* is the principal causal agent of internal fruit rot of pepper, although the closely related *Fusarium* species belonging to the *Fusarium fujikuroi* species complex (FFSC), such as *F. proliferatum*, *F. subglutinans*, and *F. verticillioides*, have also been implicated in this disease [4,6,8].

Apart from causing significant yield losses, *Fusarium* species can produce fumonisins (FBs), trichothecenes (TCs), zearalenone (ZEN), and other mycotoxins in infected plant tissues which are harmful to consumers. For example, B-series fumonisins (Figure 1), which are mainly produced by *Fusarium* species from FFSC, are the most frequently detected mycotoxins in maize, and are involved in animal and human diseases by interfering with sphingolipid metabolism. Moreover, fumonisins have been associated epidemiologically with esophageal cancer in humans in some regions of the world [16,17]. On the basis of available toxicological evidence, the International Agency for Research on Cancer (IARC) has classified fumonisins as possibly carcinogenic (Group 2B) [18]. Mycotoxin contamination in grains, vegetables, and fruit poses a serious threat to food safety.

Mycotoxins can diffuse into tissues surrounding the pathogen-infected site. The water content of fresh sweet pepper is usually higher than 90%, which contributes to the dissolution of polar compounds produced by pathogens in pepper tissues. Fumonisins, fusaric acid (FA), and moniliformin (MON) are the most common mycotoxin contaminants produced by *Fusarium* species, and migration of some of these toxins has been reported in pepper and fruit previously [19,20]. A migration study of beauvericin (BEA) and fumonisins was reported by Monbaliu et al. [19], and the results indicated the migration of fumonisins into healthy parts of the sweet pepper, while beauvericin was not detected in the tissue surrounding the lesion. Mycotoxin contaminations originating from mycotoxin-producing *Fusarium* species in pepper should be considered as an importantly sensitive food safety concern. Therefore, it is of great necessity to assess the types and levels of mycotoxin contamination in pepper and its derived products [4].

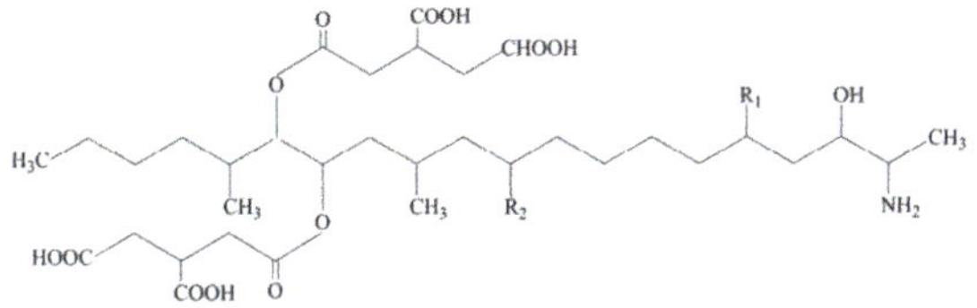

Figure	R_1	R_2
Fumonisin B_1	OH	OH
Fumonisin B_2	OH	H
Fumonisin B_3	H	OH

Figure 1. Structural formulas of B-series fumonisins.

Effective management of mycotoxin contamination in sweet pepper relies on the control of the fungal infection and requires a better understanding of *Fusarium* biology and epidemiology. To our best knowledge, there is little information on the causal agent, etiology, toxigenic potential, and geographic distribution of the *Fusarium* species involved in pepper disease in China. The objectives of this current work were: (i) To isolate and identify the causal organism from *Fusarium* genus on sweet pepper in China; (ii) to assess the potential mycotoxin profiling of the fungal pathogens; (iii) to estimate the migration behavior of mycotoxins in sweet pepper.

2. Results and Discussion

2.1. Isolation and Identification of *Fusarium* Isolates

Sweet pepper fruits were sampled from Hainan, Heilongjiang, Hunan, Shanghai, Shandong, and Zhejiang provinces in China. Following isolation from diseased pepper tissues, a total of forty-two single-spore isolates were obtained and identified as belonging to *Fusarium* genus by morphology. Two of theses strains were isolated from Hainan, one strain was isolated from Heilongjiang, five strains were isolated from Hunan, twenty-one strains were isolated from Shanghai, three strains were isolated from Shandong, and ten strains were isolated from Zhejiang (Table 1).

The purified isolates were first identified to species with morphological characteristics [21], and this was subsequently confirmed by nucleotide sequences analysis of the translation elongation factor 1-α (*TEF*-1α) genes with partial of representative strains. Of the forty-two strains, twenty-seven were identified as *F. equiseti*, ten as *F. solani*, and five as *F. fujikuroi* (Table 1). Previously, a new disease on pepper caused by *F. concentricum* was reported by our group, and the strain MUCL54697 was isolated from Hunan province, China [22].

Eleven representative strains belonging to different species were selected for *TEF-1α* gene sequencing to further confirm the morphological identification results as described before [23–25]. Obtained sequences were subjected to alignment analysis using the network service tool BLASTn of the National Center for Biotechnology Information (NCBI) database. The sequence analysis of the portion of the *TEF-1α* genes of representative strains confirmed that all the strains belonged to *Fusarium* genus. The results indicated that nucleotide sequences of three strains (Q12002, Q12003 and Q12005) showed the highest identity (>99%) with the sequence of *F. equiseti*, three (Q12029, Q12030 and Q12034) showed the highest identity (>99%) with the sequence of *F. solani*, and five (Q12038-Q12042) showed the highest identity (>99%) with the sequence of *F. fujikuroi* in the NCBI database. The molecular identification results were all identical with the morphological results. The *TEF-1α* gene sequences generated in this study were deposited in GenBank, NCBI (http://www.ncbi.nlm.nih.gov/genbank/), under accession numbers KF208617–KF208627, which is presented in Table 1.

Table 1. *Fusarium* strains isolated in this study.

Species	Strain Code	Origin	Symptom (External/Internal)	GenBank Accession No.
F. equiseti	Q12001	Shanghai	external	-
	Q12002	Shanghai	internal	KF208617
	Q12003	Shanghai	external	KF208618
	Q12004	Shanghai	external	-
	Q12005	Shanghai	internal	KF208619
	Q12006	Shanghai	external	-
	Q12007	Shanghai	external	-
	Q12008	Shanghai	internal	-
	Q12009	Shanghai	external	-
	Q12010	Hainan	external	-
	Q12011	Shandong	external	-
	Q12012	Shandong	external	-
	Q12013	Shanghai	external	-
	Q12014	Shanghai	external	-
	Q12015	Shandong	external	-
	Q12016	Helongjiang	external	-
	Q12017	Zhejiang	external	-
	Q12018	Zhejiang	internal	-
	Q12019	Zhejiang	external	-
	Q12020	Zhejiang	external	-
	Q12021	Zhejiang	external	-
	Q12022	Zhejiang	internal	-
	Q12023	Zhejiang	external	-
	Q12024	Zhejiang	external	-
	Q12025	Hunan	external	-
	Q12026	Hunan	external	-
	Q12027	Hunan	external	-
F. solani	Q12028	Shanghai	external	-
	Q12029	Shanghai	external	KF208620
	Q12030	Shanghai	external	KF208621
	Q12031	Shanghai	external	-
	Q12032	Shanghai	external	-
	Q12033	Shanghai	external	-
	Q12034	Shanghai	internal	KF208622
	Q12035	Shanghai	internal	-
	Q12036	Shanghai	external	-
	Q12037	Shanghai	external	-
F. fujikuroi	Q12038	Hainan	external	KF208623
	Q12039	Zhejiang	external	KF208624
	Q12040	Zhejiang	external	KF208625
	Q12041	Hunan	internal	KF208626
	Q12042	Hunan	external	KF208627

Among the forty-two *Fusarium* strains, all the ten *F. solani* (23.81%) strains were isolated from Shanghai, and the five *F. fujikuroi* (11.90%) strains were isolated from Hainan (one strain), Hunan (two strains), and Zhejiang (two strains). *F. equiseti* was the only species isolated from all six sampled provinces in China, and accounting for 64.29% of all *Fusarium* strains isolated (Table 1). According to our survey, *F. equiseti* was the predominant pathogen of sweet pepper fruit rot in China.

Fusarium strains were isolated from both external and internal rotten pepper fruits in this study. Of the forty-two strains, thirty-four were isolated from external rotten pepper fruits and eight strains were isolated from internal rotten pepper fruits (Table 1). For the twenty-seven *F. equiseti* strains, twenty-two were associated with external rot disease of pepper fruits and five (Q12002, Q12005, Q12008, Q12018, and Q12022) were isolated from internal rotten pepper fruits. For the ten *F. solani* and five *F. fujikuroi*, two (Q12034 and Q12035) and one strain (Q12041) were isolated from internal rotten pepper fruit, respectively. As such, *F. equiseti*, *F. solani*, and *F. fujikuroi* were the causal agents of external fruit rot of pepper in China, with *F. equiseti* being the predominant, while *F. equiseti*, *F. solani*, and *F. fujikuroi* were associated with internal fruit rot of pepper, with *F. equiseti* being the predominant. To our best knowledge, this is the first report of *F. fujikuroi*, *F. equiseti*, and *F. solani* associated with external and internal pepper fruit rot in China.

F. solani was reported as the predominant causal agent of external fruit rot of pepper in Europe and North America [7–13], which is different from China. However, it worth noting that *F. solani* is a common pathogen causing pepper fruit rot worldwide. *F. solani*, *F. lactis*, *F. proliferatum*, *F. subglutinans*, and *F. verticillioides* were reported to cause external or internal pepper fruit rot in Belgium, Canada, and United Kingdom, with *F. lactis* being the principal one [4,6,8]. In this study, *F. equiseti*, *F. solani*, and *F. fujikuroi* were found to be associated with internal pepper fruit rot, and with *F. equiseti* being the predominant. In light of the above, it is obvious that the population structure of *Fusarium* species associated with pepper fruit rot (external or internal) in China is quite different from those in surveys from Canada and Belgium [4,8,10]. Although the underlying factors for species distribution are unknown, climatic conditions (such as the annual temperature weather and humidity), hosts and their rotation, and adaptive evolution have been reported to influence the distribution of *Fusarium* species [14,26–28]. In view of the population genetic diversity and dispersal difference of the *Fusarium* pathogens, procedures for effective management of these pathogens on pepper are urgently needed.

2.2. Molecular Phylogenetics

Phylogenetic analyses were conducted on partial sequences of *TEF-1α* genes. Figure 2 shows the phylogenetic tree constructed with MEGA 5.10 [29]. As several *Fusarium* species have been reported to be the causal agents of pepper fruit rot, in addition to the nucleotide sequences obtained in this study (Table 1), corresponding sequences available in GenBank for the strains belonging to *F. concentricum*, *F. equiseti*, *F. fujikuroi*, *F. lactis*, *F. proliferatum*, *F. solani*, *F. subglutinans*, and *F. verticillioides* were retrieved and served as references.

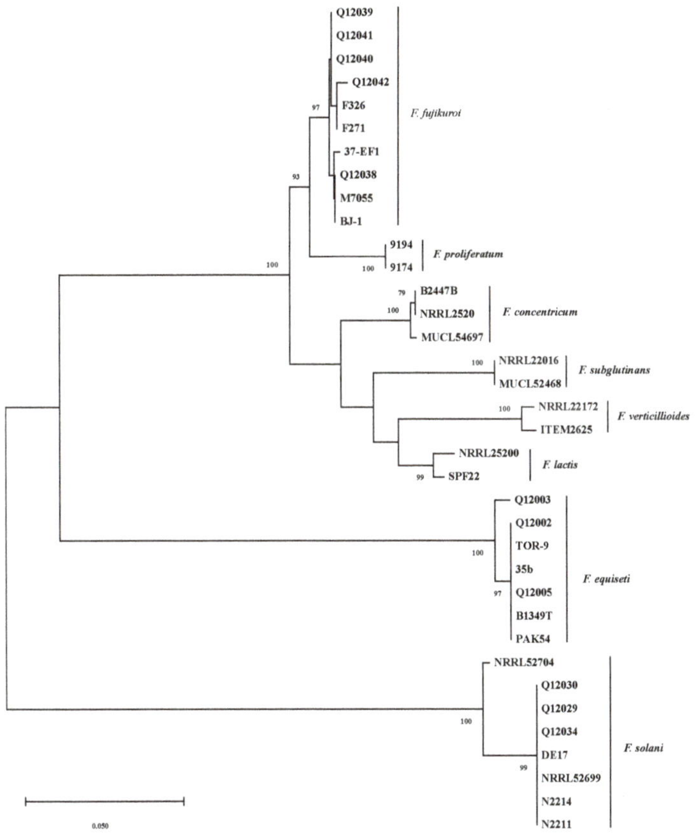

Figure 2. Phylogenetic tree inferred from alignments of *TEF-1α* sequences of *Fusarium* species by the Neighbor-Joining method with program MEGA 5.10. The numbers beside branches are the percentages of congruent clusters in 1000 bootstrap trials. Bootstrap values higher than 75% are shown.

As shown in Figure 2, bootstrap analyses of the *TEF-1α* gene partial sequences clearly separated the thirty-six *Fusarium* isolates into three major clades with a bootstrap value of 100%; the *F. equiseti* clade (seven isolates), the *F. solani* clade (eight isolates), and the third clade that was composed of the remaining twenty-one isolates belonging to *F. concentricum*, *F. fujikuroi*, *F. lactis*, *F. proliferatum*, *F. subglutinans*, and *F. verticillioides*. The six *Fusarium* species mentioned above in the third clade are all from the *F. fujikuroi* species complex (FFSC) [30], and they are relatively closer species among the species analyzed.

It is obvious that six distinct subclades were formed with >97% bootstrap support in the third clade which separated the twenty-one isolates to *F. concentricum* (three isolates), *F. fujikuroi* (ten isolates), *F. lactis* (two isolates), *F. proliferatum* (two isolates), *F. subglutinans* (two isolates), and *F. verticillioides* (two isolates) (Figure 2). Thus, the *TEF-1α* sequences can efficiently differentiate these *Fusarium* species. The *TEF-1α* sequence BLASTn and phylogenetic analysis results strongly supported the identification results of *Fusarium* strains isolated.

2.3. Multi-Mycotoxin Analysis in Pepper Fruit

For large-scale screening of mycotoxin production capabilities in pepper by the sampled *Fusarium* isolates, the well-established multi-component LC-MS/MS method was used for scanning of the 36 mycotoxins reported in agricultural products. In this multi-mycotoxin analysis, two *F. equiseti* isolates (Q12002 and Q12004), three *F. solani* isolates (Q12029, Q12034 and Q12037), four *F. fujikuroi* isolates (Q12038, Q12039, Q12040 and Q12041), and the *F. concentricum* strain MUCL54697 [22] were selected to do the inoculation experiment and assess their mycotoxin production in different sites of sweet pepper fruits (Figure 3).

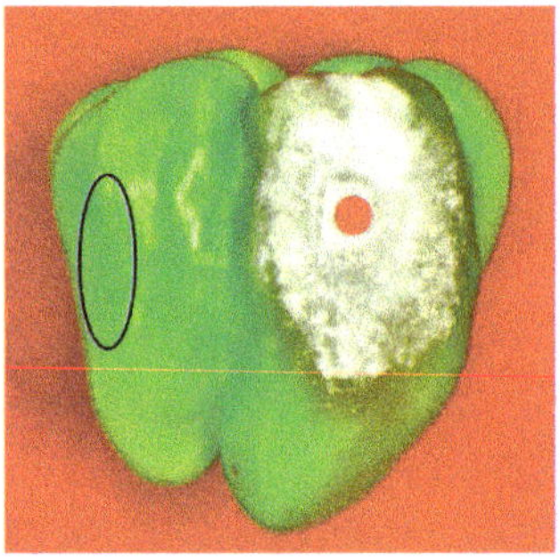

Figure 3. Inoculated pepper with the indication of inoculation site (red dot) and healthy site (black oval) for mycotoxin analysis.

Mycotoxin detection results from lesions (Figure 3, red dot) were used to do the mycotoxin profile analysis, and the results from the healthy parts (Figure 3, black oval) were used for the migration study. Mycotoxin profiles of the ten strains selected were summarized in Table 2. The multiple mycotoxin analysis resulted in the detection of BEA, FA, fumonisin B_1 (FB_1), fumonisin B_2 (FB_2), MON, and nivalenol (NIV) in pepper tissues (Figures 1 and 4). In one out of the ten isolates inoculated, none of the thirty-six mycotoxins investigated was detected. FA was the most frequently detected metabolite which was produced by nine isolates in concentrations that greatly varied from 41.44 to 10,662.36 μg/kg. BEA was produced by eight isolates with average concentrations varying between 5.20 and 1019.60 μg/kg. Both FB_1 and FB_2 were produced by the same four isolates ranging from 43.64 to 39,326.60 μg/kg and 26.96 to 3734.16 μg/kg, respectively. MON was produced by five isolates in greatly varying amounts (35.80–2439.48 μg/kg), while NIV was produced by only one isolate at a concentration of 184.16 μg/kg.

Table 2. Mycotoxins produced by selected *Fusarium* strains in sweet pepper samples.

Fusarium Species	Strain Code	Position [1]	Mycotoxins Detected (μg/kg)					
			BEA	FA	FB_1	FB_2	MON	NIV
F. equiseti	**Q12002**	IS	5.20	411.64	-	-	-	184.16
		HS	-	13.80	-	-	-	-
F. equiseti	Q12004	IS	9.12	160.32	-	-	-	-
		HS	-	-	-	-	-	-
F. solani	Q12029	IS	-	41.44	-	-	-	-
		HS	-	-	-	-	-	-
F. solani	Q12034	IS	98.48	78.98	-	-	-	-
		HS	-	-	-	-	-	-
F. solani	Q12037	IS	-	-	-	-	-	-
		HS	-	-	-	-	-	-
F. fujikuroi	Q12038	IS	153.84	10662.36	1512.48	1190.12	2439.48	-
		HS	-	592.00	45.36	31.67	193.75	-
F. fujikuroi	Q12039	IS	318.00	4870.56	1559.04	851.88	1429.76	-
		HS		130.40	41.08	24.30	172.13	-
F. fujikuroi	Q12040	IS	44.44	6522.72	43.64	26.96	151.72	-
		HS	-	874.04	-	-	-	-
F. fujikuroi	Q12041	IS	23.80	2940.72	3926.60	3734.16	1925.00	-
		HS	-	530.48	183.04	144.92	253.12	-
F. concentricum	MUCL54697	IS	1019.60	2886.08	-	-	35.80	-
		HS	-	55.64	-	-	-	-

[1] IS, Inoculation site; HS, Healthy site.

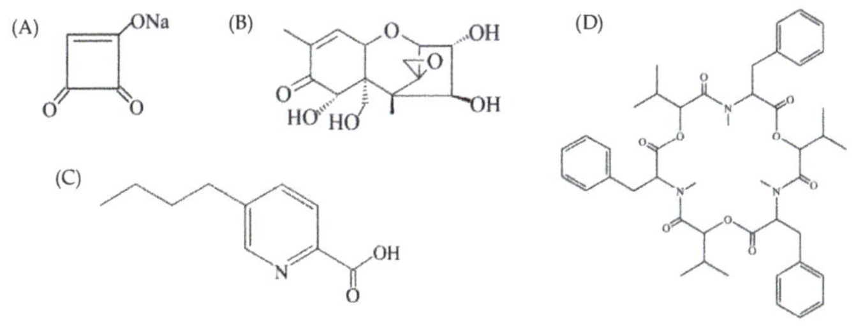

Figure 4. Structural formulas of moniliformin (**A**), nivalenol (**B**), fusariuc acid (**C**), and beauvericin (**D**).

As shown in Table 2, significantly different toxigenic profiles were observed among different species in inoculated pepper fruits. For the investigated *Fusarium* species, the most abundant of toxic metabolites were produced by *F. fujikuroi*, and all the four *F. fujikuroi* isolates can produce BEA, FA, FB_1, FB_2, and MON. With regard to the individual mycotoxin, relatively higher contents of FB_1 were generated compared to FB_2 by the same strain, which were consistent with the previously reported studies [31,32]. The ratios between the two fumonisins for individual *F. fujikuroi* strain were in the range of 1.05–1.83 in pepper lesions. Meanwhile, significant differences in fumonisin production capacities of *F. fujikuroi* strains were observed. For example, strain Q12040 produced FB_1 and FB_2 in concentrations of 43.64, 26.96 μg/kg, respectively, while large amounts of FB_1 and FB_2 were produced by isolate Q12041 (3926.60, 3734.16 μg/kg, respectively) which were about 90 and 139 times as higher than those produced by Q12040 under the same conditions. Note that similar or higher amounts of FA and MON were produced by the four *F. fujikuroi* strains when compared with FBs. For example, the amount of FA is higher than the total fumonisins (FB_1 + FB_2) produced by three out of four isolates. Strain Q12002 produced NIV, a kind of type B trichothecene, at a concentration of 184.16 μg/kg, while trichothecenes were not observed with the other strain Q12004. These two *F. equiseti* isolates showed a considerable intraspecies variation in profiles of trichothecene production, similar to results reported by Hestbjerg et al. [33]. Similarly, intraspecies variation in toxigenic profiles was also observed in

F. solani. Regarding the three *F. solani* strains, only FA was produced by strain Q12029, compared to BEA and FA (94.84, 78.98 μg/kg, respectively) that were produced by strain Q12034, while none of the thirty-six mycotoxins were detected with strain Q12037.

Large variation among strains, both in terms of their toxigenic profiles and the quantity of mycotoxins produced in pepper, was found in this study. Based on the mycotoxin profile results, it could be concluded that interspecies toxigenic profile variation appears to be a species-specific characteristic, while the intraspecies quantity variation appears to be a strain-specific characteristic.

The results of the migration study are summarized in Table 2. Among the mycotoxins detected in this study, diffusion phenomenon of FA, FB_1, FB_2, and MON from a moldy area to healthy tissues was observed in pepper fruit, while no detectable BEA and NIV were found in unaffected parts.

As shown in Table 2, FA was the most frequently detected mycotoxin in unaffected parts, with concentrations varying from 13.80 to 874.04 μg/kg. As a phytotoxin [34], the ratios of FA detected from lesions and healthy parts were in the range of 5.54–51.87. FB_1 was detected in unaffected parts with concentrations varying from 41.08 to 183.04 μg/kg. The ratios of FB_1 detected from lesions and healthy parts were in the range of 21.45–37.95. FB_2 was detected in unaffected parts with concentrations varying from 24.30 to 144.92 μg/kg and the ratios of FB_2 detected from lesions and healthy parts were similar to FB_1 (25.77–37.58). MON was detected in unaffected parts with concentrations varying from 172.13 to 253.12 μg/kg, and the ratios of the compound from lesions and healthy parts were in the range of 7.61–12.59. Migration of FB_1 and FB_2 in sweet pepper was reported by Monbaliu et al. [19], and this is the first report about the diffusion of FA and MON in sweet pepper.

Mycotoxins can persist in infected plant tissues, and depending on physical or chemical properties (solubility, polarity, hydrophilicity, molecular weight, concentration, etc.) and tissue components, might also transfer from a rotten part of the plant tissues into the surrounding sound tissues, even in the absence of fungal growth. In this study, no NIV was detected in healthy pepper tissues maybe due to the low concentration, while BEA was not detected even at a high concentration (1019.60 μg/kg). Similar results were reported by Monbaliu et al. [19] that BEA can not be detected in surrounding tissues even with an extremely high concentration, 73,800 μg/kg, in pepper lesions. As shown in Figure 4, BEA is a cyclic hexadepsipeptide that contains three D-hydroxyisovaleryl and three N-methylphenylalanyl residues in an alternating sequence [35]. As an organic and non-polar compound, BEA is insoluble in the aqueous environment. Vegetable, and sweet peppers in particular, contain >90% water, which is probably why BEA was not detected in the surrounding tissues. These results demonstrated the possible risk of mycotoxin contamination in non-infected parts of food products, and some mycotoxins can diffuse into sound tissues. Since second-quality vegetables and fruits may be used to produce derivatives such as juices, jam, etc., further studies on migration behaviors and affecting factors of different mycotoxins in various vegetables and fruits are very important to establish suitable means of protecting consumers from exposure to toxic substances [20].

3. Conclusions

Fusarium species causing pepper fruit rot (external and internal) were analyzed in this study. Altogether, forty-two isolates belonging to *F. equiseti* (27 isolates), *F. solani* (10 isolates), and *F. fujikuroi* (five isolates) were identified with *F. equiseti* being the predominant species. To our best knowledge, this is the first report of *F. fujikuroi*, *F. equiseti* and *F. solani* associated with pepper fruit rot in China. Toxigenic profiles of ten pathogens were determined in sweet peppers, and six toxic metabolites (BEA, FA, FB_1, FB_2, MON, and NIV) were detected in total. Significantly different toxigenic profiles were observed among the three *Fusarium* species. Diffusions of FA, FB_1, FB_2, and MON from lesions into the surrounding sound tissues were observed in sweet peppers, and this is the first report about the migration of FA and MON in sweet peppers. Further studies on migration behaviors and affecting factors of different mycotoxins in various vegetables and fruit should be conducted.

4. Materials and Methods

4.1. Isolation and Purification of Fusarium Strains

During the growing season, pepper fruit samples were collected from different regions in China, including Hainan, Heilongjiang, Hunan, Shandong, Shanghai, and Zhejiang provinces (Table 1). Pepper fruits with visible symptoms (external or internal when cut open) were selected for pathogen isolation. Fungi were isolated using conventional methods as follows: Symptomatic tissues (3 × 3 cm) were surface-sterilized in 0.1% $HgCl_2$ for 1 min, transferred into 70% ethanol for 30 s, then rinsed three times in sterilized distilled water, dried, and plated on 90 mm Petri dishes containing potato dextrose agar (PDA). After incubation for 3–5 days at 28 °C in the dark, colonies resembling morphologically to *Fusarium* were transferred onto new PDA. Plates were incubated at 28 °C in the dark until colonies developed, and then purified through serial transfers. No more than one strain per fruit was isolated. For each strain, a single spore culture was obtained by single-sporing as described before [36]. The pure cultures were used for the morphological and molecular characterization. Monoconidial strains were cryopreserved and maintained in tubes on PDA in the lab.

4.2. Nucleotide Maniplation

Mycelia plugs from 3-day-old PDA cultures were transferred to 50 mL of potato dextrose broth (PDB) medium and incubated with shaking (100 rpm) at 28 °C in the dark for 3 days. After incubation, mycelium was filtered through two-layered cheesecloth, washed with sterile water, then freeze-dried and ground to a fine powder using a TissueLyser II system (Qiagen Tissuelyser II, Retsch, Haan, Germany). Genomic DNA was extracted and purified using a Cetyl Trimethylammonium Bromide (CTAB) protocol as described before [37]. In brief, after homogenization, the ground power was suspended with 600 μL of CTAB lysis buffer, mixed well by shaking, and incubated at 65 °C for 1 h. After incubation, the solution was cooled at room temperature for 5 min, cellular debris were pelleted by centrifugation at 12,000 rpm for 10 min, and 500 μL of supernatant was transferred into a new tube. The supernatant was extracted with 500 μL of chloroform:isoamyl alcohol mixture (24:1, *v*/*v*). After centrifugation at 12,000 rpm for 10 min, 400 μL of aqueous phase was transferred to a fresh tube, then 400 μL of ice-cold isopropyl alcohol and 40 μL of sodium acetate (3 M, pH 5.2) were subsequently added to the samples. The tubes were mixed by gentle inversion. After incubation for 1 h at −20 °C, DNA was precipitated by centrifugation at 12,000 rpm for 10 min. The DNA sample was washed with 800 μL of pre-chilled 70% ethanol and air-dried before resuspension in 50 μL TE buffer (10 mM Tri-HCl, 0.1 mM EDTA, pH 8.0). DNA quantification and quality analysis were carried out by agarose gel electrophoresis with known DNA marker as standard.

4.3. Fusarium Strain Identification

The purified *Fusarium* strains were identified to species by morphological characteristics, and this was confirmed by *TEF-1α*gene sequence analysis of the representative strains. Methods for determining phenotypic characters and mycelial growth of *Fusarium* strains were from published protocols [21].

In order to verify the identity of *Fusarium* strains collected, DNA sequence comparisons were made for a subset of the strains using the *TEF-1α* gene, known as one of the most pertinent gene for determining the species rank in the *Fusarium* genus [23–25]. Portions of the *TEF-1α* gene were amplified with primer pair EF-1 (3′-ATGGGTAAGGA(A/G)GACAAGAC-5′) and EF-2 (3′-GGA(G/A)GTACCAGT(G/C)ATCATGTT-5′) in a thermal cycler. Polymerase chain reaction (PCR) was performed in a 50 μL reaction system afterwards [4], with minor modifications. PCR reaction mixtures contained 1× TransStar FastPfu Fly PCR SuperMix (TransGen Biotech, Beijing, China), 0.2 μM of each primer, and 50 ng of genomic DNA template. A negative control omitting the DNA template was used in every set of reactions. The thermal cycler (T100 Thermal Cycler, Bio-Rad, Hercules, CA, USA) conditions consisted of an initial denaturation step at 94 °C for 2 min, followed by 30 cycles of denaturation at 94 °C for 20 s, annealing at 58 °C for 20 s and extension at 72 °C for 30 s, then a final extension of 72 °C for 5 min. Amplified products (50 μL) were separated by electrophoresis on 1.5% (*w*/*v*) agarose gels. Gels were stained with ethidium bromide and photographed under UV light in the Bio-Imaging system (Bio-Rad, Hercules, CA USA). Fragments were excised and extracted from the gel using the QIAquick gel extraction kit (QIAGEN, Hilden, Germany) according to the manufacturer's instructions. Purified amplicons were sequenced in both directions using an ABI3730XL DNA sequencer (Applied Biosystems, Foster City, CA, USA) for each strain, and contigs were assembled with Sequencher version 4.1 program (Gene Codes Corporation). The *TEF-1α* gene sequences generated in this study were subjected to similarity searches with the BLASTn network service of NCBI nucleotide database.

4.4. Phylogenetic Analysis

Portions of the *TEF-1α* gene sequences from eleven *Fusarium* strains were generated for phylogenetic analysis in this study (Table 1). All sequences were compared with sequences of *Fusarium* species available in the GenBank database through BLASTn searches for similar sequences.

Phylogenetic analyses were conducted using MEGA v. 5.10 [29] to characterize the genetic diversity and evolutionary relationships of the strains. *TEF-1α* sequences of twenty-five fungal strains belonging to *Fusarium* genus retrieved from the NCBI database were also used as references for constructing a phylogenetic tree. In total, thirty-six sequences were analyzed, including seven *F. equiseti* strains, ten *F. fujikuroi* strains, eight *F. solani* strains, three *F. concentricum* strains, two *F. lactisi* strains, two *F. proliferatum* strains, two *F. subglutinans* strains, and two *F. verticillioides* strains. The *TEF-1α* sequences of these *Fusarium* strains were all available in NCBI nucleotide database, and detailed information about their strain code, geographic origin, and host/substrate is listed in Table 3.

Table 3. *Fusarium* strains used in phylogenetic analysis and their origins and GenBank accession numbers of *TEF-1α* genes.

Speices	Strain code	Origin	Host/Substrate	Accession number	Reference
F. concentricum	B2447B	Malaysia	Banana	KY379181	[38]
F. concentricum	MUCL54697	China	Sweet pepper	KC816735	[22]
F. concentricum	NRRL25202	Korea	Delphacidae	JF740760	[24]
F. equiseti	35b	China	Wheat	KY466715	-
F. equiseti	B1349T	China	Tomato	KM886212	-
F. equiseti	PAK54	USA	Loquat	KY523101	-
F. equiseti	Q12002	China	Sweet pepper	KF208617	This study
F. equiseti	Q12003	China	Sweet pepper	KF208618	This study
F. equiseti	Q12005	China	Sweet pepper	KF208619	This study
F. equiseti	TOR-9	Spain	Strawberry	KX215087	[39]
F. fujikuroi	37-EF1	Malaysia	Pineapple	KC584844	-
F. fujikuroi	BJ-1	China	Bletilla striata	MH263736	-
F. fujikuroi	F271	India	Rice	KM586385	-
F. fujikuroi	F326	India	Rice	KP009955	-
F. fujikuroi	M7055	China	Maize	KC964126	[40]
F. fujikuroi	Q12038	China	Sweet pepper	KF208623	This study
F. fujikuroi	Q12039	China	Sweet pepper	KF208624	This study
F. fujikuroi	Q12040	China	Sweet pepper	KF208625	This study
F. fujikuroi	Q12041	China	Sweet pepper	KF208626	This study
F. fujikuroi	Q12042	China	Sweet pepper	KF208627	This study
F. lactisi	NRRL25200	USA	*Ficus carica*	AF160272	[41]
F. lactisi	SPF22	Korea	Sweet pepper	JF411959	[5]
F. proliferatum	9174	Malaysia	Pitaya	JX869021	[42]
F. proliferatum	9194	Malaysia	Pitaya	JX869025	[42]
F. solani	DE17	Malaysia	Mangrove soil	KM096385	-
F. solani	N2211	Malaysia	Cucurbits	KT211623	-
F. solani	N2214	Malaysia	Cucurbits	KT211624	-
F. solani	NRRL52699	Colombia	Cercopidae	JF740782	[24]
F. solani	NRRL52704	USA	Tetranychidae	JF740786	[24]
F. solani	Q12029	China	Sweet pepper	KF208620	This study
F. solani	Q12030	China	Sweet pepper	KF208621	This study
F. solani	Q12034	China	Sweet pepper	KF208622	This study
F. subglutinans	MUCL52468	Belgium	Maize	HM067691	[25]
F. subglutinans	NRRL22016	USA	Maize	AF160289	[25,41,43]
F. verticillioides	ITEM2625	Slovakia	Maize	KF715264	-
F. verticillioides	NRRL22172	Germany	Maize	AF160262	[25,41,43]

All sequences were aligned initially with ClustalX software [44] and the alignments manually edited. Phylogenetic analyses of the sequences were performed with MEGA5.1 for Neighbor-joining (NJ) analysis, and Kimura-2 parameter model and pairwise deletion option for gaps were used. The reliability of the tree topologies was evaluated using bootstrap support with 1000 pseudoreplicates of the data.

4.5. Mycotoxin Production Analysis in Pepper Fruits via LC-MS/MS

Fungal strains were initially grown on PDA in 90 mm diameter Petri dishes for 7 days at 28 °C in the dark, after which they were used to inoculate pepper fruits. Mature pepper fruits were inoculated with mycelium plug as described by Van Poucke et al. [4]. After incubation, the fruit tissues from different positions, including the inoculation site and healthy site, were collected, homogenized separately, and processed for mycotoxin detection analysis. Mycotoxin detection results from lesions were used to do the mycotoxin profile analysis, and the results from the healthy parts were used for the migration study.

For each sample, 2 g of the grounded material was extracted with 8 mL extraction solvent (acetonitrile:water = 84:16, *v/v*). Multi-component analysis of mycotoxins in the inoculated samples was performed as described previously [45,46]. In total, 36 mycotoxins were included in the multi-mycotoxin analyses: Aflatoxin B_1 (AFB_1), aflatoxin B_2 (AFB_2), aflatoxin G_1 (AFG_1), aflatoxin G_2 (AFG_2), aflatoxin M_2 (AFM_2), aflatoxin M_1 (AFM_1), beauvericin (BEA), citrinin (CIT), cyclopiazonic acid (CPA), deoxynivalenol (DON), 3-acetyldeoxynivalenol (3-ADON), 15-acetyldeoxynivalenol (15-ADON), deoxynivalenol-3-glucoside (DON-3G), deepoxydeoxynivalenol (Deep-DON), diacetoxyscirpenol (DAS), fusaric acid (FA), fumonisin B_1 (FB_1), fumonisin B_2 (FB_2), fusarenon-X (FUSX), gliotoxin, HT2 toxin (HT2), moniliformin (MON), neosolaniol (NEO), nivalenol (NIV), ochratoxin A (OTA), patulin (PAT), penitrem A (PenA), sterigmatocystin (SMC), T-2 toxin (T-2), verruculogen (VER), zearalenone (ZEN), α-zearalanol (α-ZOL), β-zearalanol (β-ZOL), α-zearalenol (α-ZAL), β-zearalenol (β-ZAL), and zearalanone (ZAN). HPLC or analytical grade of acetonitrile, hexane, and other chemical agents were purchased from Merck (Darmstadt, Germany). Deionized water purified by a Milli-Q water system (Millipore, Billerica, MA, USA) was used throughout the experiments.

Author Contributions: S.W. and J.W. collected the samples; Z.Z. performed the mycotoxin analysis; S.W., S.L. and J.W. performed the experiments and analyzed the data; F.V.H. provided some protocols for isolation; writing—original draft preparation, J.W.; writing—review and editing, A.W.; supervision, A.W.

Funding: This research was funded by the National Key Research and Development Program of China (2017YFC1600304), National Natural Science Foundation of China (31871896, 31401598, and 31602124), Shanghai Agriculture Commission Basic Research Programs (2014NO.7-3-7 and 2011NO.4-3).

Conflicts of Interest: The authors declare no conflict of interest.

References

1. Vanderslice, J.T.; Higgs, D.J.; Hayes, J.M.; Block, G. Ascorbic acid and dehydroascorbic acid content of foods-as-eaten. *J. Food Compos. Anal.* **1990**, *3*, 105–118. [CrossRef]
2. Speranza, G.; Lo Scalzo, R.; Morelli, C.F.; Rabuffetti, M.; Bianchi, G. Influence of drying techniques and growing location on the chemical composition of sweet pepper (*Capsicum annuum* L., var. Senise). *J. Food Biochem.* **2019**, e13031. [CrossRef] [PubMed]
3. Qin, C.; Yu, C.S.; Shen, Y.; Fang, X.D.; Chen, L.; Min, J.M.; Cheng, J.; Zhao, S.; Xu, M.; Luo, Y.; et al. Whole-genome sequencing of cultivated and wild peppers provides insights into *Capsicum* domestication and specialization. *Proc. Natl. Acad. Sci. USA* **2014**, *111*, 5135–5140. [CrossRef] [PubMed]
4. Van Poucke, K.; Monbaliu, S.; Munaut, F.; Heungens, K.; De Saeger, S.; Van Hove, F. Genetic diversity and mycotoxin production of *Fusarium lactis* species complex isolates from sweet pepper. *Int. J. Food Microbiol.* **2012**, *153*, 28–37. [CrossRef] [PubMed]
5. Choi, H.W.; Hong, S.K.; Kim, W.G.; Lee, Y.K. First report of internal fruit rot of sweet pepper in Korea caused by *Fusarium lactis*. *Plant Dis.* **2011**, *95*, 1476. [CrossRef] [PubMed]

6. Yang, Y.; Bouras, N.; Yang, J.; Howard, R.J.; Strelkov, S.E. Mycotoxin production by isolates of *Fusarium lactis* from greenhouse sweet pepper (*Capsicum annuum*). *Int. J. Food Microbiol.* **2011**, *151*, 150–156. [CrossRef] [PubMed]
7. Fletcher, J.T. *Fusarium* stem and fruit rot of sweet peppers in the glasshouse. *Plant Pathol.* **1994**, *43*, 225–227. [CrossRef]
8. Yang, J.; Kharbanda, P.D.; Howard, R.J.; Mirza, M. Identification and pathogenicity of *Fusarium lactis*, causal agent of internal fruit rot of greenhouse sweet pepper in Alberta. *Can. J. Plant Pathol.* **2009**, *31*, 47–56. [CrossRef]
9. Howard, R.J.; Garland, J.A.; Seaman, W.L. *Disease and Pests of Vegetable Crops in Canada*, 1st ed.; The Canadian Phytopathological Society and Entomological Society of Canada: Ottawa, ON, Canada, 1994; pp. 333–336.
10. Yang, Y.; Cao, T.; Yang, J.; Howard, R.J.; Kharbanda, P.D.; Strelkov, S.E. Histopathology of internal fruit rot of sweet pepper caused by *Fusarium lactis*. *Can. J. Plant Pathol.* **2010**, *32*, 86–97. [CrossRef]
11. Utkhede, R.; Mathur, S. *Fusarium* fruit rot of greenhouse sweet peppers in Canada. *Plant Dis.* **2003**, *87*, 100. [CrossRef]
12. Utkhede, R.; Mathur, S. Internal fruit rot caused by *Fusarium subglutinans* in greenhouse sweet peppers. *Can. J. Plant Pathol.* **2004**, *26*, 386–390. [CrossRef]
13. Jarvis, W.R.; Khosla, S.K.; Barrie, S.D. *Fusarium* stem and fruit rot of sweet pepper in Ontario greenhouses. *Can. Plant Dis. Surv.* **1994**, *74*, 131–134.
14. Frans, M.; Aerts, R.; Van Laethem, S.; Ceusters, J. Environmental effects on growth and sporulation of *Fusarium* spp. causing internal fruit rot in bell pepper. *Eur. J. Plant Pathol.* **2017**, *149*, 875–883. [CrossRef]
15. Kharbanda, P.D.; Yang, J.; Howard, R.J.; Mirza, M. Internal fruit rot of greenhouse peppers caused by *Fusarium lactis*-a new disease. *Greenh. Bus.* **2006**, *5*, 11–16.
16. Chu, F.S.; Liu, G.Y. Simultaneous occurrence of fumonisin B_1 and other mycotoxins in moldy corn collected from People's Republic of China in regions with high incidences of esophageal cancer. *Appl. Environ. Microb.* **1994**, *60*, 847–852.
17. Peraica, M.; Radic, B.; Lucic, A.; Pavlovic, M. Toxic effects of mycotoxins in humans. *Bull. World Health Organ.* **1999**, *77*, 754–766. [PubMed]
18. Yazar, S.; Omurtag, G.Z. Fumonisins, trichothecenes and zearalenone in cereals. *Int. J. Mol. Sci.* **2008**, *9*, 2062–2090. [CrossRef] [PubMed]
19. Monbaliu, S.; Van Poucke, K.; Heungens, K.; Van Peteghem, C.; De Saeger, S. Production and migration of mycotoxins in sweet pepper analyzed by multimycotoxin LC-MS/MS. *J. Agric. Food Chem.* **2010**, *58*, 10475–10479. [CrossRef]
20. Restani, P. Diffusion of mycotoxins in fruits and vegetables. In *Mycotoxins in Fruits and Vegetables*, 1st ed.; Barkai-Golan, R., Paster, N., Eds.; Academic Press: San Diego, CA, USA, 2008; pp. 105–114.
21. Leslie, J.F.; Summerell, B.A. *The Fusarium Lab Manual*, 1st ed.; Blackwell Publishing: Ames, IA, USA, 2006; pp. 3–274.
22. Wang, J.H.; Feng, Z.H.; Han, Z.; Song, S.Q.; Lin, S.H.; Wu, A.B. First report of pepper fruit rot caused by *Fusarium concentricum* in China. *Plant Dis.* **2013**, *97*, 1657. [CrossRef]
23. O'Donnell, K.; Kistler, H.C.; Cigelnik, E.; Ploetz, R.C. Multiple evolutionary origins of the fungus causing Panama disease of banana: Concordant evidence from unclear and mitochondrial gene genealogies. *Proc. Natl. Acad. Sci. USA* **1998**, *95*, 2044–2049. [CrossRef]
24. O'Donnell, K.; Humber, R.A.; Geiser, D.M.; Kang, S.; Park, B.; Robert, V.A.; Crous, P.W.; Johnston, P.R.; Aoki, T.; Rooney, A.P.; et al. Phylogenetic diversity of insecticolous fusaria inferred from multilocus DNA sequence data and their molecular identification via FUSARIUM-ID and *Fusarium* MLST. *Mycologia* **2012**, *104*, 427–445. [CrossRef] [PubMed]
25. Scauflaire, J.; Gourgue, M.; Munaut, F. *Fusarium temperatum* sp. nov. from maize, an emergent species closely related to *Fusarium subglutinans*. *Mycologia* **2011**, *103*, 586–597. [CrossRef] [PubMed]
26. Ward, T.J.; Bielawski, J.P.; Kistler, H.C.; Sullivan, E.; O'Donnell, K. Ancestral polymorphism and adaptive evolution in the trichothecene mycotoxin gene cluster of phytopathogenic *Fusarium*. *Proc. Natl. Acad. Sci. USA* **2002**, *9*, 9278–9283. [CrossRef] [PubMed]
27. Jennings, P.; Coates, M.E.; Turner, J.A.; Chandler, E.A.; Nicholson, P. Determination of deoxynivalenol and nivalenol chemotypes of *Fusarium culmorum* isolates from England and Wales by PCR assay. *Plant Pathol.* **2004**, *53*, 182–190. [CrossRef]
28. Yang, L.; van der Lee, T.; Yang, X.; Yu, D.; Waalwijk, C. *Fusarium* populations on Chinese barley show a dramatic gradient in mycotoxin profiles. *Phytopathology* **2008**, *98*, 719–727. [CrossRef] [PubMed]

29. Tamura, K.; Peterson, D.; Peterson, N.; Stecher, G.; Nei, M.; Kumar, S. MEGA5: Molecular evolutionary genetics analysis using maximum likelihood, evolutionary distance, and maximum parsimony methods. *Mol. Biol. Evol.* **2011**, *28*, 2731–2739. [CrossRef]
30. Al-Hatmi, A.M.S.; Mirabolfathy, M.; Hagen, F.; Normand, A.; Stielow, J.B.; Karami-Osbo, R.; Van Diepeningen, A.D.; Meis, J.F.; De Hoog, G.S. DNA barcoding, MALDI-TOF, and AFLP data support *Fusarium ficicrescens* as a distinct species within the *Fusarium fujikuroi* species complex. *Fungal Biol.* **2016**, *120*, 265–278. [CrossRef]
31. Wulff, E.G.; Sorense, J.L.; Lubeck, M.; Nielsen, K.F.; Thrane, U.; Torp, J. *Fusarium* spp. associated with rice bakanae: Ecology, genetic diversity, pathogenicity and toxigenicity. *Environ. Microbiol.* **2010**, *12*, 649–657. [CrossRef]
32. Stepien, L.; Koczyk, G.; Waskiewicz, A. *FUM* cluster divergence in fumonisins-producing Fusarium species. *Fungal Biol.* **2011**, *115*, 112–123. [CrossRef]
33. Hestbjerg, H.; Nielsen, K.F.; Thrane, U.; Elmholt, S. Production of trichothecenes and other secondary metabolites by Fusarium culmorum and Fusarium equiseti on common laboratory media and a soil organic matter agar: An ecological interpretation. *J. Agric. Food Chem.* **2002**, *50*, 7593–7599. [CrossRef]
34. Stankovic, S.; Levic, J.; Petrovic, T.; Logrieco, A.; Moretti, A. Pathogenicity and mycotoxin production by *Fusarium proliferatum* isolated from onion and garlic in Serbia. *Eur. J. Plant Pathol.* **2007**, *118*, 165–172. [CrossRef]
35. Wang, Q.G.; Xu, L.J. Beauvericin, a bioactive compound produced by fungi: A short review. *Molecules* **2012**, *17*, 2367–2377. [CrossRef] [PubMed]
36. Qu, B.; Li, H.P.; Zhang, J.B.; Xu, Y.B.; Huang, T.; Wu, A.B.; Zhao, C.S.; Carter, J.; Nicholson, P.; Liao, Y.C. Geographic distribution and genetic diversity of *Fusarium graminearum* and *F. asiaticum* on wheat spikes throughout China. *Plant Pathol.* **2008**, *57*, 15–24. [CrossRef]
37. Wang, J.H.; Li, H.P.; Qu, B.; Zhang, J.B.; Huang, T.; Chen, F.F.; Liao, Y.C. Development of a generic PCR detection of 3-acetyldeoxynivalenol, 15-acetyldeoxynivalenol- and nivalenol-chemotypes of *Fusarium graminearum* clade. *Int. J. Mol. Sci.* **2008**, *9*, 2495–2504. [CrossRef]
38. Abd Murad, N.B.; Mohamed Nor, N.N.; Shohaimi, S.; Mohd Zainudin, N.A.I. Genetic diversity and pathogenicity of *Fusarium* species associated with fruit rot disease in banana across Peninsular Malaysia. *J. Appl. Microbiol.* **2017**, *123*, 1533–1546. [CrossRef]
39. Pastrana, A.M.; Basallote-Ureba, M.J.; Aquado, A.; Capote, N. Potential inoculum sources and incidence of strawberry soilborne pathogens in Spain. *Plant Dis.* **2017**, *101*, 751–760. [CrossRef]
40. Wang, J.H.; Zhang, J.B.; Li, H.P.; Gong, A.D.; Xue, S.; Agboola, R.S.; Liao, Y.C. Molecular identification, mycotoxin production and comparative pathogenictiy of *Fusarium temperatum* isolated from maize in China. *J. Phytopathol.* **2013**. [CrossRef]
41. Lima, C.S.; Pfenning, L.H.; Costa, S.S.; Abreu, L.M.; Leslie, J.F. *Fusarium tupiense* sp. nov., a member of the *Gibberella fujikuroi* complex that causes mango malformation in Brazil. *Mycologia* **2012**, *104*, 1408–1419. [CrossRef]
42. Masratul Hawa, M.; Salleh, B.; Latiffah, Z. Characterization and pathogenicity of *Fusarium proliferatum* causing stem rot of *Hylocereus polyrhizus* in Malaysia. *Ann. Appl. Biol.* **2013**, *163*, 269–280. [CrossRef]
43. Skovgaard, K.; Rosendahl, S.; O'Donnell, K.; Nirenberg, H.I. *Fusarium commune* is a new species identified by morphological and molecular phylogenetic data. *Mycologia* **2003**, *95*, 630–636. [CrossRef]
44. Thompson, J.D.; Gibson, T.J.; Plewniak, F.; Jeanmougin, F.; Higgins, D.G. The Clustal X windows interface: Flexible strategies for multiple sequence alignment aided by quality analysis tools. *Nucleic Acids Res.* **1997**, *25*, 4876–4882. [CrossRef]
45. Monbaliu, S.; Van Poucke, C.; Van Peteghem, C.; Van Poucke, K.; Heungens, K.; De Saeger, S. Development of a multi-mycotoxin liquid chromatography/tandem mass spectrometry method for sweet pepper analysis. *Rapid Commun. Mass Spectrom.* **2009**, *23*, 3–11. [CrossRef]
46. Zhao, Z.Y.; Yang, X.L.; Zhao, X.Y.; Chen, L.; Bai, B.; Zhou, C.Y.; Wang, J.H. Method development and validation for the analysis of emerging and traditional fusarium mycotoxins in pepper, potato, tomato, and cucumber by UPLC-MS/MS. *Food Anal. Methods* **2018**, *11*, 1780–1788. [CrossRef]

toxins

MDPI

Article

Toxin Production in Soybean (*Glycine max* L.) Plants with Charcoal Rot Disease and by *Macrophomina phaseolina*, the Fungus that Causes the Disease

Hamed K. Abbas [1,*], Nacer Bellaloui [2], Cesare Accinelli [3], James R. Smith [2] and W. Thomas Shier [4,*]

1 Biological Control of Pests Research Unit, US Department of Agriculture-Agricultural Research Service, Stoneville, MS 38776, USA

2 Crop Genetics Research Unit, US Department of Agriculture-Agricultural Research Service, Stoneville, MS 38776, USA; nacer.bellaloui@usda.gov (N.B.); rusty.smith@usda.gov (J.R.S.)

3 Department of Agricultural and Food Sciences, Alma Mater Studiorum–University of Bologna, 40127 Bologna, Italy; cesare.accinelli@unibo.it

4 Department of Medicinal Chemistry, College of Pharmacy, University of Minnesota, Minneapolis, MN 55455, USA

* Correspondence: hamed.abbas@usda.gov (H.K.A.); shier001@umn.edu (W.T.S.); Tel.: +1-662-686-5313 (H.K.A.); +1-612-624-9465 (W.T.S.)

Received: 13 September 2019; Accepted: 29 October 2019; Published: 6 November 2019

Abstract: Charcoal rot disease, caused by the fungus *Macrophomina phaseolina*, results in major economic losses in soybean production in southern USA. *M. phaseolina* has been proposed to use the toxin (-)-botryodiplodin in its root infection mechanism to create a necrotic zone in root tissue through which fungal hyphae can readily enter the plant. The majority (51.4%) of *M. phaseolina* isolates from plants with charcoal rot disease produced a wide range of (-)-botryodiplodin concentrations in a culture medium (0.14–6.11 μg/mL), 37.8% produced traces below the limit of quantification (0.01 μg/mL), and 10.8% produced no detectable (-)-botryodiplodin. Some culture media with traces or no (-)-botryodiplodin were nevertheless strongly phytotoxic in soybean leaf disc cultures, consistent with the production of another unidentified toxin(s). Widely ranging (-)-botryodiplodin levels (traces to 3.14 μg/g) were also observed in the roots, but not in the aerial parts, of soybean plants naturally infected with charcoal rot disease. This is the first report of (-)-botryodiplodin in plant tissues naturally infected with charcoal rot disease. No phaseolinone was detected in *M. phaseolina* culture media or naturally infected soybean tissues. These results are consistent with (-)-botryodiplodin playing a role in the pathology of some, but not all, *M. phaseolina* isolates from soybeans with charcoal rot disease in southern USA.

Keywords: fungi; mycotoxins; phaseolinone; LC/MS; soybean; charcoal rot disease; root infection mechanism

Key Contribution: This is the first report of a toxin being found in the tissues of soybean plants naturally infected in the field with charcoal rot disease, specifically finding (-)-botryodiplodin and not phaseolinone. This is also the first report of results consistent with some isolates of *M. phaseolina* using different toxins, other than (-)-botryodiplodin, to facilitate root infection in soybean.

---

1. Introduction

The fungus *Macrophomina phaseolina* (Tassi) Goidanich [1], also known by the teleomorph *Sclerotium bataticola* Taub. [2], is the cause of charcoal rot disease, and other named diseases, in soybeans and about 500 other crop and ornamental species in the United States and internationally [3–5]. Charcoal rot disease, also known as summer wilt, dry weather wilt, or black root disease, results in crop yield loss and seed quality deterioration in soybeans and other crops [6–11]. Charcoal rot disease is more prevalent in heat- and drought-stressed conditions [12,13]. *M. phaseolina* can spread to adjacent plants with interdigitating roots through the soil, infecting the roots and spreading throughout the infected plant through the vascular system [14,15]. *M. phaseolina* forms black spore-like mycelial structures called microsclerotia, which allow the fungus to survive over winter. These microsclerotia are the grey and black dots in the stems and roots of soybean plants that give charcoal rot disease its name [16]. Common agricultural practices such as managing planting dates, fungicide applications, and biological control have been ineffective in controlling this disease [17–23]. Despite extensive efforts to control charcoal rot disease by developing resistant soybean genotypes [24–26], currently available genotypes are still not sufficiently resistant to prevent the disease in the field, although moderately resistant genotypes have been shown to have lower levels of *M. phaseolina* in plant tissues [27–29].

The mechanism used by *M. phaseolina* to infect plants with charcoal rot disease is not yet understood, in part because of the diversity in *M. phaseolina* isolates [30–33]. *M. phaseolina* has been reported to produce toxins, including (-)-botryodiplodin and phaseolinone [34–37]. It has been proposed that a toxin may play a role in an early step of the mechanism used by *M. phaseolina* to infect susceptible plants through the roots from the soil reservoir, where the fungus normally lives, particularly over the winter [7,36].

The objective of the present study is to investigate the involvement of toxins, particularly (-)-botryodiplodin, in the charcoal rot disease of soybeans. Soybeans are selected as the subject for these studies because charcoal rot disease causes major economic losses for soybean production in the midsouthern USA (Mississippi, Arkansas, and Louisiana) [10,11,38–40]. The role(s) of toxins in root infection is investigated in these studies by assessing the production of (-)-botryodiplodin, phaseolinone, and other toxins in cell-free culture filtrates of charcoal rot disease-causing *M. phaseolina* isolates and in roots and other tissues from soybean plants naturally infected with charcoal rot disease in the field. Studies on the culture filtrates of charcoal rot disease-causing *M. phaseolina* isolates resulted in the discovery that some, but not all, isolates produce (-)-botryodiplodin, but not phaseolinone, and some isolates that do not produce (-)-botryodiplodin do produce another as yet unknown toxin(s). Studies on toxins present in soybean plant tissues provided the first demonstration of a mycotoxin known to be produced by *M. phaseolina* in soybean plant tissues naturally infected with charcoal rot disease, specifically (-)-botryodiplodin, but not phaseolinone.

2. Results and Discussion

2.1. Toxin Production in Culture by M. Phaseolina Isolates from Plants with Charcoal Rot Disease

Toxin production in culture by *M. phaseolina* isolates from many USA sites and numerous types of plant sources were examined as the toxicity of cell-free culture medium filtrates in soybean leaf disc cultures from two soybean genotypes, DS97-84-1 and DT97-4290 (Table 1). Toxicity assessments with the two genotypes exhibited a similar rank order with no substantive difference between the two, whether assessed at 50% strength or at full strength. The same cell-free culture filtrates from *M. phaseolina* isolates were also assayed by LC/MS for levels of (-)-botryodiplodin, the toxin previously [35] found associated with culture filtrates of a *M. phaseolina* isolate from a soybean plant in Mississippi with charcoal rot disease. Observed concentrations of (-)-botryodiplodin ranged from not detectable to 6.11 μg/mL (Table 1). The majority of isolates (51.4% of isolates studied) produced quantifiable levels of (-)-botryodiplodin in culture filtrates, while 37.8% of isolates studied produced trace levels (i.e., above the limit of detection (1×10^{-5} ng/μL), but less than the limit of quantitation (1×10^{-2} ng/μL), and 10.8% of isolates studied produced no detectable level of (-)-botryodiplodin in culture filtrates.

Table 1. Toxicity, color, and (-)-botryodiplodin production in cell-free culture medium filtrates from *Macrophomina phaseolina* isolates from plants exhibiting charcoal rot disease properties in various states of the USA.

			Toxicity [a] in Leaf Disc Cultures of Two Soybean Genotypes					
			DS97-84-1		DT97-4290			
Isolate	**Collection Site**	**Plant Host**	**50% Strength**	**100% Strength**	**50% Strength**	**100% Strength**	**Color [b] in One-Week Cultures**	**(-)-Botryodiplodin [c] Concentration (μg/mL)**
*Mp*001A	MS	Soybean	++	++	+	+	beige	Trace
*Mp*001B	MS	Soybean	+	+	+	+	l tan	0.19
*Mp*004	MS	Soybean	++++	++++	+++	++++	d tan	0.18
*Mp*006A	MS	Soybean	++	++	+	++	l yellow	Trace
*Mp*006B	MS	Soybean	++	+++	+	+	l tan	0.14
*Mp*007	MS	Soybean	++	+++	++	+++	beige	0.29
*Mp*008A	MS	Soybean	+	+	+	+	l yellow	0.15
*Mp*008B	MS	Soybean	++	+++	++	+++	beige	0.14
*Mp*009A	MS	Soybean	++	++	+	+	l tan	Trace
*Mp*010B	MS	Soybean	++	++	+	+	l tan	Trace
*Mp*011A	MS	Soybean	++	++	+++	+++	l tan	Trace
*Mp*144	KY	Soybean	+++	+++	++	+++	beige	0.18
*Mp*146	KY	Soybean	+++	+++	++	++	beige	0.2
*Mp*176	AR	Soybean	+	+	+	+	l yellow	0.08
*Mp*178	AR	Soybean	+++++	+++++	+++++	+++++	beige	1.64
*Mp*203	LA	Soybean	+++	+++	+++	+++	tan	Trace
*Mp*204	LA	Soybean	++	++	+	+	l tan	Trace
*Mp*214	SD	Soybean	+++	++++	+++	+++	l yellow	Trace
*Mp*220	TN	Soybean	++	++	+	+	l tan	0.17
*Mp*223	TX	Soybean	+++	+++	++++	++++	tan	0
*Mp*242	ND	Soybean	+	+	+	+	l tan	0.16
*Mp*272	MN	Soybean	++++	++++	++++	++++	l tan	Trace
*Mp*279	OK	Soybean	+++++	+++++	++++	+++++	d grey	4.03
*Mp*302	KS	Soybean	+++	+++	++	++	l tan	0.98
*Mp*305	KS	Soybean	++++	++++	+++	+++	l tan	Trace
*Mp*251	NE	Dry bean	++++	+++++	++++	+++++	tan	4.5
*Mp*228	NC	Fraser fir	+	+	+	+	l yellow	0
*Mp*264	MI	Fir	+++++	+++++	+++++	+++++	tan	6.11
*Mp*275	MN	Redwood	+++++	+++++	++++	+++++	tan	Trace
*Mp*183	FL	Strawberry	+++	++++	+++	++++	tan	0.74

Table 1. *Cont.*

			Toxicity [a] in Leaf Disc Cultures of Two Soybean Genotypes					
			DS97-84-1		DT97-4290			
Isolate	**Collection Site**	**Plant Host**	**50% Strength**	**100% Strength**	**50% Strength**	**100% Strength**	**Color [b] in One-Week Cultures**	**(-)-Botryodiplodin [c] Concentration (µg/mL)**
*Mp*315	AZ	Watermelon	++++	+++++	++++	+++++	beige	Trace
*Mp*249	GA	Unknown	+++++	+++++	++++	++++	tan	2.04
*Mp*216	Unknown	Unknown	++++	++++	+++	+++	l grey	0.31
*Mp*234	Unknown	Unknown	++++	++++	++++	++++	tan	0
*Mp*235	Unknown	Unknown	+	+	+	+	l tan	Trace
*Mp*238	Unknown	Unknown	+	+	+	+	l tan	0
*Mp*239	Unknown	Unknown	+	+	+	+	l tan	Trace

Abbreviations: *Macrophomina phaseolina, Mp*; Mississippi, MS; Kentucky, KY; Arkansas, AR; Louisiana, LA; South Dakota, SD; Tennessee, TN; Texas, TX; North Dakota, ND; Minnesota, MN; Oklahoma, OK; Kansas, KS; Nebraska, NE; North Carolina, NC; Michigan, MI; Florida, FL; Arizona, AZ; Georgia, GA; light, l; dark, d. [a] Toxicity score measured in soybean leaf disc cultures of two soybean genotypes: (i) DT97-4290, which is moderately resistant to charcoal rot disease and (ii) DS97-84-1, which is susceptible to charcoal rot disease. Toxicity was assessed qualitatively according to the following symptom rating scale: healthy tissue < a little browning around the edges of the leaf disc, + < moderate browning around the edges of the leaf disc, ++ < browning of the whole leaf disc, +++ < browning of the leaf disc with some photobleaching, ++++ < photobleaching of the whole leaf disc, +++++. [b] Color density was assessed qualitatively according to the following color density scale: whitish < light yellow < light tan < light grey < tan < beige or amber < dark tan < dark brown or dark grey < black. [c] (-)-Botryodiplodin concentrations in culture medium filtrates were measured quantitatively by LC/MS.

Whether *M. phaseolina* isolates were from trees, soybeans, melons, or other plant sources, cell-free culture filtrates were toxic in soybean leaf disc cultures, and toxicity levels varied from not detectable to very toxic (Table 1). Culture filtrates from *M. phaseolina* isolates that contained high levels of (-)-botryodiplodin (>1 μg/mL) were all very toxic in soybean leaf disc cultures, resulting in maximal or near maximal toxicity with both DT97-4290 and DS97-84-1 soybean leaf discs at 100% and 50% strength. Culture filtrates that contained intermediate levels of (-)-botryodiplodin (0.2–1.0 μg/mL) were moderately toxic in soybean leaf disc cultures. However, some other *M. phaseolina* isolate culture filtrates that contained only trace levels or even no detectable (-)-botryodiplodin were highly toxic in soybean leaf disc cultures. This observation is consistent with some disease-inducing isolates of *M. phaseolina* producing one or more toxins other than (-)-botryodiplodin. This is the first report of results supporting the hypothesis that different isolates of *M. phaseolina* may use different toxins to facilitate root infection in soybeans. Further studies are needed to determine if any of those isolates use the other toxin(s) to facilitate root infection by a mechanism analogous to the one by which (-)-botryodiplodin might facilitate root infection. Some culture filtrates from the disease-inducing isolates of *M. phaseolina* contained very little toxicity in soybean leaf disc cultures, despite the isolate being able to cause charcoal rot disease. Explanations for this observation include the possible presence of a toxin-production regulatory mechanism that suppresses toxin production by those isolates under the culture conditions used in this study, or the possibility that charcoal rot disease in soybeans may be caused by a seed-borne *M. phaseolina* endophyte that would not need a root infection mechanism or any toxins associated with it [14]. The *M. phaseolina* isolate from which phaseolinone was originally isolated [34,37] was a seed-borne endophyte.

Also included in Table 1 is an assessment of the color of week-old cultures of *M. phaseolina*. Dunlap and Bruton [41] reported that a *M. phaseolina* isolate formed pigment in an infected muskmelon (*Cucumis melo*) and in liquid culture media containing glycine and some other amino acids. Some *M. phaseolina* isolates that cause charcoal rot disease in soybeans have been observed to form large numbers of black microschlerotia under the same culture conditions that induce the production of (-)-botryodiplodin [42]. In the data in Table 1, the rank order of pigment production, as assessed qualitatively according to the color density scale used, differed substantially from the rank order of toxicity in cell-free culture filtrates as assessed in soybean leaf disc cultures at either full strength or 50% dilution and from the relative amount of (-)-botryodiplodin present as measured by LC/MS. Thus, pigment production as assessed in this study appeared to be unrelated to toxin production, consistent with the previously identified correlations not being a general phenomenon when larger numbers of *M. phaseolina* isolates are examined.

2.2. Analysis of Toxin Levels in Tissue Samples from Soybean Plants Naturally Infected with Charcoal Rot Disease

If the hyphae of a *M. phaseolina* strain that causes charcoal rot disease use a toxin(s) to create a necrotic area in the root and thereby facilitate entry into soybean plant roots from a soil reservoir, those hyphae are expected to produce a toxin(s) at least from the time the fungus detects the root in the soil until the fungal hyphae inside the plant have detected that a stable infection has been established there. Fungi that spread from plant to plant through interdigitating roots, as *M. phaseolina* does in the charcoal rot disease of soybeans, may also secrete a toxin(s) inside the roots of fully infected plants in order to create a necrotic area within the root from which hyphae may exit the plant to spread to adjacent plants. Thus, soybean plants exhibiting the symptoms of charcoal rot disease may contain a chemically and metabolically stable toxin in tissues at a level detectable by standard analytical methods such as LC/MS. If the *M. phaseolina* strain causing charcoal rot disease in a soybean plant is a constitutive (continuous) producer of the toxin, comparable levels of the toxin may be expected in all the affected tissues of diseased plants. Therefore, naturally infected soybean plants exhibiting symptoms of charcoal rot disease were collected from different infected areas in commercial soybean production fields in Mississippi in the 2004 growing season. Control soybean plants not exhibiting symptoms of charcoal rot disease were also collected. Samples of roots, leaves, stem pulp, branches, twigs, and seeds were individually extracted and analyzed by LC/MS for levels of (-)-botryodiplodin, phaseolinone, phomenone, and gigantenone (Table 2). Only (-)-botryodiplodin was detected and only in the roots of soybean plants exhibiting symptoms of charcoal rot disease, not in other tissues of diseased plants and not in the roots or any other tissues of control soybean plants not exhibiting symptoms of charcoal rot disease. This is the first report of a toxin being found in infected plant tissues associated with charcoal rot disease in soybeans. This observation would be expected if *M. phaseolina* used (-)-botryodiplodin in its mechanism for (i) initial root infection and (ii) to exit heavily infected plants in order to spread to and infect adjacent plants. However, additional studies are needed to establish a role for (-)-botryodiplodin in either the initial root infection or the root exit mechanism. No phaseolinone, phomenone, or gigantenone was found in any tissue of soybean plants with charcoal rot disease in this study. As shown in Table 3, these observations are confirmed by a similar study conducted in 2007, in which root tissue was collected from naturally infected soybean plants from commercial production fields in Mississippi and Kentucky, USA, and analyzed by LC/MS for levels of (-)-botryodiplodin, phaseolinone, phomenone, and gigantenone. As observed in the first study (Table 2), only (-)-botryodiplodin was detected in diseased roots, not phaseolinone, phomenone, or gigantenone. Again, (-)-botryodiplodin levels varied from traces to 3.14 μg/g, that is, greater than a 1000-fold concentration range. The wide range of (-)-botryodiplodin levels in charcoal rot-diseased soybean roots (Tables 2 and 3) paralleled the wide range of (-)-botryodiplodin production levels in cell-free culture filtrates of *M. phaseolina* isolates from plants with charcoal rot disease. In both experimental systems, there were a substantial number of cases in which (-)-botryodiplodin production was too low for it to be a toxin that could play a role in the pathology caused by those *M. phaseolina* strains, whether by facilitating root infection or any other mechanism.

Table 2. Mycotoxin levels in root and other tissues of soybean plants collected from soybean fields in Mississippi in 2004.

Sample Name	Charcoal Rot Disease	Soybean Tissue Type	(-)-Botryodiplodin (μg/g) [a]	Phomenone (μg/g) [a]	Gigantenone (μg/g) [a]	Phaseolinone (μg/g) [a]
RTS 999 302	Yes	Roots	0.786	0	0	0
USG 7582 306	Yes	Roots	0.13	0	0	0
DK B58-51 326	Yes	Roots	0.23	0	0	0
AG 5903 324	Yes	Roots	0.046	0	0	0
AG 5701 329	Yes	Roots	0.139	0	0	0
PGX 5703 313	Yes	Roots	0.334	0	0	0
PGY 5822 319	Yes	Roots	0.332	0	0	0
ESXVT-46 328	Yes	Roots	0.134	0	0	0
P 95 B96 301	Yes	Roots	0.006	0	0	0
P GX 5714 311	Yes	Roots	0.141	0	0	0
Garst 5812 331	Yes	Roots	0.209	0	0	0
DK 5767 32	Yes	Roots	0.061	0	0	0
All samples tested	Yes	Seeds	0	0	0	0
All samples tested	Yes	Pulp	0	0	0	0
All samples tested	Yes	Branches	0	0	0	0
All samples tested	Yes	Twigs	0	0	0	0
All samples tested	Yes	Leaves	0	0	0	0
Undiseased control [b]	No	Roots	0	0	0	0

[a] Identification and quantification of toxins in samples by LC/MS were based on one standard due to the limited amount of standards available. [b] Soybean plants of the Saline cultivar with no detectable sign of charcoal rot disease were collected from commercial fields in Mississippi. Samples of the same six tissues were taken, pooled, and extracted in the same way as tissues from diseased plants and the extracts were assayed by LC/MS in the same manner. Extracts of all undiseased soybean tissues, including roots, contained no detectable (-)-botryodiplodin or other toxin.

Table 3. Toxins in the roots of soybean plants exhibiting charcoal rot disease properties collected from commercial soybean fields in Kentucky and Mississippi in 2007.

Field and Location *	(-)-Botryodiplodin (μg/g)	Phomenone (μg/g)	Gigantenone (μg/g)	Phaseolinone (μg/g)
1 KY	0.870	0	0	0
417 MS	trace	0	0	0
1 KY	0.567	0	0	0
314 MS	3.139	0	0	0
3 KY	0.114	0	0	0
4 KY	0.115	0	0	0
2 KY	0.938	0	0	0
209 MS	0.757	0	0	0
4 KY	0.946	0	0	0
312 MS	0.703	0	0	0
210 P12 MS	trace	0	0	0

* Soybean plants exhibiting symptoms of charcoal rot disease were collected in the indicated commercial field numbers in the indicated states, brought to the laboratory, tissues harvested and stored at −20 °C until assayed. Soybean root samples had symptoms of charcoal rot and were run by LC/MS. Determination and quantification of these mycotoxins was by LC/MS based on one standard because a limited amount of these standards were available.

3. Conclusions

A wide range of (-)-botryodiplodin levels were observed in both cell-free culture medium filtrates from *M. phaseolina* isolates from plants with charcoal rot disease and in the roots, but not in the aerial parts, of soybean plants naturally infected with charcoal rot disease. Cell-free culture medium filtrates from some *M. phaseolina* isolates from plants with charcoal rot disease were strongly phytotoxic, despite containing only traces or no (-)-botryodiplodin. No phaseolinone was detected in either cell-free culture medium filtrates from *M. phaseolina* isolates or in tissues from soybean plants naturally infected with charcoal rot disease. The results of this study are consistent with some, but not all, isolates of *M. phaseolina* associated with charcoal rot disease in soybean-producing (-)-botryodiplodin. Some isolates of *M. phaseolina* cultured from soybean plants with charcoal rot disease produce no detectable (-)-botryodiplodin in culture, but do produce other unknown toxins. Further research is needed to determine what role, if any, (-)-botryodiplodin and other toxins produced by *M. phaseolina* isolates play in the root infection mechanism of the charcoal rot disease of soybeans.

4. Materials and Methods

4.1. Soybean Plant and Greenhouse Conditions

The soybean genotype DT97-4290 [28] was selected as an example of a genotype that is moderately resistant to charcoal rot disease, and the soybean genotype DS97-84-1 [43] was selected as an example of a genotype that is susceptible to charcoal rot disease. Plants were germinated in trays with vermiculite, and the seedlings of each genotype were transplanted into six soil-filled 9.45 L pots, each containing four plants of the same genotype. During the growth period, the soil water potential of the plants was maintained at approximate field conditions, 15 to −20 kPa. Six pots, each containing four plants, were used for each genotype. The greenhouse temperature was set to 34 °C for the day cycle and 28 °C for the night cycle. Light intensity ranged from that of sunny to cloudy days. Plants were harvested during the vegetative stage.

4.2. *M. phaseolina* Culture Sources

The collection locations and plant hosts of the 37 cultures of *M. phaseolina* used in the study are presented in Table 1. Some *M. phaseolina* cultures were isolated from infected plant tissues in the Abbas laboratory in 2013 using the method of Mengistu et al. [4,25], while other cultures were provided by colleagues from their collections, particularly G.L. Sciumbato, Mississippi State University.

4.3. Preparation of Cell-Free Culture Extracts

Potato dextrose broth (PDB) was prepared by boiling 200 g of peeled potatoes, straining them through a cheesecloth, and adding 20 g of dextrose per liter of water. PDB (150 mL) was placed in 500 mL Erlenmeyer flasks, covered with cotton plugs, autoclaved for 15 min, and allowed to cool to room temperature. Upon cooling, each flask was inoculated with three to four plugs of *M. phaseolina* isolate and placed on an Innova 40 Benchtop Incubator Shaker (New Brunswick Scientific Co., Inc., Edison, NY, USA) for seven days at 128 rpm, 28 °C. The color change of each culture after one week of incubation was observed and recorded according to the following color density scale: whitish < light yellow < light tan < light grey < tan < beige or amber < dark tan < dark brown or dark grey < black.

After seven days of incubation, the culture medium was passed through Whatman No.1 filter paper into a plastic beaker. The filtrate was then filtered through an 0.45 μm membrane filter in a disposable filter unit (Nalgene Company, Rochester, NY, USA, Size 250 mL cellulose nitrate CN Filter Unit) using a laboratory vacuum to achieve a cell-free filtrate that was stored at −20 °C until used.

4.4. Toxicity of Cell-Free Filtrates of M. phaseolina Culture Media in Soybean Leaf Disc Cultures

The toxicity of *M. phaseolina* culture filtrates was assessed by rating the appearance of soybean leaf discs from two genotypes (DT97-4290, which is moderately resistant to charcoal rot, and DS97-84-1, which is susceptible) after four to five days in half (50%) and full strength (100%) cell-free culture filtrates, *M. phaseolina* isolates were grown on potato dextrose agar (PDA) for seven days at 28 °C. True mature leaves with no signs of damage were harvested from 3- to 4-week-old soybean plants, and 4 mm discs were cut from the leaves using a sterile cork borer (No.4). Three leaf discs were placed in each well of sterile 24-well tissue culture trays with low evaporative lids (Becton Dickinson and Company, Franklin Lakes, NJ, USA) containing 1.5 mL of culture filtrate in triplicate at two concentrations (50% and 100%). The trays were then incubated in a growth chamber at 25 °C under continuous light for 96 h. The discs were observed for signs of toxic effects after 24, 48, 72, and 96 h. Toxicity was assessed qualitatively according to the following symptom rating scale: healthy tissue < a little browning around the edges of the leaf disc, + < moderate browning around the edges of the leaf disc, ++ < browning of the whole leaf disc, +++ < browning of the leaf disc with some photobleaching, ++++ < photobleaching of the whole leaf disc, +++++.

4.5. Toxin Standards for LC/MS Analyses

The structures of toxins measured in this study are presented in Figure 1. (±)-Botryodiplodin was synthesized, as described in the accompanying manuscript [44], as a white powder with purity over 98%. A stock solution of (±)-botryodiplodin (1000 ng/μL) was prepared in chloroform. Working standards were prepared in the concentration range 1.0×10^{-5} ng/μL to 40 ng/μL in ethyl acetate. Gigantenone and phomenone were gifts from Gary A. Strobel, Montana State University, Bozeman, MT. Phaseolinone was synthesized (Figure 2) from a sample of the phomenone (6.5 mg, 0.0246 mmole) dissolved in 1 mL chloroform and mixed with a 1.2 molar excess of m-chloroperoxybenzoic acid (Acros Organics, 0.029 mmole, 7.15 mg of 70% pure material) and pyridine (4.7 μL, 4.6 mg, 0.058 mmole) dissolved in 200 μL chloroform. The mixture was incubated for 1 h at −10 °C with stirring and then allowed to warm to room temperature overnight. The reaction mixture was diluted with ether, extracted twice with water, once with 1N HCl to remove pyridine, twice with saturated sodium bicarbonate-brine solution to remove product m-chlorobenzoic acid and unreacted m-chloroperoxybenzoic acid, dried over anhydrous sodium sulfate, and evaporated in vacuo. The product (7.5 mg) gave a single peak at *m/e* 281 (phaseolinone + H^+) in LC/MS analysis under the conditions described below, with no detectable phomenone starting material at *m/e* 265. A single peak was observed in LC/MS for the phaseolinone preparation, even though the reaction conditions would be expected to produce a mixture of phaseolinone and epi-phaseolinone, presumably because the two forms were not resolved under the liquid chromatography conditions used.

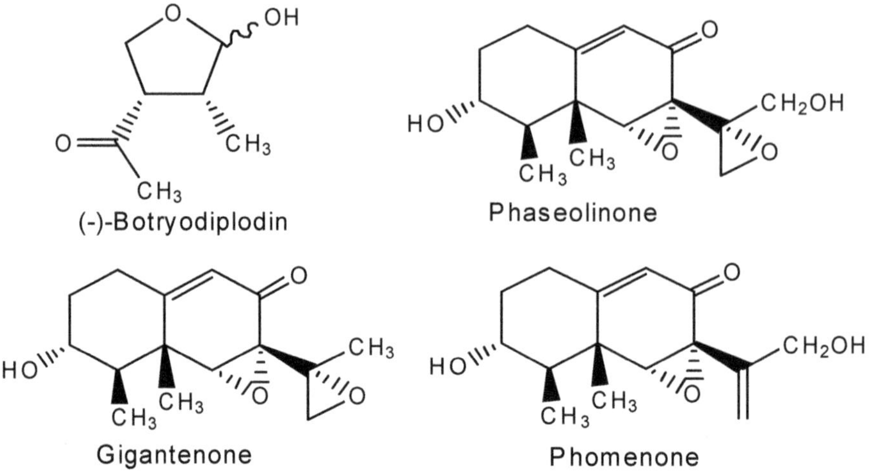

Figure 1. Chemical structures of the toxins measured by LC/MS in *M. phaseolina* culture media and soybean root tissues.

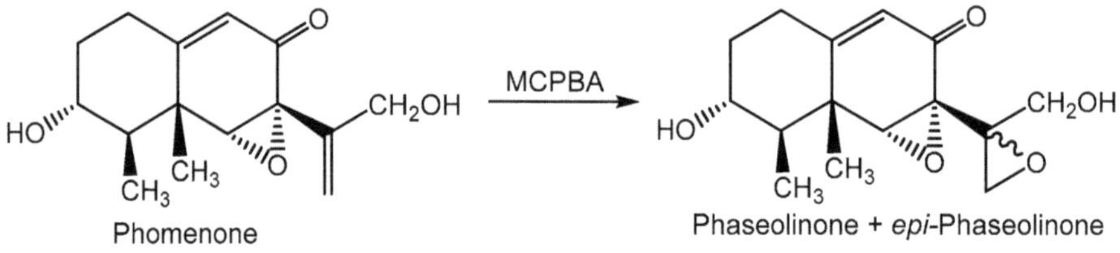

Figure 2. The chemical reaction used in the semi-synthesis of the LC/MS standard phaseolinone from the natural toxin phomenone. MCPBA = meta-chloroperoxybenzoic acid.

4.6. Preparation of Plant Tissue and M. phaseolina Culture Medium Extracts for LC/MS Analyses

Soybean root and other tissue samples were cleaned of adherent earth, dried in an oven at 45 °C for two to three days, and ground to the consistency of flour using a Stain Laboratory Mill Grinder, Model M-2 (Fred Stein Laboratories, INC., Atchison, Kansas, USA). Ethyl acetate (10 g) was added to 50 g of each sample, shaken for 1 h, filtered through filter paper (Whatman No.1), and transferred to vials for analysis by LC/MS as described below. *M. phaseolina* culture medium cell-free filtrate samples were extracted with ethyl acetate in a 1:1, *v:v* ratio on a vortex mixer for 1 min and allowed to separate into two distinct layers. The ethyl acetate layer was transferred to vials for analysis by LC/MS.

4.7. LC/MS Analysis

LC/MS analyses of toxin samples obtained prior to 2007 were conducted on a Thermo Finnigan LCQ Advantage instrument coupled to a Thermo Finnigan Surveyor MS and a Thermo Finnigan Surveyor MS Pump (Thermo Electron Corporation, West Palm Beach, FL, USA). After 2007, a more advanced and upgraded LTQ XL Ion Trap Mass Spectrometer, Finnigan Surveyor Autosampler, and Finnigan Surveyor MS Pump (Thermo Scientific, West Palm Beach, FL, USA) were used. Analyses were carried out in positive scan mode at ambient temperature using a Waters Nova-Pak C18 column, a 10 µL partial loop injection, and mobile phases (A) 1% acetic acid in methanol, (B) water, and (C) methanol at a flow rate of 500 µL/min. The analysis occurred over 25 min using a gradient of 20% A and 80% B for 12 min, then 20% A, 5% B, and 75% C for 3 min, and then back to 20% A and 80% B for the duration of the 25 min. The analysis utilized the following scan events of a full scan from *m/e* 100 to 300. The confirmation of (-)-botryodiplodin used three masses: *m/e* 127, 145, and 109. The limit of detection (LOD) was 1×10^{-5} μg/mL and the limit of quantitation (LOQ) was 0.01 μg/mL. The LOQ was based on the regression of the standards used for analysis. The full scan run of phomenone, gigantenone, and phaseolinone was from *m/e* 100 to 500, and their confirmations were identified by using *m/e* 265, 265, and 281, respectively.

4.8. Statistical Analysis

The analysis of variance was performed on toxin concentration data using the PROC GLM procedure in SAS Version 9.22 (Cary, NC, USA, 2010). Means were separated by Fisher's Least Significant Difference test with $p \leq 0.05$ level of significance.

Author Contributions: Conceptualization, H.K.A., N.B., C.A., J.R.S., W.T.S.; methodology, H.K.A., W.T.S.; validation, H.K.A.; investigation, H.K.A., W.T.S.; resources, H.K.A., W.T.S.; data curation, H.K.A., W.T.S.; writing—original draft preparation, H.K.A., W.T.S.; writing—review and editing, H.K.A., N.B., C.A., J.R.S., W.T.S.; visualization, W.T.S.; supervision, H.K.A.; project administration, H.K.A.; funding acquisition, H.K.A., W.T.S.

Funding: This research was funded by the Mississippi Soybean Promotion Board, grant numbers 34-2016 and 34-2017.

Acknowledgments: The authors are grateful to Alemah Butler, Bobbie J. Johnson (retired), Jeremy Kotowicz, and Vivek H. Khambhati for their technical assistance. Also, the authors are grateful for G.L. Sciumbato (retired) for supplying cultures and plant samples. Trade names are used in this publication solely for the purpose of providing specific information. The mention of trade names or commercial products in this publication is solely for the purpose of providing specific information and does not imply recommendation or endorsement by the United States Department of Agriculture.

Conflicts of Interest: All authors declare no conflict of interest.

References

1. Dhingra, O.D.; Sinclair, J.B. Location of *Macrophomina phaseoli* on soybean plants related to culture characteristics and virulence. *Phytopathology* **1973**, *63*, 934–936. [CrossRef]
2. Holliday, P.; Punithalingam, E. *Macrophomina Phaseolina*; No. 275; Descriptions of Pathogenic Fungi and Bacteria; CMI: Kew, Surrey, UK, 1970.
3. Ghosh, T.; Biswas, M.K.; Guin, C.; Roy, P. A review on characterization, therapeutic approaches and pathogenesis of *Macrophomina phaseolina*. *Plant Cell Biotechnol. Mol. Biol.* **2018**, *19*, 72–84.
4. Mengistu, A.; Ray, J.D.; Smith, J.R.; Paris, R.L. Charcoal rot disease assessment of soybean genotypes using a colony-forming unit index. *Crop Sci.* **2007**, *47*, 2453–2461. [CrossRef]
5. Wyllie, T.D. Macrophomina phaseolina—Charcoal rot. In *World Soybean Research: Proceedings of the World Soybean Research Conference*; Hill, L.D., Ed.; Interstate Printers and Publishers Inc.: Danville, IL, USA, 1976; pp. 482–484.
6. Bellaloui, N.; Mengistu, A.; Paris, R.L. Soybean seed composition in cultivars differing in resistance to charcoal rot (*Macrophomina phaseolina*). *J. Agric. Sci.* **2008**, *146*, 667–675. [CrossRef]
7. Bellaloui, N.; Mengistu, A.; Zobiole, L.H.S.; Shier, W.T. Resistance to toxin-mediated fungal infection: Role of lignins, isoflavones, other seed phenolics, sugars and boron in the mechanism of resistance to charcoal rot disease in soybean. *Toxin Rev.* **2012**, *31*, 16–26. [CrossRef]
8. Bowen, C.R.; Schapaugh, W.T., Jr. Relationship among charcoal rot infection, yield, and stability estimates in soybean blends. *Crop Sci.* **1989**, *29*, 42–46. [CrossRef]
9. Gupta, G.K.; Sharma, S.K.; Ramteke, R. Biology, epidemiology and management of the pathogenic fungus *Macrophomina phaseolina* (Tassi) Goid with special reference to charcoal rot of soybean (*Glycine max* (L.) Merrill). *J. Phytopathol.* **2012**, *160*, 167–180. [CrossRef]
10. Wrather, J.A. Soybean disease loss estimates for the southern United States, 1974 to 1994. *Plant Dis.* **1995**, *79*, 1076–1079.
11. Wrather, J.A.; Koenning, S.R. Estimates of disease effects on soybean yields in the United States 2003–2005. *J. Nematol.* **2006**, *38*, 173–180.
12. Illinois Soybean Association. *Ideas that Elevate*; Research report; Illinois Soybean Association: Bloomington, IL, USA, 2010; pp. 2–16.

13. Smith, G.S.; Wyllie, T.D. Charcoal rot. In *Compendium of Soybean Diseases*, 4th ed.; Hartman, G.L., Sinclair, J.B., Rupe, J.C., Eds.; APS Press, The American Phytopathological Society: St. Paul, MN, USA, 1999; pp. 29–31.
14. Gangopadhyay, S.; Wyllie, T.D.; Luedders, V.D. Charcoal rot disease of soybean transmitted by seeds. *Plant Dis. Rep.* **1970**, *54*, 1088–1091.
15. Kaiser, W.J.; Horner, G.M. Root rot of irrigated lentils in Iran. *Can. J. Bot.* **1980**, *58*, 2549–2556. [CrossRef]
16. Abawi, G.S.; Pastor-Corrales, M.A. *Root Rots of Beans in Latin America and Africa; Diagnosis, Research Methodologies and Management Strategies*; International Center for Tropical Agriculture (CIAT): Palmira, Cali, Columbia, 1990; p. 114.
17. Francl, L.J.; Wyllie, T.D.; Rosenbrock, S.M. Influence of crop rotation on population density of *Macrophomina phaseolina* in soil infested with *Heterodora glycines*. *Plant Dis.* **1988**, *72*, 760–764. [CrossRef]
18. Ghaffar, A.; Zentmyer, G.A.; Erwin, D.C. Effect of organic amendments on severity of *Macrophomina phaseolina* root rot of cotton. *Phytopathology* **1969**, *59*, 1267–1269.
19. Mueller, J.D.; Short, B.J.; Sinclair, J.B. Effect of cropping history, cultivar, and sampling date on the internal fungi of soybean roots. *Plant Dis.* **1985**, *69*, 520–523. [CrossRef]
20. Rothrock, C.S.; Kirkpatrick, T.L. The influence of winter legume cover crops on soilborne plant pathogens and cotton seedling diseases. *Plant Dis.* **1995**, *79*, 167–171. [CrossRef]
21. Siddiqui, Z.A.; Mahmood, I. Biological control of *Meloidogyne incognita* race 3 and *Macrophomina phaseolina* by *Paecilomyces lilacinus* and *Bacillus subtilis* alone and in combination in chickpea. *Fund. Appl. Nematol.* **1993**, *16*, 215–218.
22. Todd, T.C. Soybean planting date and maturity effects on *Hetrodera glycines* and *Macrophomina phaseolina* on southeastern Kansas. *Suppl. J. Nematol.* **1993**, *25*, 731–737.
23. Wyllie, T.D.; Scott, D.H. (Eds.) Charcoal rot of soybean-current status. In *Soybean Diseases of the North Central Region*; American Phytopathological Society: St. Paul, MN, USA, 1988; pp. 106–113.
24. Kendig, S.R.; Rupe, J.C.; Scott, H.D. Effect of irrigation and soil water stress on densities of *Macrophomina phaseolina* in soil and roots of two soybean cultivars. *Plant Dis.* **2000**, *84*, 895–900. [CrossRef]
25. Mengistu, A.; Arelli, P.A.; Bond, J.P.; Shannon, G.J.; Wrather, A.; Rupe, J.B.; Chen, P.; Little, C.R.; Canaday, C.H.; Newman, M.A.; et al. Evaluation of soybean genotypes for resistance to charcoal rot. *Plant Health Prog.* **2011**. [CrossRef]
26. Smith, G.S.; Carvil, O.N. Field screening of commercial and experimental soybean cultivars for their reaction to *Macrophomina phaseolina*. *Plant Dis.* **1997**, *81*, 363–368. [CrossRef]
27. Mengistu, A.; Ray, J.D.; Smith, J.R.; Arelli, P.R.; Bellaloui, N.; Chen, P.; Shannon, G.; Boykin, D. Effect of charcoal rot on selected putative drought tolerant soybean genotypes and yield. *Crop Prot.* **2018**, *105*, 90–101. [CrossRef]
28. Paris, R.L.; Mengistu, A.; Tyler, J.M.; Smith, J.R. Registration of soybean germplasm line DT97-4290 with moderate resistance to charcoal rot. *Crop Sci.* **2006**, *46*, 2324–2325. [CrossRef]
29. Smith, J.R.; Ray, J.D.; Mengistu, A. Genotypic differences in yield loss of irrigated soybean attributable to charcoal rot. *J. Crop Improv.* **2018**, *32*, 781–800. [CrossRef]
30. Dhingra, O.D.; Sinclair, J.B. Variation among isolates of *Macrophomina phaseoli* (*Rhizoctonia bataticola*) from the same soybean plant. *Phytopathology* **1972**, *62*, S1108.
31. Jana, T.K.; Singh, N.K.; Koundal, K.R.; Sharma, T.R. Genetic differentiation of Charcoal rot pathogen, *Macrophomina phaseolina*, into specific groups using URP-PCR. *Can. J. Microbiol.* **2005**, *51*, 159–164. [CrossRef]
32. Mayék-Pérez, N.; López-Castañeda, C.; González-Chavira, M.; Garcia-Espinosa, R.; Acosta-Gallegos, J.; de la Vega, O.M.; Simpson, J. Variability of Mexican isolates of *Macrophomina phaseolina* based on pathogenesis and AFLP genotype. *Physiol. Mol. Plant Pathol.* **2001**, *59*, 257–264. [CrossRef]
33. Reyes-Franco, M.C.; Hernández-Delgado, S.; Beas-Fernández, R.; Medina-Fernández, M.; Simpson, J.; Mayek-Pérez, N. Pathogenic and genetic variability within *Macrophomina phaseolina* from Mexico and other countries. *J. Phytopathol.* **2006**, *154*, 447–453. [CrossRef]
34. Dhar, T.K.; Siddiqui, K.A.I.; Ali, E. Structure of phaseolinone, a novel phytotoxin from *Macrophomina phaseolina*. *Tetrahedron Lett.* **1982**, *23*, 5459–5462.
35. Ramezani, M.; Shier, W.T.; Abbas, H.K.; Tonos, J.L.; Baird, R.E.; Sciumbato, G.L. Soybean charcoal rot disease fungus *Macrophomina phaseolina* in Mississippi produces the phytotoxin, (-)-botryodiplodin, but no detectable phaseolinone. *J. Nat. Prod.* **2007**, *70*, 128–129. [CrossRef]

36. Shier, W.T.; Abbas, H.K.; Baird, R.E.; Ramezani, M.; Sciumbato, G.L. (-)-Botryodiplodin, a unique ribose-analog toxin. *Toxin Rev.* **2007**, *26*, 343–386. [CrossRef]
37. Siddiqui, K.A.I.; Gupta, A.K.; Paul, A.K.; Banerjee, A.K. Purification and properties of a heat-resistant exotoxin produced by *Macrophomina phaseolina* (Tassi) Goid in culture. *Experientia* **1979**, *35*, 1222–1223. [CrossRef]
38. Wrather, J.A.; Anderson, T.R.; Arsyad, D.M.; Tan, Y.; Ploper, L.D.; Porta-Puglia, A.; Ram, H.H.; Yorinori, J.T. Soybean disease loss estimates for the top ten soybean-producing countries in 1998. *Can J. Plant Pathol.* **2001**, *23*, 115–121. [CrossRef]
39. Wrather, J.A.; Stienstra, W.C.; Koenning, S.R. Soybean disease loss estimates for the United States from 1996 to 1998. *Can J. Plant Pathol.* **2001**, *23*, 122–131. [CrossRef]
40. Wrather, J.A.; Koenning, S.R.; Anderson, T.R. Effect of diseases on soybean yields in the United States and Ontario (1999–2002). *Plant Health Prog.* **2003**. [CrossRef]
41. Dunlap, J.R.; Bruton, B.D. Pigment biosynthesis by *Macrophomina phaseolina*: The glycine–specific requirement. *Trans. Br. Mycol. Soc.* **1986**, *86*, 111–115. [CrossRef]
42. Shier, W.T.; Abbas, H.K.; Kotowicz, J.K.; Khambhati, V. Induction of simultaneous (-)-botryodiplodin release, microschlerotia formation and enhanced hyphal branching in *Macrophomina phaseolina*. *Mycotoxin Res.* in preparation.
43. Shultz, J.L.; Ray, J.D.; Smith, J.R. Mapping two genes in the purine metabolism pathway of soybean. *DNA Seq.* **2008**, *19*, 264–269. [CrossRef]
44. Abbas, H.K.; Bellaloui, N.; Butler, A.M.; Nelson, J.L.; Abou-Karam, M.; Shier, W.T. Botryodiplodin, a toxin produced by the charcoal rot disease fungus, *Macrophomena phaseolina*, induces phytotoxic responses in soybean (*Glycine max* L.) that are of types that could be used to facilitate root infection. *Toxins* **2019**, submitted.

toxins

MDPI

Article

Phytotoxic Responses of Soybean (*Glycine max* L.) to Botryodiplodin, a Toxin Produced by the Charcoal Rot Disease Fungus, *Macrophomina phaseolina*

Hamed K. Abbas [1,*], Nacer Bellaloui [2], Alemah M. Butler [1], Justin L. Nelson [3], Mohamed Abou-Karam [3] and W. Thomas Shier [3,*]

1 Biological Control of Pests Research Unit, US Department of Agriculture-Agricultural Research Service, Stoneville, MS 38776, USA; Alemah.Butler@sanofi.com

2 Crop Genetics Research Unit, US Department of Agriculture-Agricultural Research Service, Stoneville, MS 38776, USA; nacer.bellaloui@usda.gov

3 Department of Medicinal Chemistry, College of Pharmacy, University of Minnesota, Minneapolis, MN 55455, USA; nels6685@umn.edu (J.L.N.); m_aboukaram@yahoo.com (M.A.-K.)

* Correspondence: hamed.abbas@usda.gov (H.K.A.); shier001@umn.edu (W.T.S.); Tel.: +1-662-686-5313 (H.K.A.); +1-612-624-9465 (W.T.S.)

Received: 13 September 2019; Accepted: 18 December 2019; Published: 1 January 2020

Abstract: Toxins have been proposed to facilitate fungal root infection by creating regions of readily-penetrated necrotic tissue when applied externally to intact roots. Isolates of the charcoal rot disease fungus, *Macrophomina phaseolina*, from soybean plants in Mississippi produced a phytotoxic toxin, (−)-botryodiplodin, but no detectable phaseolinone, a toxin previously proposed to play a role in the root infection mechanism. This study was undertaken to determine if (−)-botryodiplodin induces toxic responses of the types that could facilitate root infection. (±)-Botryodiplodin prepared by chemical synthesis caused phytotoxic effects identical to those observed with (−)-botryodiplodin preparations from *M. phaseolina* culture filtrates, consistent with fungus-induced phytotoxicity being due to (−)-botryodiplodin, not phaseolinone or other unknown impurities. Soybean leaf disc cultures of Saline cultivar were more susceptible to (±)-botryodiplodin phytotoxicity than were cultures of two charcoal rot-resistant genotypes, DS97-84-1 and DT97-4290. (±)-Botryodiplodin caused similar phytotoxicity in actively growing duckweed (*Lemna pausicostata*) plantlet cultures, but at much lower concentrations. In soybean seedlings growing in hydroponic culture, (±)-botryodiplodin added to culture medium inhibited lateral and tap root growth, and caused loss of root caps and normal root tip cellular structure. Thus, botryodiplodin applied externally to undisturbed soybean roots induced phytotoxic responses of types expected to facilitate fungal root infection.

Keywords: botryodiplodin; root infection mechanism; root toxicity; *Macrophomina phaseolina*; hydroponic culture

Key Contribution: Botryodiplodin was observed to be phytotoxic in cultured leaf discs from soybean genotypes susceptible or resistant to charcoal rot disease, but the phytotoxic response was greatest in susceptible genotypes. Botryodiplodin was shown to be phytotoxic when applied externally to intact *Lemna pausicostata* plantlets. Botryodiplodin treatment of undisturbed soybean seedling roots in hydroponic culture resulted in loss of root tips, creating a lesion of a type that may facilitate root infection.

1. Introduction

Charcoal rot is a plant disease caused by the fungus, *Macrophomina phaseolina* (Tassi) Goid [1], in over 500 commercially-important plant species ranging from ornamental plants to trees to major food and fiber crops, including soybean (*Glycine max* L. (Merr.)). An example of the impact of charcoal rot disease on agriculture was provided by attempts to establish commercial natural rubber production with guayule (*Parthenium argentatum* Gray) in the arid southwest region of the US as an alternative to imported material from the rubber tree (*Hevea brasiliensis*) [2]. Guayule rubber production was only competitive when plants were grown close enough together that the roots interdigitated, under which conditions charcoal rot could spread from plant to plant destroying the crop [3]. Because charcoal rot is favored by hot, dry conditions [4], it is a climate-impacted plant disease that is predicted to be an increasingly important agronomic problem going forward, given that climate change is predicted to result in hotter, drier conditions in the majority of the world [5].

Research on (−)-botryodiplodin as a food contaminant has mainly focused on its production by the blue cheese fungus, *Penicillium roqueforti* [6,7]. (−)-Botryodiplodin production by *P. paneum* in bread and silage is also a concern [8,9]. Concerns about (−)-botryodiplodin as a possible contaminant in Roquefort cheese and other foods have led to extensive studies of its possible toxic effects in mammalian systems [10]. Because *M. phaseolina* is known to produce (−)-botryodiplodin and to be present in seeds as an endophyte, contamination of food items such as tofu and vegetable oil by (−)-botryodiplodin is a concern [10]. However, studies on foods and feeds impacted by charcoal rot disease have not been reported.

Although soybean cyst nematode is the major cause of soybean yield losses most years in most parts of the US, charcoal rot has traditionally been the most economically-important disease of soybean in the mid-southern region of the US (i.e., in Arkansas, Mississippi, and Louisiana) [11–15]. However, rising average temperatures and increased prevalence of drought have made the disease an increasingly important cause of yield losses during hot, dry growing seasons in all but northern parts of the US and other parts of the world [16]. Extensive studies have been carried out attempting to use selective breeding to develop soybean genotypes that are resistant to charcoal rot, but this approach has yielded only tolerant or moderately resistant genotypes [17,18]. Attempts to use various agronomic techniques to prevent the disease have also failed, so research on charcoal rot continues [17,19].

The mechanism used by *M. phaseolina* to infect soybean plants from the soil reservoir is poorly understood. *M. phaseolina* enters plants through the roots, then spreads through conductive tissues, reducing conduction volume, plant weight, and height, as well as reducing seed quality and quantity [16,20]. Inside plant tissues, *M. phaseolina* produces microsclerotia that appear as gray to black dots in and on stems and leaves and serve as reproductive structures that survive over winter in soil or as endophytes in the infested seed [21]. Fungi are widely believed to gain admission to plant roots from the soil by either (i) physical penetration of tissue; or (ii) secretion of toxins that kill plant tissue locally, creating a necrotic region through which fungal hyphae can easily propagate [19,22–24]. The mechanism(s) used by toxins to create localized necrosis in plant roots is not well understood, but two possible mechanisms are (i) secretion of hydrolytic enzymes or toxins that induce activation of endogenous hydrolytic enzymes; and (ii) secretion of toxins that specifically kill dividing meristematic cells near root tips, which creates necrotic tissue in a place that provides convenient access to the plant's vascular system through which the fungus can spread throughout the plant [19].

M. phaseolina has been reported to produce several mycotoxins that are candidates for toxin-mediated initiation of infection by generating a necrotic zone. These mycotoxins include phaseolinone [25], botryodiplodin [26], and patulin, because the *M. phaseolina* genome contains genes for its biosynthetic enzymes [27]. Siddiqui et al. (1979) [25] identified phaseolinone in culture extracts of pathogenic *M. phaseolina* isolated as an endophyte of mung bean. Dhar et al. (1982) [28] proposed the structure of the isolated toxin to be an epoxidized analog of a known phytotoxin, phomenone, which is part of an extensive family of phytotoxic eremophilane sesquiterpenoid (C-15) toxins produced by numerous plant pathogenic fungi [29]. Phaseolinone has been synthesized by Kitahara et al. (1991) [30] by conversion of another known eremophilane sesquiterpenoid toxin, phomenone. A series of 12 eremophilane analogs, including synthetic phaseolinone, were shown to be phytotoxic, producing either green islands on monocot leaves or necrotic lesions on dicots [29,31].

Ramezani et al. (2007) [32] and Abbas et al. (2019) [33] found no detectable phaseolinone in culture extracts of *M. phaseolina* isolated from infected soybean plants in the Mississippi Delta region of the southern USA. Bioassay-guided fractionation of the extracts led to the isolation of a different, known mycotoxin, botryodiplodin, which was first isolated by Sen Gupta et al. (1966) [26] from culture filtrates of *Botryodiplodia theobromae* Pat. (syn. *Lasiodiplodia theobromae* (Pat.) Griffon & Maubl), a cellulolytic fungus first isolated in 1944 from mildewed tent fabric in India, and subsequently shown to be a plant pathogen in many economically-important crops in the tropics and sub-tropics around the world [34].

The objectives of the present study were to investigate the identity of the phytotoxin produced by *M. phaseolina* isolates from Mississippi soybeans with charcoal rot disease as botryodiplodin, and to characterize some botryodiplodin root toxicity properties that could enable it to play a role in the initial stages of the soybean root infection mechanism of *M. phaseolina*.

2. Results and Discussion

2.1. Synthesis of (±)-Botryodiplodin

Chemically synthesized (±)-botryodiplodin exhibited potent phytotoxicity in each of a series of experimental systems, including *L. pausicostata* axenic cultures (Figure 1), soybean leaf discs in culture (Figures 2 and 3), and soybean seedling roots in hydroponic (Figure 4) and sand (Figure 5) culture. One explanation for the observation [32] that bioassay-guided fractionation of phytotoxicity produced by *M. phaseolina* isolates that cause charcoal rot disease in Mississippi soybeans yielded (-)-botryodiplodin, but no detectable phaseolinone, was that the toxin preparations contained a small percentage of either phaseolinone or another unknown, but the potent toxin that was responsible for the observed phytotoxicity. Phaseolinone was proposed by Siddiqui et al. (1979) [25] to mediate infection in charcoal rot disease based on its isolation from culture filtrates of an *M. phaseolina* endophyte from mung beans in India. When a phytotoxin is purified from nature, it is never 100% pure, so that it is always possible that the phytotoxicity may actually reside in a highly toxic impurity, rather than in the major component of the preparation. Chemical synthesis is one approach that can provide evidence that the major component of the preparation is the actual toxin. Chemical synthesis of a toxin is unlikely to produce the same impurities as found in material purified from nature. Even if the impurities in the two types of preparations are both toxic, they are unlikely to induce identical pathology in all toxicity tests. Therefore, identical phytotoxic properties are unlikely to be observed in synthetic and natural preparations of a toxin, if the activities of either are due to a highly active impurity. At least seven syntheses of botryodiplodin have been reported, since the initial success by McCurry & Abe (1973) [35]. None of these syntheses could conceivably produce phaseolinone or any other eremophilane sesquiterpenoid as a by-product. Although the method used in this study to synthesize (±)-botryodiplodin was selected because it involved only five steps using simple, standard chemistry and low cost reagents, it also could not conceivably produce phaseolinone or any other eremophilane sesquiterpenoid as a contaminant. Antibacterial activity was the first biological activity identified for (-)-botryodiplodin [26], and the easiest to assay. Chemically synthesized (±)-botryodiplodin was shown to exhibit antibacterial activity indistinguishable from that of (−)-botryodiplodin purified from *M. phaseolina* cultures [32] (data not shown). In addition, (±)-botryodiplodin induced phytotoxic responses indistinguishable from those induced by (−)-botryodiplodin, when compared in duckweed (*L. pausicostata*) plantlet cultures and soybean leaf discs in culture (see below). Identical activity of (±)-botryodiplodin and (−)-botryodiplodin is consistent with extensive studies on the mechanism of action of (−)-botryodiplodin by Moule et al. (1981a; 1981b; 1982) [36–38], which indicated that the toxin acts by chemical reactions in cell nuclei that covalently cross-link proteins to DNA, and not by interacting with a chiral binding site on any enzyme or receptor that might require an optically active form. Although (+)-botryodiplodin has been prepared by chemical synthesis [39], its biological activity, or the lack thereof, has not been reported by these investigators or others. More extensive structural alterations of botryodiplodin in the form of epimers have been reported to be inactive in the case of 4-*epi*-botryodiplodin [40]. Félix et al. (2019) [41] observed that cytotoxicity of 3-*epi*-botryodiplodin measured in Vero monkey kidney cells and 3T3 mouse fibroblast cultures was 0–5% of the cytotoxicity of botryodiplodin. However, in a leaf puncture assay in young tomato plant leaves, 3-*epi*-botryodiplodin produced a much larger lesion with different morphology than botryodiplodin, but similar to the lesion produced by botryodiplodin acetate. Thus, the possibility that (+)-botryodiplodin might be an inactive diluent in the (±)-botryodiplodin preparations used in this study, cannot be rigorously excluded, but if it were inactive, all conclusions drawn would be the same, with reported (−)-botryodiplodin activities occurring at half the stated concentrations.

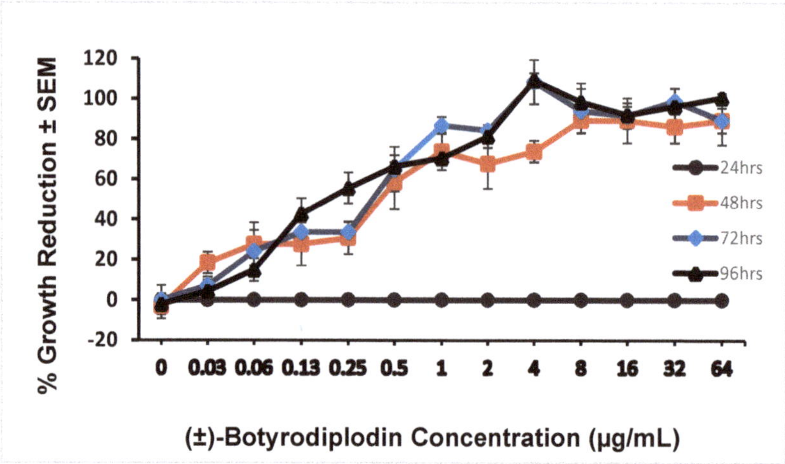

Figure 1. Inhibition of duckweed (*Lemna pausicostata*) plantlet growth in axenic cultures containing a range of concentrations of (±)-botryodiplodin in the culture medium. Duckweed growth was measured as percent inhibition of frond production ± SEM relative to controls not treated with toxin. Phytotoxicity was assessed at 24 h (●), 48 h (■), 72 h (♦), and 96 h (▲). The full toxic response was observed by 48 h (IC_{50} = 0.22 µg/mL); that is, the percent growth reduction at 48, 72, and 96 h were not significantly different from each other, but all were significantly greater than that at 24 hours, $p < 0.05$, multiple linear regression analysis.

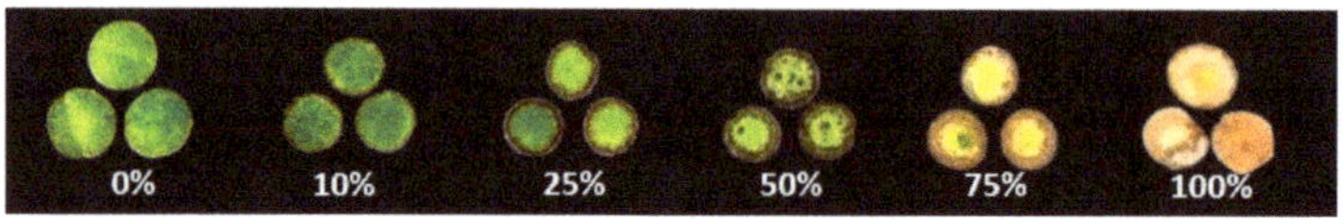

Figure 2. Phytotoxicity rating scale used to determine the percent severity of (±)-botryodiplodin phytotoxicity on soybean leaf discs, in which 0% = healthy tissue; 10% = slight browning around the edges of the leaf disc; 25% = moderate browning around the edges of the leaf disc; 50% = browning around the edges of the leaf disc with slight bleaching; 75% = extensive browning of the leaf disc with bleaching; and 100% = complete bleaching of the leaf disc.

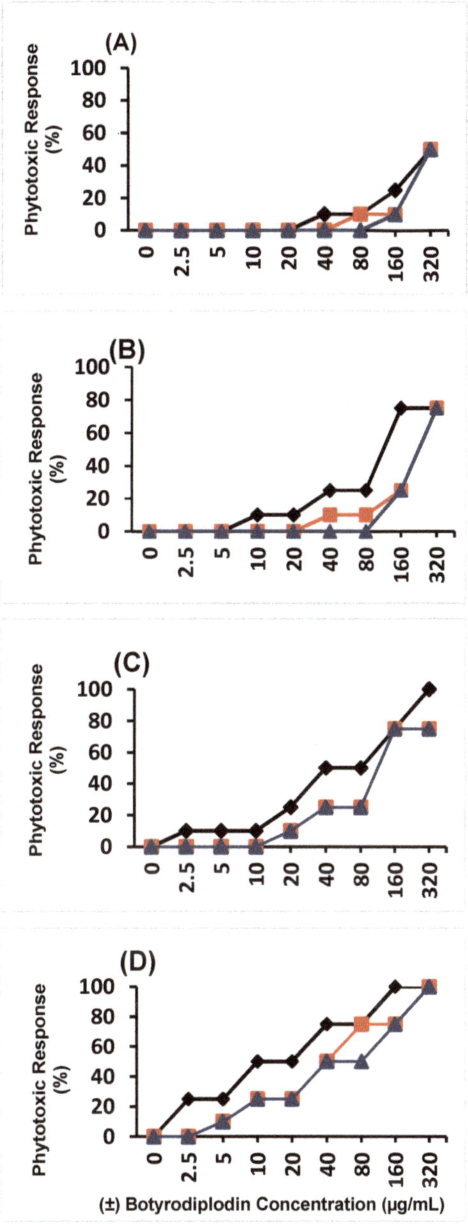

Figure 3. Phytotoxicity effects of (±)-botryodiplodin in cultured leaf discs from three different soybean genotypes, DT97-4290 (▲), which was released as a charcoal rot disease resistant genotype, Saline (♦) and DS97-84-1 (■). The phytotoxic response is shown at (**A**) 24 h, (**B**) 48 h, (**C**) 72 h and (**D**) 96 h. The phytotoxicity rating scale is described in Figure 2. Saline was significantly ($p < 0.05$, multiple regression) more susceptible to the phytotoxic effects of (±)-botryodiplodin than DS97-84-1 and DT97-4290 at each time point. Results are the mean of three replicates.

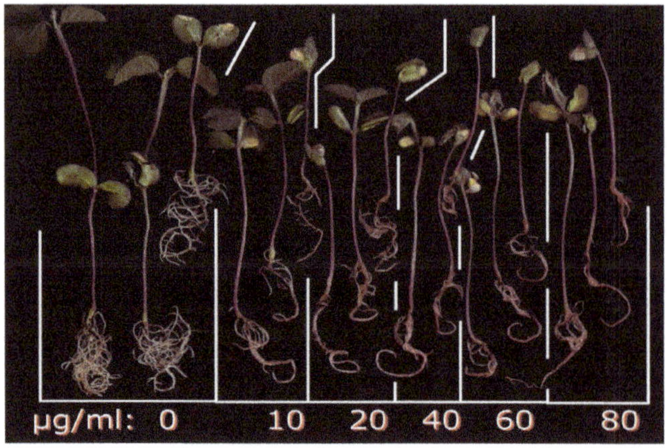

Figure 4. Effects of various (±)-botryodiplodin concentrations (0 to 80 µg/mL) in hydroponic culture medium on soybean seedlings. A reduced number of lateral roots and discoloration occurred at all (±)-botryodiplodin concentrations tested.

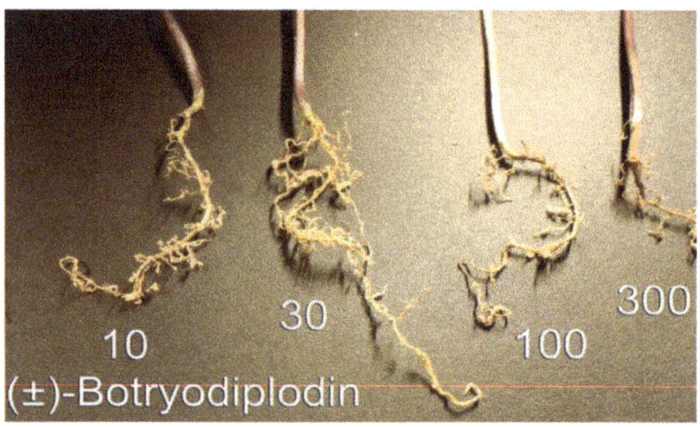

Figure 5. Soybean seedling roots treated with a range of concentrations of (±)-botryodiplodin (10 to 300 µg/mL) in sand culture served as controls for unsupported soybean seedling roots in hydroponic culture. A reduced number of lateral roots and discoloration occurs at higher concentrations of (±)-botryodiplodin.

The simplest explanation for differences in the type of toxin produced in culture by endophytic *M. phaseolina* isolated from mung beans in India [25] and pathogenic *M. phaseolina* isolated from soybeans in Mississippi [32] is that the isolate studied by Siddiqui et al. (1979) [25] produced both phaseolinone and (−)-botryodiplodin, whereas only (−)-botryodiplodin was produced by the Mississippi isolates [10]. Production of multiple, structurally dissimilar mycotoxins by a single fungus has been well-documented [42], and there are numerous examples in the scientific literature of regional variations in mycotoxin production by the same species of fungus [43,44].

2.2. Phytotoxicity of (±)-Botryodiplodin in Lemna Pausicostata (Duckweed) Cultures

A series of studies were initiated to determine if botryodiplodin possesses properties useful for a mycotoxin to play a role in mediating root infection by *M. phaseolina* from a soil reservoir. Specifically, to be an effective mediator of root infection, a toxin must be able to kill undisturbed, actively growing root tissue in the absence of an insect, nematode, or other vector that physically damages root tissue. Root cells killed by the toxin should create a necrotic region, preferably one that would provide fungal hyphae with facile access to the plant vascular system. A toxin-mediated fungal root infection mechanism should be able to facilitate tissue entry in the absence of fungal structures such as appressoria [45] that enable fungal cells to physically penetrate plant leaf tissue in the absence of a vector.

(±)-Botryodiplodin (0 to 64 μg/mL) dissolved in the culture medium of parallel axenic cultures of the aquatic plant of *Lemna pausicostata* (duckweed) induced a phytotoxic response in intact, growing plantlets floating on the surface of the culture medium over a 96-hour period (Figure 1) that was indistinguishable from the phytotoxic response to (−)-botryodiplodin prepared as described by Ramezani et al. (2007) [32]. Phytotoxicity was measured as percent growth reduction measured by the number of plantlet fronds produced relative to parallel control cultures not treated with (±)-botryodiplodin. Additional phytotoxicity occurred as a formation of necrotic tissue with light brownish color around the edges of the fronds and some bleaching progressing to 100% growth inhibition, 100% mortality, and complete bleaching. No detectable toxicity was observed at 24 hours, because growth was measured as frond number and more time than that was needed for a plantlet to generate a new frond under conditions used. However, the full extent of toxicity was observed at 48 hours with IC_{50} = 0.22 μg/mL. The dose-response curves at 72 hours (IC_{50} = 0.19 μg/mL) and 96 hours (IC_{50} = 0.18 μg/mL) were not significantly different from each other (Pearson's $r = 0.993$, $p = 0.601$, multiple linear regression analysis), or from that at 48 hours (Pearson's $r = 0.994$, $p = 0.995$ at 72 hr; r = 0.984, $p = 0.874$ at 96 hrs, multiple linear regression analysis).

Phytotoxicity of (±)-botryodiplodin was determined in leaf discs from charcoal rot tolerant and susceptible soybean genotypes. (±)-Botryodiplodin (0 to 320 μg/mL) in culture medium for 96 hours induced the same phytotoxic response in soybean leaf discs cut from mature leaves of three- to four-week old soybean seedlings as observed with (-)-botryodiplodin [32], specifically progressive browning (necrosis) around the edges of the leaf disc and bleaching (light-induced loss of chlorophyll) progressing to complete browning of the leaf disc and 100% bleaching. (±)-Botryodiplodin phytotoxicity was compared in leaf discs from the following three genotypes: DT97-4290, which was released as a charcoal rot disease resistant soybean genotype; and two others that are considered susceptible to charcoal rot disease, DS97-84-1 and Saline. The percent severity of phytotoxic responses was quantitated at 24, 48, 72, and 96 hours using the rating scale given in Figure 2. At each time period, Saline was significantly ($p < 0.05$, multiple regression) more susceptible to the phytotoxic effects of (±)-botryodiplodin than DS97-84-1 and DT97-4290. While DS97-84-1 was more susceptible to (±)-botryodiplodin than DT97-4290 at some times, the differences were not significant. At 24 hours (Figure 3A), phytotoxicity was observed only at the highest (±)-botryodiplodin concentrations with IC_{50} values of 320 μg/mL for each of Saline, DS97-84-1, and DT97-4290, respectively. At 48 hours, (Figure 3B) phytotoxicity was observed at lower (±)-botryodiplodin concentrations with IC_{50} values of 136 μg/mL for Saline and 272 μg/mL for DS97-84-1 and DT97-4290. At 72 hours (Figure 3C), substantial phytotoxicity was observed at progressively lower (±)-botryodiplodin concentrations with IC_{50} values of 59.5 μg/mL for Saline and 132 μg/mL for DS97-84-1 and DT97-4290. At 96 hours (Figure 3D), substantial phytotoxicity was observed at much lower (±)-botryodiplodin concentrations with IC_{50} values of 14.9, 38.5, and 42.9 μg/mL for Saline, DS97-84-1 and DT97-4290, respectively. The observation that the three soybean genotypes examined in the study exhibited susceptibility to the phytotoxic effects of (±)-botryodiplodin in the order Saline > DS97-84-1 > DT97-4290 is consistent with the charcoal rot tolerance reported for genotype DT97-4290 [18] resulting from a change expressed in multiple tissues, including leaf tissue. Given that the level of resistance expressed by genotype DT97-4290 is not sufficient to prevent charcoal rot disease and infection by *M. phaseolina* [18], subsequent studies focused on investigating root-specific responses believed to be associated with initial infection.

2.3. Root Toxicity of (±)-Botryodiplodin in Soybean Seedlings

Studies on root toxicity of (±)-botryodiplodin used soybean seedlings in hydroponic culture with the toxin being added to culture medium bathing only the roots. Soybean seedlings in hydroponic culture were treated for four days with a range of (±)-botryodiplodin concentrations (10 to 80 μg/mL) in the nutrient solution bathing the roots. Control seedlings produced abundant lateral roots during the hydroponic culture period. The addition of (±)-botryodiplodin to the nutrient solution reduced lateral root production even at 10 μg/mL, the lowest concentration tested in initial trials (Figure 4). Inhibition of root growth by (±)-botryodiplodin treatment was quantified by the dry weight relative to that of control plants exposed to 0 μg/mL (±)-botryodiplodin. There was significantly greater toxicity to lateral roots than to tap roots ($p < 0.05$, regression analysis) (Figure 6). (±)-Botryodiplodin exposure resulted in about an eight-fold reduction in lateral root growth, but only in about a two-fold reduction in tap root growth. There was significant reduction in tap root growth at the highest (±)-botryodiplodin concentrations tested (≥40 μg/mL), but the IC_{50} (23.5 μg/mL) was 5.6-fold higher than the IC_{50} for lateral roots (4.2 μg/mL), which exhibited significant ($p < 0.05$, Student's *t*-test) reduction in lateral root growth at ≥5 μg/mL (Figure 6). Thus, botryodiplodin caused toxicity to undisturbed soybean roots when applied externally, which is a property expected for a toxin capable of playing a role in facilitating fungal root infection from a soil reservoir (Figures 4 and 6).

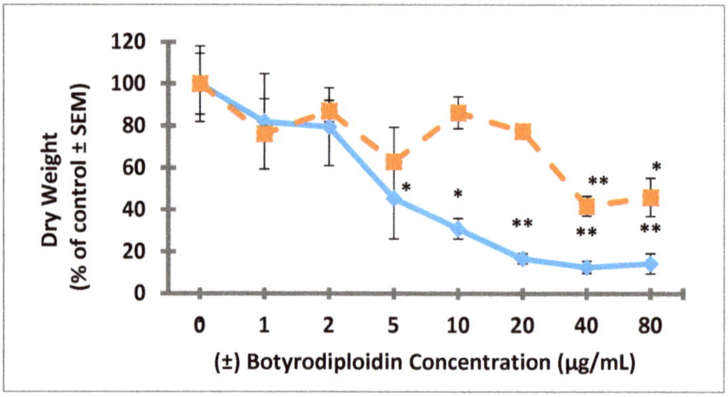

Figure 6. Inhibitory effects of various (±)-botryodiplodin concentrations in hydroponic culture medium (0 to 80 μg/mL) on lateral soybean seedling root growth (—◊—) with inhibition at IC_{50} = 4.2 μg/mL (100% dry weight = 11.5 ± 2.1 mg), and on tap root growth (- - - ■ - - -) with inhibition at IC_{50} = 23.5 μg/mL (100% dry weight = 13.8 ± 2.0 mg). Root growth presented on the vertical axis was measured as dry weight of excised lateral or tap roots after (±)-botryodiplodin exposure for 96 h at room temperature in continuous light. Results are the mean of three replicates ± SEM. * Significantly reduced soybean root growth at $p < 0.05$; ** significantly reduced soybean root growth at $p < 0.01$ (Student's *t*-test).

A set of experiments exposing soybean seedling roots to (±)-botryodiplodin in sand culture was conducted to eliminate the possibility that physical contact of soybean roots with solid soil particles might induce or maintain a protective layer on roots. Seedlings germinated in soil were transplanted to sand culture, acclimatized, and then the roots exposed to (±)-botryodiplodin (10, 100, and 300 μg/mL) dissolved in fresh culture medium (Figure 5). (±)-Botryodiplodin treatment resulted in greatly reduced lateral root production, particularly at the higher concentrations. There was no indication that the sand used in the sand culture system interfered with phytotoxicity either by adsorption of toxin on silica surfaces, or by interfering with conduct of the experiment either by preventing continuous visual monitoring of toxin-induced damage or causing root damage when washing sand away.

Pink to red discoloration of exposed roots occurred at the highest (±)-botryodiplodin concentration (300 μg/mL) in sand culture (Figure 5), and at the higher concentrations tested in liquid hydroponic culture (Figure 4), with the darkest coloration at the highest concentration (80 μg/mL). Formation of pigment by reaction of botryodiplodin with protein and other amines has been observed numerous times [26,35,39,46,47]. The (±)-botryodiplodin used in the present study has been shown to react with proteins, amino acids, and a wide variety of other amines to give red to yellow pigments [48]. Given that soybean seedlings have been reported to express proteins such as nutrient and water transporters on root surfaces [49], the pink to red pigment observed on soybean seedling roots treated with (±)-botryodiplodin in hydroponic culture (Figures 4 and 5) may have formed by a similar reaction with root surface proteins.

The production of abundant lateral roots by soybean seedlings under the stationary hydroponic conditions used in this study (Figures 4 and 6) presumably results from disruption of oxygen and ethylene exposure to roots, which has been shown in *Arabidopsis thaliana* to be genetically defined and environmentally regulated [50,51]. Soybean has similar ethylene receptors and associated regulatory gene products [52], which provides an explanation for the well-documented occurrence of lateral root production by soybean when soil becomes waterlogged [53,54]. In plant root growth, cell division occurs solely in meristematic regions near root caps, and root extension primarily results from subsequent cell elongation. Botryodiplodin has been shown to target DNA synthesis and dividing cells in a wide variety of biological systems, including bacteria [26,55], fungi [56], yeast [26], plants [32], and mammalian cells [35,37,57–59]. A phytotoxin such as (−)-botryodiplodin, which kills dividing cells, would be expected to target meristematic tissue near the tips of both tap and lateral roots. The higher reduction in lateral root growth (~eight-fold) than in tap root growth (~two-fold) by (±)-botryodiplodin (Figure 6) is consistent with the toxin acting on meristematic tissue, which makes up a larger percentage of total tissue weight in small lateral roots than it does in the larger tap root.

Soybean seedlings growing in hydroponic culture with roots exposed to (±)-botryodiplodin (15 μg/mL) in culture medium (Figure 7) resulted in the loss of the root cap and meristematic tissue without involvement of a vector or physical injury, and were consistent with the toxin targeting dividing cells in the meristem. Similar loss of the root cap and meristematic tissue occurred at the higher (±)-botryodiplodin concentrations tested (35 and 80 μg/mL). Additional studies are needed to determine how rapidly the root tip loss occurs at various (±)-botryodiplodin concentrations.

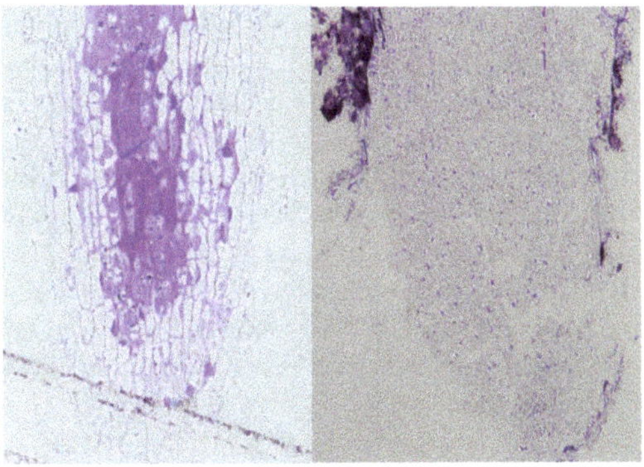

Figure 7. Light micrographs of root tips of soybean seedlings after four days in hydroponic culture in 10% Villagarcia medium in water with no (±)-botryodiplodin (left panel, 400×) or with (±)-botryodiplodin (15 μg/mL) (right panel, 200×).

Thus, (±)-botryodiplodin applied externally to undisturbed soybean roots induced phytotoxic responses of a type expected to facilitate fungal root infection. An example of a plausible root infection mechanism involving the observed responses of soybean root to (±)-botryodiplodin could involve hyphae of a fungus like *M. phaseolina* propagating outward from a plant-derived nutrient source through the soil in all directions until hyphae detect the presence of a root tip, stimulating release of (−)-botryodiplodin. The released (−)-botryodiplodin would be expected to cause loss of the root tip and exposure of the vascular system that should facilitate the propagation of fungal hyphae into the vascular system and subsequently throughout the plant [19]. However, additional studies will be needed to confirm that targeting of root tip meristematic cells is involved in the actual root infection mechanism used by *M. phaseolina* in charcoal rot disease of soybeans in the field.

3. Conclusions

The toxin, botryodiplodin, produced by *M. phaseolina*, the fungus that causes charcoal rot disease in many plant species, is phytotoxic in soybean leaf disc cultures and in actively growing *Lemna pausicostata* plantlet cultures. Botryodiplodin exposed to undisturbed roots of soybean seedlings in hydroponic culture results in a root tip destruction response that would facilitate fungal infection of the root.

4. Materials and Methods

4.1. Preparation of (±)-Botryodiplodin

(±)-Botryodiplodin was selected for use in these studies, because it is readily synthesized chemically in larger amounts than were available by fermentation [32]. The mechanism of action of botryodiplodin has been extensively studied by Moule et al. [36–38], who provided evidence for non-enzymatic (i.e., chemical) crosslinking of DNA to protein. There have been no reports of botryodiplodin binding specifically to a chiral binding site on any enzyme or receptor. A non-enzymatic mechanism of action for botryodiplodin would result in phytotoxicity of synthetic (±)-botryodiplodin being equivalent to that of fermentation-derived (−)-botryodiplodin. The (±)-botryodiplodin used in this study was synthesized by preparing α-methyl-α-angelicalactone, using a modification of the method of Helberger et al. (1949) [60], followed by its conversion to the final product using four steps that are included in the synthetic method developed by Mukaiyama et al. (1974) [61] (Figure 8). Briefly, α-methyllevulinic acid (**1**) (500 mg) (TCI America, Portland, OR, USA), was treated with phosphoric acid (1% wt/wt) and subjected to vacuum distillation at 120–130 °C and ~40 Torr to provide α-methyl-α-angelicalactone (**2**) in approximately 80% yield. The product was treated under argon with boron trifluoride etherate and formaldehyde generated in situ by thermal degradation of paraformaldehyde. The reaction was quenched with $NaHCO_3$ aqueous solution and extracted into dichloromethane. The product, (±)-cis-α-methyl-β-acetyl-γ-butyrolactone (**3**), was purified by chromatography on silica gel in diethyl ether:hexane 4:1 and crystallized from hexane. The ketone group of **3** was blocked with ethanethiol in the presence of zinc chloride and the product **4** extracted into dichloromethane and purified by chromatography on silica gel in diethyl ether:hexane 4:1. Reduction of **4** with diisobutylaluminium hydride in tetrahydrofuran at −78 °C yielded the diethanethiol derivative of (±)-botryodiplodin (**5**), which was purified by chromatography on silica gel using a 5% to 20% diethyl ether:hexane gradient. Unblocking of lactol **5** in acetone containing 1% water, $CuCl_2$ and CuO was accomplished at room temperature in 30–60 minutes. (±)-Botryodiplodin (**6**) was extracted from the reaction mixture into dichloromethane and purified by chromatography on silica gel using ether:hexane 4:1 followed by re-chromatography on silica gel using dichloromethane:methanol 20:1 to yield 116 mg (20.9% overall yield) at a purity of >98% based on thin layer chromatography and nuclear magnetic resonance spectroscopy. The (±)-botryodiplodin (**6**) exhibited ^1H nuclear magnetic resonance spectroscopy values and thin layer chromatographic R_f values identical to those reported in the literature [39,62] and those obtained in this laboratory with (−)-botryodiplodin purified from cultures of *M. phaseolina* [32], except that (±)-botryodiplodin was not optically active.

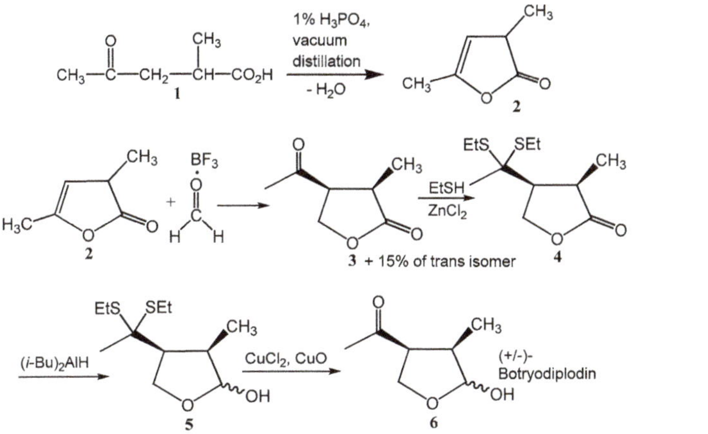

Figure 8. Chemical synthesis of (±)-botryodiplodin.

4.2. Assay of Antibacterial Activity of Botryodiplodin

The biological activity level of (±)-botryodiplodin was confirmed using antibacterial activity, the type of activity used to guide the initial isolation of (−)-botryodiplodin by Sen Gupta et al. (1966) [26], and the most easily measured of its numerous reported biological activities, including antifungal [56], phytotoxic [25,32], anti-cancer [37,57], mutagenic [36], and antifertility [58] activities. Antibacterial activity was compared on samples of (±)-botryodiplodin, prepared as described above, and (−)-botryodiplodin purified as described by Ramezani et al. (2007) [32] from culture filtrates of *M. phaseolina* isolated from a soybean plant with charcoal rot disease in Mississippi. Antibacterial activity was measured by serial dilution from 20 to 0.1 µg/mL in Mueller-Hinton broth in triplicate in the wells of a 96-well tray using (±)-botryodiplodin and (−)-botryodiplodin samples sterilized by dissolution at 10 mg/mL in 95% ethanol. The wells were inoculated with an actively growing culture of *Bacillus subtilis*, strain 1a1, isolated in this laboratory from lawn soil and shown to be susceptible to all antibiotics in a 28-member panel except thiostrepton. Trays were cultured overnight at 37 °C and bacterial growth estimated as the OD at 600 nm in a plate reader (BioTek Instruments Synergy HT, Winooski, VT, USA).

4.3. Plant Growth and Environmental Conditions

Soybean genotypes DT97-4290 (moderately resistant to charcoal rot) [18], DS97-84-1 and Saline [63] (both of which are susceptible to charcoal rot) were grown in the greenhouse. Seeds were planted and germinated in flat trays of vermiculite, and similarly sized seedlings were transplanted into 9.45 L pots filled with a silt loam soil (24% sand, 54% silt, and 22% clay with 1.3% organic matter) pH 6.5, 17 cmol/kg cation exchange capacity. Plants were watered as needed to maintain soil water potential at field capacity, i.e., between −15 to −20 kPa. Four pots were used for each soybean genotype, and three plants were grown in each pot. Greenhouse conditions were about 34 °C ± 8 °C during the day and approximately 28 °C ± 6 °C at night with a photosynthetic photon flux density of about 850–2100 $\mu mol \cdot m^{-2}\ s^{-1}$, as measured by Quantum Meter (Spectrum Technologies, Inc., Aurora, IL, USA). The range of light intensity reflects the range from a cloudy day (850 $\mu mol \cdot m^{-2}\ s^{-1}$) to a sunny day (2100 $\mu mol \cdot m^{-2}\ s^{-1}$). The source of lighting in the greenhouse was a mixture of natural and artificial lights. Plant leaves were harvested during the vegetative phase of growth.

4.4. Phytotoxicity of (±)-Botryodiplodin in Soybean Leaf Discs

Dose-response curves were obtained for phytotoxic responses to a range of (±)-botryodiplodin concentrations by triplicate cultures of three soybean leaf discs. Leaf discs cut from healthy leaflets from true mature leaves of 3- to 4-week-old plants of each of the three soybean types were used to determine the phytotoxicity of (±)-botryodiplodin. All leaves were harvested in the laboratory and three soybean leaf discs measuring 4-mm diameter were cut with a sterile cork borer (#4) and placed in sterile 24-well tissue culture plates with low evaporative lids (Becton Dickinson and Company, Franklin Lakes, NJ). (±)-Botryodiplodin solutions in water (1.5 mL) over a range of concentrations (0, 2.5, 5.0, 10, 20, 40, 80, 160, and 320 μg/mL) were added to the wells of plates in triplicate. Leaf discs were incubated in a growth chamber at 25 °C under continuous visible light for 96 h and examined for signs of phytotoxicity after 24, 48, 72, and 96 h using the following symptom rating scale: Healthy tissue, 0%; a narrow zone of brown (necrotic) tissue forming around the edges of the leaf disc, 10%; a substantial zone of brown tissue forming around the edges of the leaf disc, 25%; brown tissue throughout the leaf disc, 50%; brown tissue throughout the leaf disc with bleaching, 75%; complete bleaching of the leaf disc, 100% (Figure 2).

4.5. *Phytotoxicity of (±)-Botryodiplodin in Duckweed Plant Cultures*

Dose-response curves were obtained for phytotoxic responses to a range of (±)-botryodiplodin concentrations by triplicate cultures of three-frond duckweed plantlets. Cultures containing three duckweed (*Lemna pausicostata* Helgelm.) plantlets were used to bioassay phytotoxicity, as described by Tanaka et al. (1993) [64], with some modification. Briefly, three duckweed plantlets containing three fronds each were transferred from a laboratory maintenance culture with clean forceps to each well of a sterile 24-well tissue culture plate with a low evaporation lid. Aliquots (1.5 mL) of culture medium containing a range of (±)-botryodiplodin concentrations (0, 0.03, 0.06, 0.13, 0.25, 0.5, 1, 2, 4, 8, 16, 32, and 64 μg/mL) were added in triplicate to the wells of culture plates. Duckweed plants were subsequently incubated in a growth chamber at 25 °C under continuous light for 96 hr. Duckweed plantlets were observed for signs of phytotoxicity after 24, 48, 72, and 96 hr. Growth was measured as addition of fronds in treated cultures relative to control cultures not treated with (±)-botryodiplodin. No additional fronds being produced in a treated culture was scored as 100% inhibition of growth.

4.6. *Hydroponic Culture of Soybean Seedlings*

The effects of (±)-botryodiplodin on soybean root growth were investigated in soybean seedlings germinated from a commercial soybean seed variety assumed to be charcoal rot-susceptible (Kansas Soybean Commission, Topeka, KS, USA) in autoclaved soil and grown under continuous light to the cotyledon stage (VC, 4–7 cm). Seedling roots were washed free of soil particles and transplanted to hydroponic growth medium. Seedlings were grown under hydroponic conditions for four days before use in root toxicity assays in individual 16 × 100 mm glass tubes containing 5 mL of a mixture of 90% distilled water and 10% Villagarcia medium [65]. The Villagarcia medium used consisted of distilled water (999 mL) containing $CaSO_4.2H_2O$ (690 mg), KH_2PO_4 (34 mg), KNO_3 (200 mg), $MgSO_4.7H_2O$ (61 mg), and 1 mL of 1000-fold concentrated microsolute nutrient solution containing $FeSO_4.7H_2O$ (50 mg), KCl (14 mg), H_3BO_4 (5.7 mg), $MnSO_4.H_2O$ (1.5 mg), $ZnSO_4.7H_2O$ (2.6 mg), $CuSO_4.5H_2O$ (0.45 mg), and $(NH_4)_6Mo_7O_{24}$ (2.1 mg). Seedlings were held in place by the tube walls and maintained with roots covered with medium added daily as needed. Seedlings placed under sand culture conditions were grown four days in 5 mL of washed, sterile sand, which was added after the seedling was placed in the tube and kept soaked with 10% (*v*/*v*) Villagarcia medium in water added daily as needed.

4.7. *Root Toxicity of (±)-Botryodiplodin in Soybean Seedlings in Hydroponic Culture*

Dose-response curves were obtained for phytotoxic responses to a range of (±)-botryodiplodin concentrations by the roots of groups of three soybean seedlings cultured individually in hydroponic medium. Soybean seedlings were grown in continuous light for four days at room temperature in 5 mL of hydroponic growth medium consisting of 10% Villagarcia medium and 90% water in individual 16 × 100 mm glass tubes, using the walls of the glass tubes to hold the seedlings upright.

The medium was withdrawn from seedling cultures with a Pasteur pipet, replaced by fresh medium containing a range of (±)-botryodiplodin concentrations in triplicate in three individual glass tubes (0 to 300 μg/mL in an initial range-finding assay, and 0 to 80 μg/mL in subsequent studies), and cultured for an additional four days at room temperature in continuous light. Root growth was quantified by removing seedlings from the culture tubes and washing the roots with a stream of deionized water from a wash bottle. Roots were excised at the stem line with a scalpel. Lateral roots were cut from the tap roots and the two root types dried separately overnight under vacuum in a desiccator over Drierite desiccant at room temperature. Lateral and tap roots were weighed separately on a sensitive balance (Mettler Toledo UMX2 Ultra-Microbalance, Mettler-Toledo International, Columbus, Ohio), and the dry weights of triplicate samples plotted as mean ±standard error versus (±)-botryodiplodin concentration.

4.8. Light Micrographs of Soybean Seedling Roots Exposed to (±)-Botryodiplodin in Hydroponic Culture

Soybean (commercial variety) seedlings were established in hydroponic culture as described above, then transplanted to individual new 16 × 100 mm glass tube containing 5 ml of (±)-botryodiplodin (0, 15, 35, and 80 μg/ml) in 10% Villagarcia medium and 90% water. Seedlings were incubated at room temperature for 4 days with continuous light, at which time control seedlings in 0 μg/ml (±)-botryodiplodin had abundant lateral roots. Seedlings in 15 μg/ml (±)-botryodiplodin had substantially reduced numbers of lateral roots and seedlings in 35 and 80 μg/ml (±)-botryodiplodin had stunted roots stained pink. An Xacto knife was used to cut the roots off at slightly above where the root begins. The excised roots were placed in labeled glass scintillation vials filled to the top with Karnovsky's fixative [66]. Root samples were embedded in resin and thick-sectioned on an Ultracut UCT microtome (Leica, Buffalo Grove, IL, USA) using a diamond knife. Sections were collected on glass slides, stained with toluidine blue, and imaged using bright-field light microscopy on an Eclipse 90i (Nikon Inc., Melville, NY, USA) with a D2-Fi2 color camera running Nikon Elements software.

4.9. Data Analysis

Phytotoxic responses were quantified as IC_{50} values (the concentration of (±)-botryodiplodin that causes 50% of the maximal toxic response) determined graphically by interpolation on plots of toxic response versus log (±)-botryodiplodin concentration prepared using the graphing package included in Microsoft Excel 2010. Statistical analyses (correlation analysis, multiple linear regression analysis, Student's *t*-test) were conducted using the statistical package included in Microsoft Excel 2010. $p \leq 0.05$ was considered significant.

Author Contributions: Conceptualization, H.K.A. and W.T.S.; Formal analysis, A.M.B. and W.T.S.; Funding acquisition, H.K.A.; Investigation, H.K.A., N.B., A.M.B., J.L.N., M.A.-K. and W.T.S.; Project administration, H.K.A.; Writing—original draft, H.K.A.; Writing—review & editing, N.B., A.M.B., J.L.N., M.A.-K. and W.T.S. All authors have read and agree to the published version of the manuscript. All authors have read and agreed to the published version of the manuscript.

Funding: This work was supported in part by the Mississippi Soybean Promotion Board and the Mississippi State University Special Research Initiatives grants program.

Acknowledgments: The authors are grateful to Bobbie J. Johnson (retired), Jeremy Kotowicz, and Vivek H. Khambhati for their technical assistance. Trade names are used in this publication solely for the purpose of providing specific information. Mention of a trade name, propriety product, or specific equipment does not constitute a guarantee or warranty by the USDA-ARS and does not imply approval of the named product to exclusion of other similar products.

Conflicts of Interest: All authors declare no conflict of interest.

References

1. Holiday, P.; Punithalingam, E. *Macrophomina phaseolina. No. 275 in CMI (Commonweath Mycological Institute), Descriptions of Pathogenic Fungi and Bacteria*; Commonweath Mycological Institute: Kew Surrey, UK, 1970.
2. Ray, D.T.; Coffelt, T.A.; Dierig, D.A. Breeding guayule for commercial production. *Ind. Crop. Prod.* **2005**, *22*, 15–25. [CrossRef]

3. Kuti, J.O.; Schading, R.L.; Latigo, G.V.; Bradford, J.M. Differential responses of guayule (*Parthenium argentatum*) genotypes to culture filtrate and toxin from *Macrophomina Phaseolina*. *J. Phytopath.* **1997**, *145*, 305–311. [CrossRef]
4. Wyllie, T.D. Macrophomina phaseolina Charcoal rot. In *World Soybean Research, Proceedings of the World Soybean Research Conference*; Hill, L.D., Ed.; Interstate Printers and Publishers Inc.: Danville, IL, USA, 1976; pp. 482–484.
5. Medhaug, I.; Stolpe, M.B.; Fischer, E.M.; Knutti, R. Reconciling controversies about the 'global warming hiatus'. *Nature* **2017**, *545*, 41–47. [CrossRef] [PubMed]
6. Dubey, M.K.; Aamir, M.; Kaushik, M.S.; Khare, S.; Meena, M.; Singh, S.; Upadhyay, R.S. PR toxin-biosynthesis, genetic regulation, toxicological potential, prevention and control measures, Overview and challenges. *Front. Pharmacol.* **2018**, *9*, 288. [CrossRef]
7. Moreau, S.; Lablache-Combier, A.; Biguet, J.; Foulon, C.; Delfosse, C. Botryodiploidin, a mycotoxin produced by a strain of *Penicillium roqueforti*. *J. Org. Chem.* **1982**, *47*, 2358–2359. [CrossRef]
8. Nielsen, K.F.; Sumarah, M.W.; Frisvad, J.C.; Miller, J.D. Production of metabolites from the *Penicillium roqueforti* complex. *J. Agric. Food Chem.* **2006**, *54*, 3756–3763. [CrossRef]
9. O'Brien, M.; Nielsen, K.F.; O'Kiely, P.; Forristal, P.D.; Fuller, H.T.; Frisvad, J.C. Mycotoxins and other secondary metabolites produced in vitro by *Penicillium paneum* Frisvad and *Penicillium roqueforti* Thom isolated from baled grass silage in Ireland. *J. Agric. Food Chem.* **2006**, *54*, 9268–9276. [CrossRef]
10. Shier, W.T.; Abbas, H.K.; Baird, R.E.; Ramezani, M.; Sciumbato, G.L. (-)-Botryodiplodin, a unique ribose-analog toxin. *Toxin Rev.* **2007**, *26*, 343–386. [CrossRef]
11. Wrather, J.A.; Anderson, T.R.; Arsyad, D.M.; Tan, Y.; Ploper, L.D.; Porta-Puglia, A.; Ram, H.H.; Yorinori, J.T. Soybean disease loss estimates for the top ten soybean-producing countries in 1998. *Can. J. Plant. Pathol.* **2001**, *23*, 115–121. [CrossRef]
12. Wrather, J.A.; Koenning, S.R.; Anderson, T.R. Effect of diseases on soybean yields in the United States and Ontario (1999–2002). *Plant. Health Prog.* **2003**, *4*, 24. [CrossRef]
13. Wrather, J.A.; Koenning, S.R. Estimates of disease effects on soybean yields in the United States 2003–2005. *J. Nematol.* **2006**, *38*, 173–180. [PubMed]
14. Wrather, J.A.; Stienstra, W.C.; Koenning, S.R. Soybean disease loss estimates for the United States from 1996 to 1998. *Can. J. Plant. Pathol.* **2001**, *23*, 122–131. [CrossRef]
15. Wrather, J.A. Soybean disease loss estimates for the southern United States, 1974 to 1994. *Plant. Dis.* **1995**, *79*, 1076–1079.
16. Mengistu, A.; Wrather, A.; Rupe, J.C. *Charcoal Rot. Compendium of Soybean Diseases and Pests*, 5th ed.; Hartman, G.L., Rupe, J.C., Sikora, E.J., Domier, L.L., Davis, J.A., Steffey, K.L., Eds.; American Phytopathology Society: Saint Paul, MN, USA, 2015; pp. 67–69.
17. Mengistu, A.; Reddy, K.N.; Zablotowicz, R.M.; Wrather, A.J. Propagule densities of *Macrophomina phaseolina* in soybean tissue and soil as affected by tillage, cover crop, and herbicides. *Plant. Health Prog.* **2009**, *10*, 28. Available online: https://www.plantmanagementnetwork.org/pub/php/research/2009/soybean/ (accessed on 23 December 2019). [CrossRef]
18. Paris, R.L.; Mengistu, A.; Tyler, J.M.; Smith, J.R. Registration of soybean germplasm line DT97-4290 with moderate resistance to charcoal rot. *Crop. Sci.* **2006**, *46*, 2324–2325. [CrossRef]
19. Bellaloui, N.; Mengistu, A.; Zobiole, L.H.S.; Shier, W.T. Resistance to toxin-mediated fungal infection, Role of lignins, isoflavones, other seed phenolics, sugars and boron in the mechanism of resistance to charcoal rot disease in soybean. *Toxin Rev.* **2012**, *31*, 16–26. [CrossRef]
20. Bellaloui, N.; Mengistu, A.; Paris, R.L. Soybean seed composition in cultivars differing in resistance to charcoal rot (*Macrophomina phaseolina*). *J. Agric. Sci.* **2008**, *146*, 667–675. [CrossRef]
21. Gangopadhyay, S.; Wyllie, T.D.; Luedders, V.D. Charcoal rot disease of soybean transmitted by seeds. *Plant. Dis. Rep.* **1970**, *54*, 1088–1091.
22. Ichinose, Y.; Taguchi, F.; Mukaihara, T. Pathogenicity and virulence factors of Pseudomonas syringae. *J. Gen. Plant. Pathol.* **2013**, *79*, 285–296. [CrossRef]
23. Mihail, J.D. *Macrophomina. Methods for Research on Soilborne Phytopathogenic Fungi*; Singleton, L., Mihail, J.D., Rush, C.M., Eds.; The American Phytopathological Society, APS Press: Paul, MN, USA, 1992; pp. 134–136.
24. Oku, H. *Plant. Pathogenesis and Disease Control*; Lewis Publishers: Boca Raton, FL, USA, 1994.

25. Siddiqui, K.A.I.; Gupta, A.K.; Paul, A.K.; Banerjee, A.K. Purification and properties of a heat-resistant exotoxin produced by *Macrophomina phaseolina* (Tassi) Gold in culture. *Experentia* **1979**, *35*, 1222–1223. [CrossRef]
26. Sen Gupta, R.; Chandran, R.R.; Divekar, P.V. Botryodiplodin, a new antibiotic from *Botryodiplodia theobromae*. I. Production, isolation, and biological properties. *Indian J. Exp. Biol.* **1966**, *4*, 152–153.
27. Islam, M.S.; Haque, M.S.; Islam, M.M.; Emdad, E.M.; Halim, H.; Hossen, Q.M.M.; Hossain, M.Z.; Ahmed, B.; Rahim, S.; Rahman, M.S.; et al. Tools to kill, Genome of one of the most destructive plant pathogenic fungi *Macrophomina phaseolina*. *BMC Genom.* **2012**, *13*, 493. [CrossRef] [PubMed]
28. Dhar, T.K.; Siddiqui, K.A.I.; Ali, E. Structure of phaseolinone, a novel phytotoxin from *Macrophomina phaseolina*. *Tetrahedron Lett.* **1982**, *23*, 5459–5462.
29. Bunkers, G.; Kenfield, D.; Strobel, G.; Sugawara, F. Structure-activity relationships of the eremophilanes produced by *Drechslera gigantea*. *Phytochem* **1990**, *29*, 1471–1474. [CrossRef]
30. Kitahara, T.; Kiyota, H.; Kurata, H.; Mori, K. Synthesis of oxygenated eremophilanes, gigantenone, phomenone and phaseolinone, phytotoxins from pathogenic fungi. *Tetrahedron* **1911**, *47*, 1649–1654. [CrossRef]
31. Sugawara, F.; Hallock, Y.F.; Bunkers, G.D.; Kenfield, D.S.; Strobel, G.; Yoshida, S. Phytoactive eremophilanes produced by the weed pathogen *Drechslera gigantea*. *Biosci. Biotechnol. Biochem.* **1993**, *57*, 236–239. [CrossRef] [PubMed]
32. Ramezani, M.; Shier, W.T.; Abbas, H.K.; Tonos, J.L.; Baird, R.E.; Sciumbato, G.L. Soybean charcoal rot disease fungus *Macrophomina phaseolina* in Mississippi produces the phytotoxin, (-)-botryodiplodin, but no detectable phaseolinone. *J. Nat. Prod.* **2007**, *70*, 128–129. [CrossRef]
33. Abbas, H.K.; Bellaloui, N.; Accinelli, C.; Smith, J.R.; Shier, W.T. Toxin production in soybean (*Glycine max* L.) plants with charcoal rot disease and by *Macrophomina phaseolina*, the fungus that causes the disease. *Toxins* **2019**, *11*, 645. [CrossRef]
34. Goos, R.D.; Cox, E.A.; Stotzky, G. *Botryodiplodia theobromae* and its association with *Musa* species. *Mycologia* **1961**, *53*, 262–277. [CrossRef]
35. McCurry, P.M.; Abe, K. Stereochemistry and synthesis of the antileukemic agent botryodiplodin. *J. Am. Chem. Soc.* **1973**, *95*, 5824–5825. [CrossRef]
36. Moule, Y.; Decloitre, F.; Hamon, G. Mutagenicity of the mycotoxin botryodiplodin in the *Salmonella typhimurium*/microsomal activation test. *Environ. Mutagen.* **1981**, *3*, 287–291. [CrossRef] [PubMed]
37. Moule, Y.; Douce, C.; Moreau, S.; Darracq, N. Effects of the mycotoxin botryodiplodin on mammalian cells in culture. *Chem.-Biol. Interact.* **1981**, *37*, 155–164. [CrossRef]
38. Moule, Y.; Renauld, F.; Darracq, N.; Douce, C. DNA-protein cross-linking by the mycotoxin, botryodiplodin, in mammalian cells. *Carcinogen* **1982**, *3*, 211–214. [CrossRef] [PubMed]
39. Rehnberg, N.; Magnusson, G. Total synthesis of (-)- and (+)-botryodiplodin and (+)- and (-)-epibotryodiplodin. *Acta Chem. Scand.* **1990**, *44*, 377–383. [CrossRef]
40. Fujimoto, Y.; Kamiya, M.; Tsunoda, H.; Ohtsubo, K.; Tatsuno, T. Recherche toxicologique des substances métaboliques de *Penicillium carneo-lutescens*. *Chem. Pharm. Bull.* **1980**, *28*, 1062–1066. [CrossRef]
41. Félix, C.; Salvatore, M.M.; DellaGreca, M.; Ferreira, V.; Duarte, A.S.; Salvatore, F.; Naviglio, D.; Gallo, M.; Alves, A.; Esteves, A.C.; et al. Secondary metabolites produced by grapevine strains of *Lasiodiplodia theobromae* grown at two different temperatures. *Mycologia* **2019**, *111*, 466–476. [CrossRef]
42. Bhatnagar, D.; Payne, G.A.; Cleveland, T.E.; Robens, J.F. Mycotoxins, Current Issues in USA. In *Meeting the Mycotoxin Menace*; Barug, H., van Egmond, H.P., Lopez-Garcia, R., van Osenbruggen, W.A., Visconti, A., Eds.; Wageningen Academic Publishers: Wageningen, The Netherlands, 2004; pp. 17–47.
43. Horn, B.W.; Dorner, J.W. Regional differences in production of aflatoxin B_1 and cyclopiazonic acid by soil isolates of *Aspergillus flavus* along a transect within the United States. *Appl. Environ. Microbiol.* **1999**, *65*, 1444–1449. [CrossRef]
44. Shier, W.T. On the origin of antibiotics and mycotoxins. *Toxin Rev.* **2011**, *30*, 6–30. [CrossRef]
45. Ryder, L.S.; Talbot, N.J. Regulation of appressorium development in pathogenic fungi. *Curr. Opin. Plant. Biol.* **2015**, *26*, 8–13. [CrossRef]
46. Dunlap, J.R.; Bruton, D.B. Pigment biosynthesis by *Macrophomina phaseolina*. The glycine-specific requirement. *Trans. Br. Mycol. Soc.* **1986**, *86*, 111–115. [CrossRef]

47. Renault, F.; Moreau, S.; Lablache-Combier, A.; Tiffon, B. Botryodiplodin: A mycotoxin from *Penicillium roqueforti*, Reaction with amino-pyrimidines, amino-purines and 2′-deoxynucleosides. *Tetrahedron* **1985**, *41*, 955–962. [CrossRef]
48. Alam, S.; Abbas, H.K.; Okunowu, W.O.; Kotowicz, J.; Butler, A.M.; Shier, W.T. Development of an in-culture assay for detecting production of the mycotoxin (-)-botryodiplodin by *Macrophomina phaseolina*. In preparation.
49. Brechenmacher, L.; Lee, J.; Sachdev, S.; Song, Z.; Nguyen, T.H.N.; Joshi, T.; Oehrle, N.; Libault, M.; Mooney, B.; Xu, D.; et al. Establishment of a protein reference map for soybean root hair cells. *Plant. Physiol.* **2009**, *149*, 670–682. [CrossRef] [PubMed]
50. Lewis, D.R.; Negi, S.; Sukumar, P.; Muday, G.K. Ethylene inhibits lateral root development, increases IAA transport and expression of PIN3 and PIN7 auxin efflux carriers. *Development* **2011**, *138*, 3485–3495. [CrossRef]
51. Negi, S.; Ivanchenko, M.G.; Muday, G.K. Ethylene regulates lateral root formation and auxin transport in *Arabidopsis thaliana*. *Plant. J.* **2008**, *55*, 175–187. [CrossRef]
52. Niu, Y.; Chen, M.; Xu, Z.; Li, L.; Chen, X.; Ma, Y. Characterization of ethylene receptors and their interactions with GmTPR-A novel tetratricopeptide repeat protein (TPR) in soybean (*Glycine max* L.). *J. Integr. Agric.* **2013**, *12*, 571–581. [CrossRef]
53. Drew, M.C. Soil aeration and plant root metabolism. *Soil Sci.* **1992**, *154*, 259–268. [CrossRef]
54. Jackson, M.B.; Drew, M.C. The effect of flooding on growth and metabolism of herbaceous plants. In *Physiological Ecology, A Series of Monographs, Texts and Treatises*; Kozlowski, T.T., Ed.; Academic Press: Cambridge, MA, USA, 1984; pp. 47–128.
55. Roy, R.; Bhattacharya, G.; Siddiqui, K.A.I.; Bhadra, R. A new antileishmanial compound, phaseolinone. *BioChem. Biophys. Res. Commun.* **1990**, *168*, 43–50. [CrossRef]
56. Sturdikova, M.; Fuskova, A.; Proksa, B.; Fuska, J. Relationships between structure and biological activities of the antibiotic PSX-1 (botryodiplodine). *Biology (Bratisl. Slovak.)* **1988**, *43*, 233–238.
57. Fuska, J.; Fuskova, A. The in vitro-in vivo effect of antibiotic PSX-1 on lympholeukemia L-5178. *J. Antibiot. (Tokyo)* **1976**, *29*, 981–982. [CrossRef]
58. Chakraborty, S.; Lala, S. Assessment of the antifertility effect of phaseolinone, an antileishmanial agent, in male rats. *Contraception* **1998**, *58*, 183–191. [CrossRef]
59. Fuska, J.; Kuhr, I.; Nemec, P.; Fuskova, A. Antitumor antibiotics produced by *Penicillium stipitatum*. *J. Antibiot (Tokyo)* **1974**, *27*, 123–127. [CrossRef] [PubMed]
60. Von Helberger, J.H.; Ulubay, S.; Civelekoglu, H. EIN EINFACHES VERFAHREN ZUR GEWINNUNG VON ALPHA-ANGELICALACTON UND UBER DIE HYDRIERENDE SPALTUNG SAUERSTOFFHALTIGER RINGE. *ANNALEN DER CHEMIE-JUSTUS LIEBIG.* **1949**, *561*, 215–220. (In German) [CrossRef]
61. Mukaiyama, T.; Wada, M.; Hanna, J. A convenient synthesis of the antibiotic botryodiplodin. *Chem. Lett.* **1974**, *3*, 1181–1184. [CrossRef]
62. Nouguier, R.; Gastaldi, S.; Stien, D.; Bertrand, M.; Villar, F.; Andrey, O.; Renaud, P. Synthesis of (±)- and (-)-botryodiplodin using stereoselective radical cyclizations of acyclic esters and acetals. *Tetrahedron Asymmetry* **2003**, *14*, 3005–3018. [CrossRef]
63. Owen, P.A.; Nickell, C.D.; Noel, G.R.; Thomas, D.J.; Frey, K. Registration of 'Saline' Soybean. *Crop. Sci.* **1994**, *34*, 1689. [CrossRef]
64. Tanaka, T.; Abbas, H.K.; Duke, S.O. Structure-dependent phytotoxicity of fumonisins and related compounds in a duckweed bioassay. *Phytochem* **1993**, *33*, 779–785. [CrossRef]
65. Villagarcia, M.R.; Carter, T.E.; Rufty, T.W.; Niewoehner, A.S.; Jennette, M.W.; Arrellano, C. Genotypic rankings for aluminum tolerance of soybean roots grown in hydroponics and sand culture. *Crop. Sci.* **2001**, *41*, 1499–1507. [CrossRef]
66. Sheehan, D.; Hrapchak, B. *Theory and Practice of Histotechnology*, 2nd ed.; Battelle Press: Columbus, OH, USA, 1980; pp. 330–331.

toxins

MDPI

Article

Ergochromes: Heretofore Neglected Side of Ergot Toxicity

Miroslav Flieger [1], Eva Stodůlková [1], Stephen A. Wyka [2], Jan Černý [3], Valéria Grobárová [3], Kamila Píchová [1], Petr Novák [1], Petr Man [1], Marek Kuzma [1], Ladislav Cvak [4], Kirk D. Broders [2] and Miroslav Kolařík [1,*]

1 Laboratory of Fungal Genetics and Metabolism, Institute of Microbiology of the Czech Academy of Sciences, Vídeňská 1083, CZ-14220 Prague, Czech Republic
2 Department of Bioagricultural Sciences and Pest Management, Colorado State University, Fort Collins, CO 80523, USA
3 Department of Cell Biology, Faculty of Science, Charles University, Viničná 7, CZ-128 00 Prague, Czech Republic
4 TEVA Czech Ind, CZ-74770 Opava, Czech Republic
* Correspondence: mkolarik@biomed.cas.cz; Tel.: +420-296-442-332

Received: 25 June 2019; Accepted: 23 July 2019; Published: 25 July 2019

Abstract: Ergot, fungal genus *Claviceps*, are worldwide distributed grass pathogens known for their production of toxic ergot alkaloids (EAs) and the great agricultural impact they have on both cereal crop and farm animal production. EAs are traditionally considered as the only factor responsible for ergot toxicity. Using broad sampling covering 13 ergot species infecting wild or agricultural grasses (including cereals) across Europe, USA, New Zealand, and South Africa we showed that the content of ergochrome pigments were comparable to the content of EAs in sclerotia. While secalonic acids A–C (SAs), the main ergot ergochromes (ECs), are well known toxins, our study is the first to address the question about their contribution to overall ergot toxicity. Based on our and published data, the importance of SAs in acute intoxication seems to be negligible, but the effect of chronic exposure needs to be evaluated. Nevertheless, they have biological activities at doses corresponding to quantities found in natural conditions. Our study highlights the need for a re-evaluation of ergot toxicity mechanisms and further studies of SAs' impact on livestock production and food safety.

Keywords: mycotoxins; ergot alkaloids; ergochromes; secalonic acid; food safety; cereals; tetrahydroxanthones; *Claviceps*

Key Contribution: Ergot alkaloids (EAs) were considered as the only factor responsible for the ergot toxicity. We showed—using the robust sample size—that ergochromes are similarly abundant as ergot alkaloids and possess high toxicity to human cells. Thus, their importance for human and animal health should be further investigated.

1. Introduction

Ergot, the genus *Claviceps* (Ascomycota: Hypocreales) includes obligate plant parasitic fungi that develop in the ovary of grasses (including cereals), sedges, and rushes and form sclerotia containing toxins. The famous rye ergot, *Claviceps purpurea*, is a member of the section *Claviceps* which is specified by the production of highly toxic ergopeptines [1]. Recently it has been shown, that *C. purpurea sensu lato* (*s. l.*) is a complex of four cryptic species with different host grass spectra. While common land grasses are often infected by both *C. purpura sensu stricto* (*s. s.*) and *C. humidiphila*, cereal crops seem to be infected by just *C. purpurea s. s.* In the Palearctic region, these two species are the most important from an agricultural point of view [2,3]. Furthermore, recent findings suggest further cryptic diversification among North American *C. purpurea s. l.* specimens and their impacts on agricultural remains uncertain [4].

Ergot poisoning causes ergotism in humans and livestock. Most of the research related with ergotism has been focused on the ergot alkaloids (EAs) as these are among the most important natural pharmaceuticals and toxins in human history [5,6]. There is still some pharmaceutical research being conducted on EAs, however, research into their toxic effects on human health have relatively diminished. Humans are no longer at risk of ergotism in most of the world due to advanced seed cleaning and food screening for the presence of EAs. However, there has been a resurgence of research interested in the toxicoses of livestock or wild animals in recent years which has brought to light the substantial challenge of elucidating alkaloid-induced effects of animal responses to exposure [7,8]. Currently, the EU Scientific Panel on Contaminants in the Food Chain of the European Food Safety Authority (EFSA) recommended 12 priority alkaloids for monitoring in food and feed, all of which are grouped in the ergopeptines produced by *C. purpurea s. l.*

A recent review by Klotz [9] detailed the collective knowledge on ergotism and fescue toxicoses of livestock. He noted the complexity of this area of research as EA toxicity is affected by changes in alkaloid concentrations, proportions, and availability as well as individual's genetic predispositions, prior exposures, and ambient environments. This led to the overall conclusion that the impacts of EAs on livestock, especially convulsive (neurological and abortogenic) symptoms are not caused by the sole action of a single toxin, but rather the combined impact and synergistic action of multiple EAs derived from *Claviceps* and *Epichloë* species [9,10]. While most of the available data of EAs effects on animals both address the symptoms and define the problem, there is still a lack of research on other fungal metabolites and their potential harmful effects on livestock and humans.

In *C. purpurea s. l.*, the average EAs content in sclerotia varies between studies and ranges from 0.01–1.3 mg/g [11–16] to 2.88–7.26 mg/g [17], with individual values rarely reaching 5–10 mg/g (d/w) [12,16,18]. In addition to EAs, *C. purpurea* produces many other secondary metabolites. Most have been identified and inspected for toxicity while others have still eluded proper examination, with no research on their effects on livestock [10]. In addition, some of these other metabolites are produced in greater quantity than the heavily researched EAs. Ergot sclerotia can contain 1–2% of pigments, predominantly yellow biphenyl pigments called ergochromes (ECs) [19], which typically reach 5 mg/g of the sclerotia dry weight [20]. The main ECs of ergot are secalonic acids A–C (SAA, SAB, SAC), whereas related ergoflavin, ergochrysin A, B and chrysergonic acid are produced in negligible amounts. Other minor pigments, such as anthraquinone derivates endocrocin and clavorubin, are present [21]. Secalonic acids D–F were described from various moulds and lichens [22,23]. Secalonic acids exhibit various biological activities with the best studied secalonic acid D (SAD) showing mutagenic, teratogenetic, and cytotoxic activity [24–26]. Strong biotoxic activity against animals, plants, or microbial cells was also documented in secalonic acid A [27,28], F [29], and G [30].

Surprisingly, across the distribution of ergot species, the quantity and environmental role of ECs are still unknown, despite their proved activity against mammalian cells. There is currently no knowledge on the effect of ECs on livestock or how synergistic actions of ECs with other ECs or EAs affect their toxicity on livestock or humans. Therefore, we pose the following question: Could ECs represent an important and so-far neglected part of ergot toxicity? For that purpose, we quantified ECs content across a large set of ergot sclerotia and present the basic cytotoxicity assays on human cell lines.

2. Results

2.1. Ergot Alkaloids and Ergochromes Content

Three major SAA, SAB, and SAC and two minor ECs, endocrocin, and ergochrysin were identified in sclerotia. The average content of all SAs and EAs across all 111 samples was 4.08 mg/g (SD 4.39) and 3.58 mg/g (SD 2.46), respectively (Table 1, Figures 1 and 2, Table S1). These values were statistically not different (paired t-test, $p = 0.3$) and moderately, but significantly correlated (Figure 3, Pearsson coefficient 0.46, two tailed *t*-test, $p < 0.001$). The SAs content and proportion differed substantially between species and between European and North American (NA) populations of *C. purpurea s.s. Claviceps arundinis* and *C. humidiphila* contained significantly more SAs than EAs and had the highest content of all SAs among analyzed species. The dominance of SAs over EAs was also found in *C. capensis*, *C. macroura*, *C. monticola*, *C. pazoutovae*, and *C. fimbristylidis* (not tested for significance due to the low sample size). The opposite ratio was found in *C. purpurea* (all sample set), *C. spartinae* (significant different in both cases), *C. cyperi*, and *C. nigricans* (not tested for significance). European *C. purpurea s. s.* population had similar content of SAs and EAs, whereas the NA population had significantly more EAs than SAs (Table 1, Figure 2, Table S1). Both populations differed significantly in SAs (Mann-Whitney test, $p < 0.005$), but not in EAs content. The spectrum of SAs was shown to have an obvious chemotaxonomic value which separates European *C. purpuera* and *C. spartinae* (SAA as a dominant and often single secalonic acid), from the NA *C. purpurea* (SAC dominant, followed by SAB and SAA) and *C. arundinis* (SAB dominant, followed by SAC) and *C. humidiphila* (SAB dominant, SAC minor) (Figure 4, Table S1).

Table 1. Concentration summary of ergochromes and ergot alkaloids in *Claviceps* spp. sclerotia. Content in dry sclerotia is expressed as minimum-average (standard deviation)-maximum. The category of other species includes: *Claviceps* sp. 1, sp. 2, *C. capensis*, *C. cyperi*, *C. fimbristylidis*, *C. macroura*, *C. monticola*, *C. nigricans*, and *C. pazoutovae* (Table S1).

Taxon	# Samples	Total Secalonic Acids (mg/g)	Endocrocin, Ergochrysin (µg/g)	EAs (mg/g)
C. purpurea—Europe	13	1.66–5.05 (4.87)–17.96	0.00–17.51 (29.64)–97.58	0.00–2.69 (1.65)–5.17
C. purpurea—NA	46	0.02–1.91 (1.43)–6.33	0.00–3.13 (13.75)–84.82	0.02–2.96 (1.99)–9.71
C. purpurea—all	61	0.02–2.59 (2.81)–17.96	0.00–6.09 (18.96)–97.58	0.00–3.03 (2.03)–9.71
C. humidiphila	15	2.56–7.54 (6.04)–20.90	0.00–14.96 (16.07)–50.31	1.70–4.77 (2.38)–10.16
C. arundinis	13	3.70–9.67 (5.08)–20.23	0.00–50.28 (34.18)–126.93	2.18–5.32 (2.77)–12.87
C. spartinae	7	1.67–2.29 (0.49)–3.15	0.00–56.84 (68.65)–205.13	1.55–4.20 (1.42)–6.07
other spp.	15	0.03–2.66 (1.93)–6.50	0.00	0.00–1.77 (3.20)–11.99
all samples	111	0.02–4.08 (4.39)–20.90	0.00–9.01 (24.55)–205.13	0.00–3.57 (2.46)–12.87

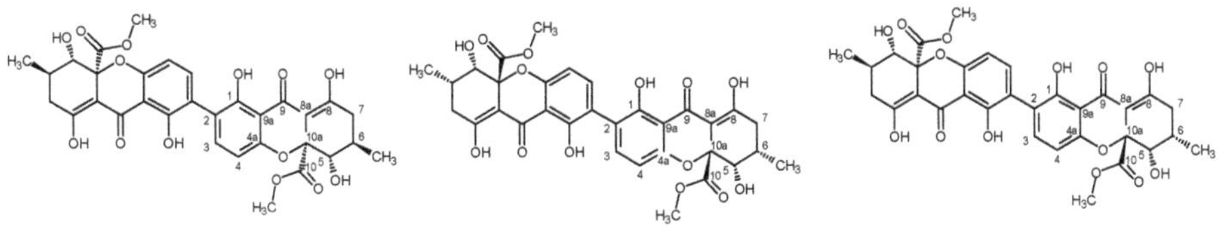

secalonic acid A secalonic acid B secalonic acid C

Figure 1. Structures of the main ergochromes from this study, secalonic acid A–C.

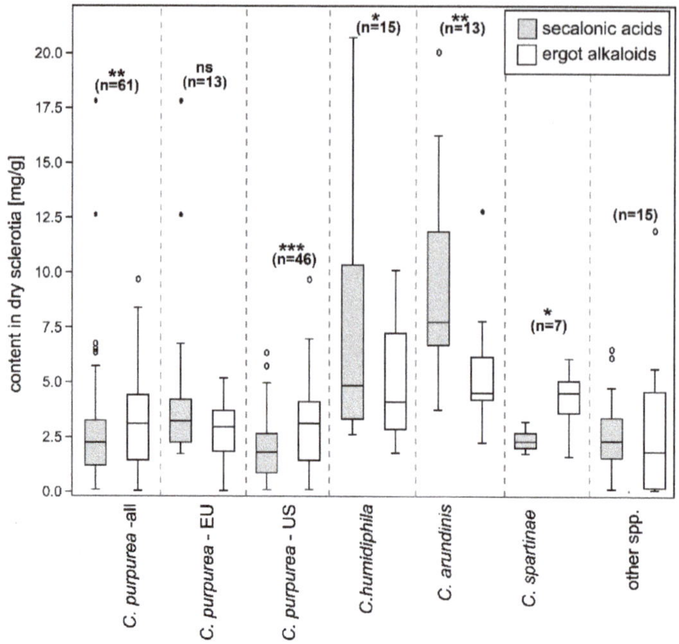

Figure 2. Box plot graph summarizing the total content of secalonic acids and ergot alkaloids in the dry sclerotia. The category of other species includes: *Claviceps* sp. 1, sp. 2, *C. capensis*, *C. cyperi*, *C. fimbristylidis*, *C. macroura*, *C. monticola*, *C. nigricans*, and *C. pazoutovae* (Table S1). *** $p < 0.001$, ** $p < 0.01$, * $p < 0.05$, ns—not significant, in the Wilcoxon Signed Rank test.

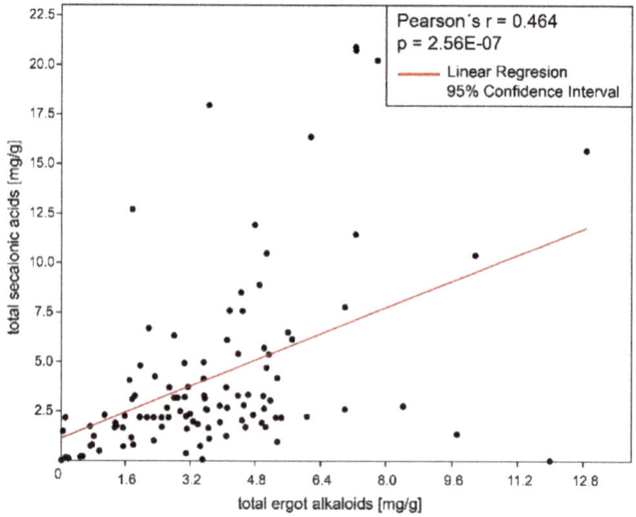

Figure 3. Linear regression of total secalonic acid (SAA, SAB, SAC) and ergot alkaloid content in sclerotia.

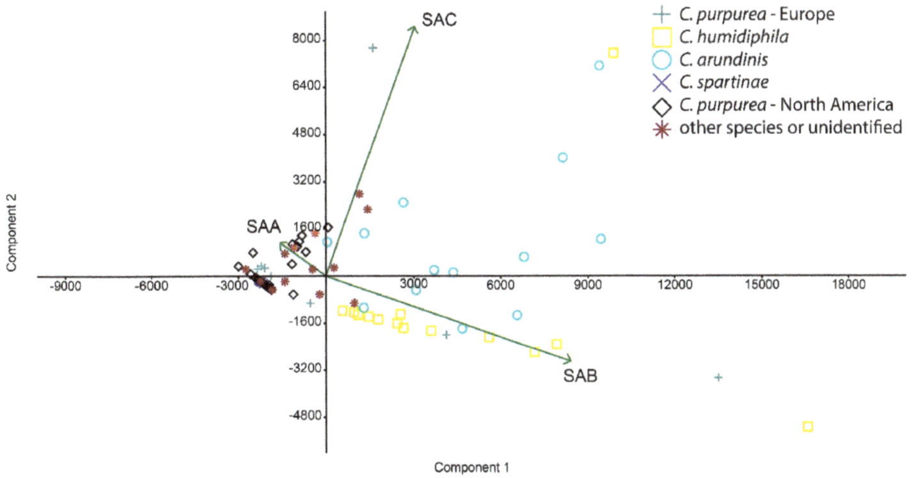

Figure 4. Principal component analysis showing relatedness of samples based on content of SAA, SAB, and SAC. PCA (Principal Component Analysis) axis 1 and 2 explained 76.3% and 16.1%, respectively.

2.2. *Biological Activity In Vitro*

Studied compounds were tested using cancer-derived Jurkat (Figure 5) and HeLa cell lines along with primary skin-derived fibroblasts (Figure 6). Toxicity tests on Jurkat cells (24 h exposure, Figure 5) showed that endocrocin (anthraquinone) did not cause apoptosis or cell death even in extremely high concentrations (LD50 705.5 μg/mL). The toxicity of ergoxanthine (LD50 142.0 μg/mL) and ergochrysin (LD50 118.8 μg/mL) was lower in comparison to SAs and EAs. Toxicity after 24 h exposure to SAA, SAB, SAC, and EA began at the lowest tested concentration (0.75 μg/mL), with 12 (EAs) and 25 (SAs) μg/mL resulting in 50%, and 50 (EAs) and 100 (SAs) μg/mL resulting in 100% of dead or apoptotic cells in all variants. The fraction of apoptotic and dead cells only slightly differed between these compounds, with EAs (LD50 13.5 μg/mL) showing the highest toxicity, followed by SAA (LD50 19.8 μg/mL), SAB (LD50 35.9 μg/mL), and SAC (LD50 36.5 μg/mL). For SAA + EAs (LD50 12.8 μg/mL) and SAB + SAC + EAs (LD50 15.4 μg/mL) neutral to synergistic effects on the number of dead cells could be observed.

Strong effects including changes in morphology and cell contact was observed in human primary fibroblasts and HeLa cells. At concentrations above 25 μg/mL cells incubated with SAA, SAB, SAC, and EA stopped dividing and showed loose stress fibers which started to detach. Striking effects on cellular morphology could be detected using Mitotracker probe (Figure 6). In the case of secalonic acid, concentrations above 12 μg/mL elicited rounded mitochondria with extremely high positivity in greater than 50% of fibroblasts and 100% of HeLa cells, indicating modulation of mitochondrial function, namely proton gradient value. In contrast, specific effects of ergotamine to both HeLa (100% affected cells above 50 μg/mL) and fibroblasts (25 μg/mL) caused the formation of swollen vacuolar structures. We can estimate that these swollen structures (not acidic—negative for Lysotracker probe) could stand for more than half of the cellular volume. Representative data for SAA and ergotamine treatments (various concentrations and simultaneous detection of actin cytoskeleton, mitochondria, and nuclei) are shown as Figure S1.

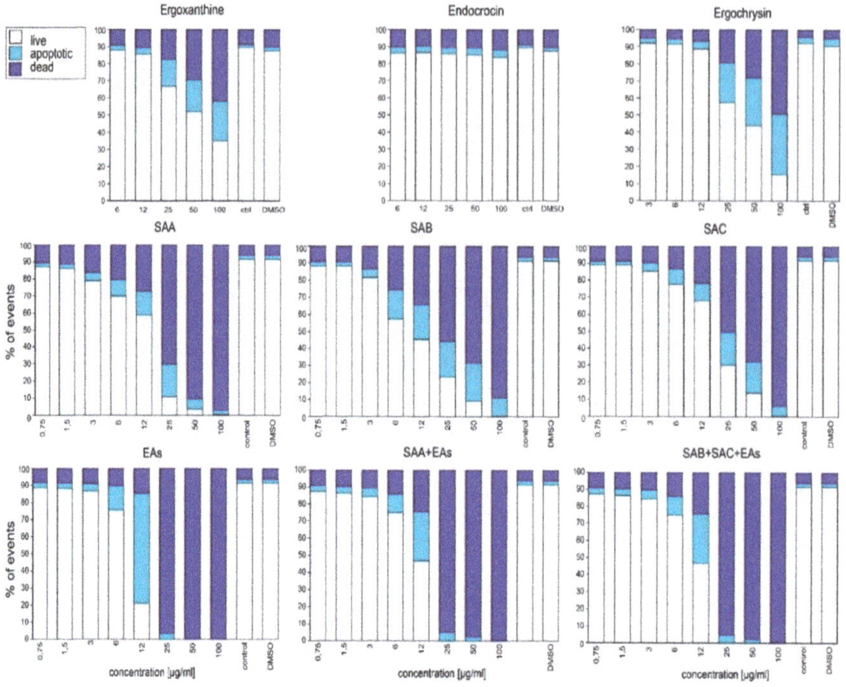

Figure 5. Live, Apoptotic, and dead cell events in Jurkat cells after 24 h incubation. Representative toxicity values for endocrocin, ergochromes, ergotamine, and the combinations of SAs and ergotamine. Combinations reflect the mixtures of SAs and EAs found in the real sclerotia. Cells are shown as events detected by flow cytometry and expressed in percentages (total amount of cells = 100% of events).

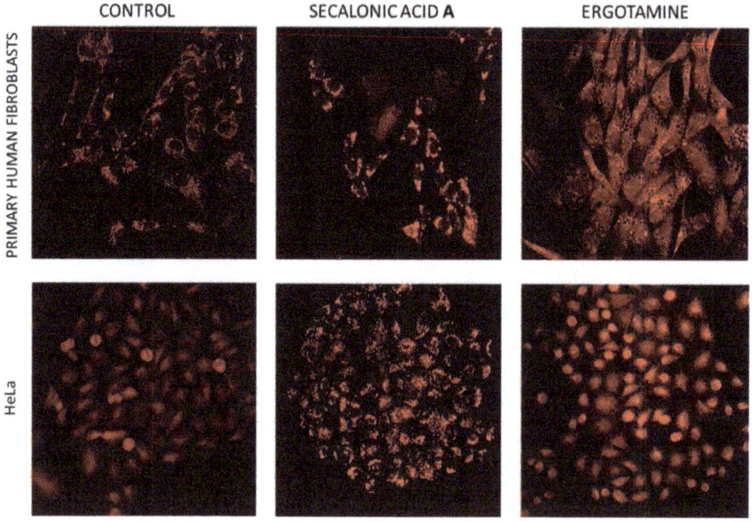

Figure 6. Mitochondrial architecture and Mitotracker positivity in HeLa cells and primary skin-derived fibroblasts. Cell cultures grown on glass cover slips were treated for 24 h with 12 µg/mL secalonic acid A or ergotamine and in vivo incubated with MitoTracker® Red CMXRos. Magnification 20×.

3. Discussion

3.1. Ergochrome Quantity and Distribution Across the Species

Ergochrome production in ergot fungi seems to be limited to the section *Claviceps* [1]. This section, represented by *C. purpurea s. l.*, is the most widely distributed section of the genus *Claviceps* and infects the largest number of host plants [1,2]. Due to its cosmopolitan distribution with over 400 potential hosts, including many economically important crops such as rye, wheat, triticale, and barley, the EFSA has selected *C. purpurea s. l.* to be the focus of chemical analysis for food safety concerns [7]. Among the members of *C. purpurea s. l.*, only *C. purpurea s. s.* and *C. humidiphila* infect cereals or cultivated and wild forage grasses and thus have an agricultural importance. *Claviceps cyperi*, infecting *Cyperus* spp. is distributed only in South Africa and is a known causal agent of ergotism in cattle [31]. *Claviceps arundinis* (mostly on *Phragmites*, *Mollinia*, or *Leymus arenarius*) and *C. spartinae* (*Spartina*, *Distichlis*) can be very common in their particular habitats, but their grass hosts are not significantly grazed by animals [2,3,32,33]. Populations of others, i.e., Paleartic *C. nigricans* (*Eleocharis*, *Scirpus*) or South African *Claviceps capensis* (*Ehrharta*), *C. fimbristylidis* (*Fimbristylis*), *C. pazoutovae* (*Ehrharta* and *Stipa*), *C. macroura* (*Cenchrus*), or *C. monticola* (*Brachypodium*) are rare in abundance and their hosts have low palatability [34,35].

Three major combinations of SAs in sclerotium were found and their mutual ratios have taxonomic value. Franck [36] analyzed three *C. purpurea* sclerotia from rye and found SAA as the dominant SA, followed by SAB and SAC, which is concordant with our data for SAs in European *C. purpurea s. s.* Concerning the total content of ECs, the only reliable publication reports 5 mg/g [20] which fully corresponds with our results. Besides SAs, other pigments were also found in several samples (*C. arundinis*, *C. humidiphila*, and *C. spartinae*) but in negligible quantity. The observed quantity of endocrocin (maximum 205 μg/g) corresponds with Franck [20] which reports maximal values of 40 μg/g (Table 1, Table S1).

Based on our data, the total EAs and SAs content in sclerotia was significantly correlated and the amount of toxic compounds in a single sclerotium is thus cumulative. This correlation also shows that measuring EAs can be used to some extent as a proxy for SAs abundance. It is already known that the pigment content of sclerotia is proportional to its alkaloid content and thus a pigments quantification (namely clavorubrin) can provide a method for measuring the samples' toxicity [37,38].

Both toxin groups are metabolically independent, but their production in sclerotia is contemporary and seems to be regulated by the same stimuli (phosphate level) [39], which can explain the observed correlation. Fungal pigments typically have a light protection role, and this ability is also expected in the case of ECs [39]. Contrary to this, EAs are light sensitive [40] and the correlation between the contents of EAs and SAs could also just be a consequence of light induced degradation of EAs in the sclerotia with primary lower contents of pigments (SAs).

3.2. Ecological Role of SAs

From an ecological point of view, SAs can contribute to ergot toxicity (see below) and are thus involved in the protective mutualism known in *C. purpurea s. l.* [41]. SAs can play an important role in the protection of the sclerotia against light or in antibiosis (resistance to microbial attacks). In particular, SAB showed activity against *Bacillus megaterium*, *Escherichia coli*, and *Microbotryum violaceum* [42], and SAA showed antibiotic activity against *Bacillus subtilis*, *Piricularia oryzae* [27], *Microccocus luteus* (MIC 4–8 μg/mL), and *Enterococcus faecalis* (MIC 32 μg/mL) [43]. SAA is also a highly potent non-host specific phytotoxine acting as a possible virulence factor of *Pyrenophora terrestris* [28]. Interestingly, the whole section *Claviceps*, which is unique due to the presence of ECs, also has an extraordinary broad host range [1]. This suggests that ECs could potentially play some role in the virulence cycle, but are surely not essential for it, as was shown in infections test with mutant *C. purpurea* strains with blocked ECs synthesis [39].

3.3. Ergochromes Toxicity and Significance

The main aim of this study was to determine the quantity of ECs produced by *C. purpurea* and other members of the section *Claviceps* to help assess their potential role in ergotism pathogenicity. The effort to control the toxicosis of forage and human food has generally been successful; however, there has been a resurgence of research interested in the toxicosis of livestock due to increased ergot abundance in recent years [44] and continual reports of ergotism on livestock.

While many researchers continue to focus on compounds that possess the tetracyclic ergoline ring of ergot alkaloids, we showed that so far neglected SAs are equally abundant as alkaloids and have similar toxicity to cell cultures. While our data shows the essential first step, further research into the toxicity of SAs is needed to elucidate their real impact on human and animal health. Understanding the connection of SAs to ergotism might help explain some of the unexplained aspects of egotism. Klotz [9] published a thorough review of the inconsistent nature and occurrence of ergotism in livestock. While his review only covered the toxicosis of *Claviceps*-derived ergotamine and ergocristine and *Epichloë*-derived ergovaline, he was still able to determine that the impacts of alkaloids on livestock are not caused by the sole action of a single toxin but rather the combined impact and synergistic action of multiple alkaloids. This was evident as many researchers were generally unsuccessful in replicating the complete effects of ergotism by introducing individual or even combinations of multiple alkaloids to livestock. For example, individual applications of ergovaline and ergotamine and combined applications of ergocornine, ergocryptine, and ergocristine were unable to produce gangrenous ergotism or fescue foot in all of the exposed livestock [45–48]. Similar inconclusive results were also observed for other aspects of ergotism such as fat necrosis and male-specific effects [9]. Such inconsistencies might be the results of concentration levels, alkaloid proportions, isomeric forms, accumulation, as well as individual's genetic predispositions, prior exposures, and ambient environments.

Therefore, SAs might represent a missing piece in the larger picture of ergotism on livestock. A few experiments on living animals were conducted with SAs. The major compound of ergot sclerotia, SAA, is lethal to mice at the peritoneal injected doses 50–100 mg/kg [27]. In another study, SAA caused edema and inflammation in rats after the intraperitoneal application of 12.5–50 mg/kg [49]. This toxicity is comparable to well recognized toxin SAD which LD50 for mice in intraperitoneal injection was reported as 42 mg/kg [50] or in a range of 26.5–51.7 mg/kg [24]. Teratogenic effects were observed in rats injected with SAD and teratogenic activity started at doses of 5 mg/kg body weight [25,51]. Data from humans are missing, but it is known that SAD produces cleft palate as the only malformation in fetal mice which is of potential relevance to human health [52]. Furthermore, SAs have various biological effects at non-toxic doses. SAA at the concentrations 0.15–0.75 mg/kg injected peritoneally to mice affect the metabolism of dopaminergic neurons [53,54].

In cases of cell line cultures, the toxicity to cancer cells is much higher than for normal cells. SAA is toxic against cultured mouse (IC50 = 0.5 µg/mL, [55]) or human leukemia cells (ED50 = 3.5 µg/mL, [43]). These values roughly correspond to the LD50 ranging between 20–37 µg/mL found in SAA-SAC for Jurkat cells in our study. The IC50 for murine melanoma cells was 1.8 µg/mL for SAA and 0.18 µg/mL for SAD, but to affect healthy keratinocytes a 3.5× (SAA) or 13× (SAD) higher concentration was needed [56]. SAD is also cytotoxic against various carcinoma cell lines at very low concentrations (IC50 = 0.05–0.76 ug/mL) and its mechanism of function is the best studied among all ECs [57].

Thus, the question is whether SAs of ergot origin can negatively affect animal health. The only available data are for SAD, and optical antipode of SAA, which have very similar toxicity to animal models and potentially have the same mode of action [58]. Whereas, at the intraperitoneal application, the LD50 for SAD and SAA ranges between 25–37 mg/kg (applied one times) while there is an 11-fold lower sensitivity when introduced by an oral route in mice [59]. Thus, an LD50 of around 400 mg/kg body weight can be close to toxicity values found in field conditions. Scenarios accounting for repeated applications of sublethal doses increase the toxicity by approximately three times as toxic effects of SAD were found to be cumulative in a five-day feeding experiment, which indicates that the toxin can be accumulated within the organism [59]. The question, what is the exposition of livestock to SAs under natural conditions, remains unanswered. In EAs the lowest save doses (no-observed-adverse-effect levels) are 0.22–0.60 mg/kg body weight per day [7]. Concerning the fact that SAs and EAs have very similar concentrations in ergot, we can expect that animals encounter similar doses. Based on our above review, the lethal toxicity of SAs is more than 125 times lower than in EAs and their importance in the acute intoxication can play a role in case of highly contaminated fodder only. Nevertheless, SAs have various biological activities in much lower doses (i.e., 0.15 mg/kg injected peritoneally, [53,54]) corresponding to expositions in natural conditions.

3.4. Mode of Action

SAs exhibit various bioactivities, generally cytotoxic and cytostatic. SAD and SAF exhibit antitumor activity in low micromolar ranges, including induction of cell cycle arrest in G1 or induction of apoptosis [60,61]. The molecular mechanism behind the antitumor selectivity and toxicity remain putative. Opposite to cytotoxic effects, SAA applications in a Parkinson's disease mouse model protected against dopaminergic neuron death [53]. The best studied SA, SAD, exhibited various modes of cytotoxicity towards multidrug resistance cells due to induction of ABCG2 degradation via calpain-1 activation [57]. Our observations agree with this general view that particular bioactivities are cell type dependent (in our case leukemic cell line, adenocarcinoma, and primary human fibroblasts) in terms of effective concentrations and particular phenotypes (proliferative block, loss of stress fibres, proportion of apoptotic cells). The hallmark physiological and morphological changes in all cell types treated with SAs was transformation of the typical mitochondrial network to isolated rounded mitochondria with extremely high positivity for Mitotracker probe, indicating interference with mitochondrial function. For example, electron-transport chain functions and proton gradient levels. This is in agreement with previously published results that SAD uncoupled the oxidative phosphorylation in isolated rat mitochondria [62]. Another indication, that mitochondria could be the cellular target for SAs is based on the observation that SAA protects dopaminergic neurons from 1-methyl-4-phenylpyridinium induced cell death via the mitochondrial apoptotic pathway [54].

4. Conclusions

Despite the fact that ergochromes do not play a significant role in acute toxicity of ergot, the complexity of the secondary metabolites produced by *Claviceps* species including secalonic acids points to a more complex fungus-grazing animal interaction. Grazing animals consuming ergotised grasses are constantly exposed to doses of secondary metabolite mixtures that can have a profound biological effect on their physiology or development. This publication is focused on the major secondary metabolite family, SAs, which can offer the tempting explanation to the complex ecological interaction between the herbivore and the fungus. Historically, the major body of research was focused on the ergot alkaloids. The observation that *Claviceps* secondary metabolome is much more diverse than anticipated, providing new research direction. Future research needs to examine metabolism, absorption, and excretion of SAs to determine their potential in short term versus long term toxicosis. For example, the described effect of SAs on mitochondria (temping molecular mechanism behind the bioactivity) indicating high interference with function needs detailed studies to be understood completely. These research directions are essential to understand ergotism itself in its complexity and to help determine whether forage and human food contaminated with *Claviceps purpurea* should be monitored for the control of ECs content, as proposed in this publication.

5. Materials and Methods

5.1. Specimens Analyzed

The analyzed sclerotia (n = 111) covers material from four continents. All 13 agriculturally and environmentally important ergot species producing ergochromes, were collected from the wild as well as cultivated grasses and cereals; i.e., *C. purpurea s.s.* (collections from Europe, North America,

New Zealand), *C. humidiphila* (Europe), *C. arundinis* (Europe), *C. nigricans* (Europe), *C. spartinae* (Europe), *C. cyperi*, *C. fimbristylidis*, *C. macroura*, *C. monticola*, *C. pazoutovae*, (all from South Africa), and two undescribed *Claviceps* sp. (USA, New Zealand). Materials originated from previous studies [2,34,63] or were collected during the course of this study (Table 1, Table S1). Sclerotia were identified using the ITS rDNA sequence barcode. DNA from sclerotia was isolated using the fast NaOH protocol [64] for European samples or using the PowerPlant Pro DNA Isolation Kit (MoBio/Qiagen) for US/NZ samples. PCR and sequencing of the ITS barcode was performed according to Pažoutova et al. [2]. DNA and chemical analyses were done from the same sclerotium in the case of larger sclerotia. In cases of very small sclerotia, chemical analysis was performed from the whole sclerotium and DNA based identification was completed using a sclerotium collected from the same or adjacent grass spiclet.

5.2. Sample Preparation, Extraction, and HPLC Analyses

Pulverized sclerotia (1–10 mg) were mixed with extraction mixture dichloromethane and concentrated ammonia (500:1, *v:v*, 0.5–2.0 mL) and gently stirred for 1 h. Supernatant was separated by centrifugation and kept in the freezer until use. The same HPLC instrumentation and method as published earlier [1] was used for the analysis of EAs and ECs in sclerotia of all *C. purpurea s.s.* analyzed.

5.3. Ergot Alkaloids and Ergochromes Identification and Quantification

5.3.1. General Workflow

Identification of EAs was based on retention time which was compared with standard compounds and UV–VIS spectra of individual compounds. Secalonic acids A, B, and C, were isolated and identified using UV–VIS spectra, FTMS, NMR, and optical rotation. The isolated compounds were used as chromatographic standards for quantification of their content in individual sclerotia. Further isolated ECs were determined as endocrocin and ergochrysin by the same procedures as used for the SAs. In both cases the data obtained were in agreement with previously published data [20].

5.3.2. FTMS

Samples were measured using 15T solariX FTMS equipped with an ESI/MALDI ion source and ParaCell (Bruker Daltonics, Billerica MA). The analysis was performed using an electrospray ionization (ESI) in a positive ion mode as described in Flieger et al. [65] with the following differences: The collision energy was kept at −15.5 V, the mass range for MS data acquisition started at *m/z* 150 a.m.u., resulting in a resolution of 250,000 at *m/z* 400. The detailed FTMS data for SAA-SAC are presented in Figure S2.

5.3.3. NMR

NMR spectra were measured on a Bruker Avance III 600 MHz spectrometer (600.23 MHz for 1H, 150.93 MHz for ^{13}C) in CD3CN (20 and 30 °C). Residual signals of solvent were used as an internal standard (at 20 °C: δ_H 1.941, δC 1.41, at 30 °C: δ_H 1.936, δ_C 1.35). NMR experiments: ^{1}H NMR, ^{13}C NMR, COSY, ^{1}H-^{13}C HSQC, ^{1}H-^{13}C HMBC, and ROESY were performed as described in Stodůlková et al. [66]. Detailed NMR data of the identified compounds are provided in Table S2 (^{13}C NMR) and Table S3 (^{1}H NMR).

5.3.4. Quantification of Ergot Alkaloids and Ergochromes

A standard solution of quantified compounds, i.e., ergotamine and ergochrysin, were prepared in methanol and SAA in acetone at final concentrations of 31.75, 62.5, 125, 250, 500, and 1000 μg mL^{-1}. The calibration graphs were constructed by plotting the integrated peak areas of individual compounds versus concentration. The following linear regression equations and correlation coefficients were obtained: Ergotamine; y = 5298.3x, R^2 = 0.9994, UV = 315nm; secalonic acid A; y = 14537x + 6452, R^2 = 0.9995, UV = 315nm; ergochrysin; y = 6205.7x − 2015, R^2 = 0.9991, UV = 315nm.

5.4. Biological Activity Testing

For toxicity studies, immortalized T-lymphocyte-derived cancer cell line Jurkat was cultivated in 96-well plates at a density of 2×10^5 cells in a final volume of 300 μL of RPMI1640 (LONZA, USA). Cells were treated with different concentrations of SAs, ergoxanthin, endocrocin, ergotamine, and a combination of SAA and ergotamine (1:1) and SAB, SAC, and ergotamine (0.5:0.5:1) (Figure 5). Cells cultured in RPMI1640 and in RPMI1640 with only DMSO were only used as negative controls. After the incubation (24 h), cells were washed in PBS containing 0.02% gelatine and 0.01% sodium azide (Sigma-Aldrich, St. Louis, MO, USA). Hoechst 33258-stained cells were analyzed with the FACS LSRII instrument (BD Biosciences, San Jose, CA, USA) and FlowJo 10.5.3 software (Tree Star, Ashland, OR, USA).

For fluorescent microscopy adenocarcinoma cell line HeLa and primary human skin-derived fibroblasts were used. Cells were cultivated in DMEM medium with 10% FCS (Gibco, Invitrogen, Grand Island, NY, USA) and seeded on glass cover slips (up to density 50%) in 24-well plates. Cells treated with different concentrations of tested compounds were cultured in DMEM, wells supplemented with only DMSO were used as negative controls. After 24 h incubation, cells were incubated (10 min, Lysotracker® Red, or MitoTracker® Red CMXRos (Molecular Probes-Invitrogen, Carlsbad, CA, USA) and fixed (3.7% paraformaldehyde in PBS, 20 min, RT), permeabilized (0.1% Triton X-100 in PBS), blocked (1% BSA in PBS), and stained with Phalloidin-Alexa Fluor®488. All fluorescent dyes were from Molecular Probes (Invitrogen Carlsbad, CA, USA). Morphological observations were performed using Olympus IX71microscope equipped with DP70 camera 20× objective. Nuclei were stained and specimens mounted using Fluoroshield DAPI (Sigma Aldrich).

5.5. Statistical Analysis

Data were visualized on PCA (Principal Component Analysis). The normality of the data was tested using Chi-squared test and the correlation between SAs and EAs production was done using the linear Pearson test. A non-parametric Wilcoxon signed rank test was used to test the null hypothesis of no difference in the EAs and ECs concentrations within the particular species or population. Non parametric Mann-Whitney test or parametric paired *t*-test was used to compare EAs and SAs content between populations or across all samples. These statistical analyses were done using the PAST 3.25 software [66]. The LC_{50} values of tested compounds were calculated using probit analysis [67,68] using Microsoft Excell® Professional Plus 2013 software (Microsoft Corp., Redmond, WA, USA).

Supplementary Materials: The following are available online at http://www.mdpi.com/2072-6651/11/8/439/s1, Table S1: List of analyzed ergot samples and the content of ergochromes and ergot alkaloids, Table S2: ^{13}C NMR data for secalonic acid A–C, Table S3: ^{1}H NMR data for secalonic acid A–C, Figure S1: Cell cultures grown on glass cover slips were treated for 24 h with secalonic acid A or ergotamine and in vivo incubated with MitoTracker® Red CMXRos, fixed, permeabilized, and labeled with Phalloidin-Alexa Fluor®488, Figure S2: FTMS data for secalonic acid A–C.

Author Contributions: Conceptualization, M.K. (Miroslav Kolařík) and M.F.; methodology, M.F., J.Č., and M.K. (Miroslav Kolařík); resources, M.K. (Miroslav Kolařík), S.A.W., K.D.B., J.Č., and M.F.; investigation, E.S., K.P., S.A.W., P.N., M.K. (Marek Kuzma), P.M., and V.G.; formal analysis, M.F., M.K. (Miroslav Kolařík), and J.Č.; validation, M.F., M.K., and J.Č.; writing—original draft preparation, M.K. and S.A.W.; writing—review & editing, M.K., S.A.W., M.F., and J.Č.; funding acquisition, M.K. (Miroslav Kolařík), K.D.B.

Funding: This research was funded by the Czech Science Foundation (GAČR), grant number 13-00788S and by European Regional Development Funds, grant number CZ.1.05/1.1.00/02.0109 BIOCEV. Stephen A. Wyka and Kirk D. Broders were supported by American Malting Barley Assoc. Grant No. 17037621.

Conflicts of Interest: The authors declare no conflict of interest.

References

1. Píchová, K.; Pažoutová, S.; Kostovčík, M.; Chudíčková, M.; Stodůlková, E.; Novák, P.; Flieger, M.; van der Linde, E.; Kolařík, M. Evolutionary history of ergot with a new infrageneric classification (Hypocreales: Clavicipitaceae: *Claviceps*). *Mol. Phylogen. Evol.* **2018**, *123*, 73–87. [CrossRef] [PubMed]
2. Pažoutová, S.; Pešicová, K.; Chudíčková, M.; Šrůtka, P.; Kolařík, M. Delimitation of cryptic species inside *Claviceps purpurea*. *Fungal Biol.* **2015**, *119*, 7–26. [CrossRef] [PubMed]
3. Negård, M.; Uhlig, S.; Kauserud, H.; Andersen, T.; Høiland, K.; Vrålstad, T. Links between genetic groups, indole alkaloid profiles and ecology within the grass-parasitic *Claviceps purpurea* species complex. *Toxins (Basel)* **2015**, *7*, 1431–1456. [CrossRef] [PubMed]
4. Shoukouhi, P.; Hicks, C.; Menzies, J.G.; Popovic, Z.; Chen, W.; Seifert, K.A.; Assabgui, R.; Liu, M. Phylogeny of Canadian ergot fungi and a detection assay by real-time polymerase chain reaction. *Mycologia* **2019**, *111*, 493–505. [CrossRef] [PubMed]
5. Arroyo-Manzanares, N.; Gámiz-Gracia, L.; García-Campaña, A.M.; Diana Di Mavungu, J.; De Saeger, S. Ergot alkaloids: Chemistry, biosynthesis, bioactivity, and methods of analysis. In *Fungal Metabolites*; Mérillon, J.-M., Ramawat, K.G., Eds.; Springer: Berlin, Germany, 2017; pp. 887–929.
6. Young, C.A.; Schardl, C.L.; Panaccione, D.G.; Florea, S.; Takach, J.E.; Charlton, N.D.; Moore, N.; Webb, J.S.; Jaromczyk, J. Genetics, genomics and evolution of ergot alkaloid diversity. *Toxins (Basel)* **2015**, *7*, 1273–1302. [CrossRef]
7. EFSA. Scientific opinion on ergot alkaloids in food and feed. *EFSA J.* **2012**, *10*, 158. [CrossRef]
8. Belser-Ehrlich, S.; Harper, A.; Hussey, J.; Hallock, R. Human and cattle ergotism since 1900: Symptoms, outbreaks, and regulations. *Toxicol. Ind. Health* **2013**, *29*, 307–316. [CrossRef]
9. Klotz, J. Activities and effects of ergot alkaloids on livestock physiology and production. *Toxins (Basel)* **2015**, *7*, 2801–2821. [CrossRef]
10. Bauer, J.I.; Gross, M.; Cramer, B.; Wegner, S.; Hausmann, H.; Hamscher, G.; Usleber, E. Detection of the tremorgenic mycotoxin paxilline and its desoxy analog in ergot of rye and barley: A new class of mycotoxins added to an old problem. *Anal. Bioanal. Chem.* **2017**, *409*, 5101–5112. [CrossRef]
11. Miedaner, T.; Dänicke, S.; Schmiedchen, B.; Wilde, P.; Wortmann, H.; Dhillon, B.; Geiger, H.; Mirdita, V. Genetic variation for ergot (*Claviceps purpurea*) resistance and alkaloid concentrations in cytoplasmic-male sterile winter rye under pollen isolation. *Euphytica* **2010**, *173*, 299–306. [CrossRef]
12. Mulder, P.; Van Raamsdonk, L.; Van Egmond, H.; Van Der Horst, T.; De Jong, J. Dutch survey ergot alkaloids and sclerotia in animal feeds. In *Report/RIKILT 2012*; Institute of Food Safety: Wageningen, The Netherlands, 2012; Available online: http://edepot.wur.nl/234699 (accessed on 24 July 2019).
13. Franzmann, C.; Wächter, J.; Dittmer, N.; Humpf, H.-U. Ricinoleic acid as a marker for ergot impurities in rye and rye products. *J. Agric. Food Chem.* **2010**, *58*, 4223–4229. [CrossRef] [PubMed]
14. Appelt, M.; Ellner, F.M. Investigations into the occurrence of alkaloids in ergot and single sclerotia from the 2007 and 2008 harvests. *Mycotoxin Res.* **2009**, *25*, 95–101. [CrossRef] [PubMed]
15. Fajardo, J.; Dexter, J.; Roscoe, M.; Nowicki, T. Retention of ergot alkaloids in wheat during processing1, 2. *Cereal Chem.* **1995**, *72*, 291–298.
16. Pažoutová, S.; Olšovská, J.; Linka, M.; Kolínská, R.; Flieger, M. Chemoraces and habitat specialization of *Claviceps purpurea* populations. *Appl. Environ. Microbiol.* **2000**, *66*, 5419–5425. [CrossRef] [PubMed]
17. Aboling, S.; Drotleff, A.; Cappai, M.; Kamphues, J. Contamination with ergot bodies (*Claviceps purpurea* sens ulato) of two horse pastures in Northern Germany. *Mycotoxin Res.* **2016**, *32*, 207–219. [CrossRef] [PubMed]
18. Uhlig, S.; Vikøren, T.; Ivanova, L.; Handeland, K. Ergot alkaloids in Norwegian wild grasses: A mass spectrometric approach. *Rapid Commun. Mass Spectrom.* **2007**, *21*, 1651–1660. [CrossRef] [PubMed]
19. Stoll, A.; Renz, J.; Brack, A. Über gelbe Farbstoffe im Mutterkorn. 11. Mitteilung über antibakterielle Stoffe. *Helv. Chim. Acta* **1952**, *35*, 2022–2034. [CrossRef]
20. Franck, B. Structure and biosynthesis of the ergot pigments. *Angew. Chem. Int. Ed. Engl.* **1969**, *8*, 251–260. [CrossRef]
21. Buchta, M.; Cvak, L. Ergot alkaloids and other metabolites of the genus *Claviceps*. In *Ergot: The Genus Claviceps*; Křen, V., Cvak, L., Eds.; Harwood Academic Publishers: Amsterdam, The Netherlands, 1999; pp. 173–200.

22. Masters, K.-S.; Bräse, S. Xanthones from fungi, lichens, and bacteria: The natural products and their synthesis. *Chem. Rev.* **2012**, *112*, 3717–3776. [CrossRef]
23. Wezeman, T.; Bräse, S.; Masters, K.-S. Xanthone dimers: A compound family which is both common and privileged. *Nat. Prod. Rep.* **2015**, *32*, 6–28. [CrossRef]
24. Ciegler, A.; Hayes, A.W.; Vesonder, R.F. Production and biological activity of secalonic acid D. *Appl. Environ. Microbiol.* **1980**, *39*, 285–287. [PubMed]
25. Reddy, C.; Reddy, R.; Hayes, A.; Ciegler, A. Teratogenicity of secalonic acid D in mice. *J. Toxicol. Environ. Health A* **1981**, *7*, 445–455. [CrossRef] [PubMed]
26. Zhang, J.-Y.; Tao, L.-Y.; Liang, Y.-J.; Yan, Y.-Y.; Dai, C.-L.; Xia, X.-K.; She, Z.-G.; Lin, Y.-C.; Fu, L.-W. Secalonic acid D induced leukemia cell apoptosis and cell cycle arrest of G1 with involvement of GSK-3β/β-catenin/c-Myc pathway. *Cell Cycle* **2009**, *8*, 2444–2450. [CrossRef] [PubMed]
27. Yamazaki, M.; Maebayshi, Y.; Miyaki, K. The isolation of secalonic acid A from *Aspergillus ochraceus* cultured on rice. *Chem. Pharm. Bull. (Tokyo)* **1971**, *19*, 199–201. [CrossRef] [PubMed]
28. Steffens, J.C.; Robeson, D.J. Secalonic acid A, a vivotoxin in pink root-infected onion. *Phytochemistry* **1987**, *26*, 1599–1602. [CrossRef]
29. Andersen, R.; Buechi, G.; Kobbe, B.; Demain, A.L. Secalonic acids D and F are toxic metabolites of *Aspergillus aculeatus*. *J. Org. Chem.* **1977**, *42*, 352–353. [CrossRef]
30. Elsaid, A.; Sallam, A.; Ashour, A.; Ebrahim, W.; Lahloub, M.F.; Saad, H.-E. Biologically active metabolites from *Penicillium* sp., An endophyte isolated from *Glaucium arabicum*. *J. Am. Sci.* **2016**, *12*, 33–41. [CrossRef]
31. Naude, T.W.; Botha, C.; Vorster, J.H.; Roux, C.; van der Linde, E.; van der Walt, S.I.; Rottinghaus, G.; van Jaarsveld, L.; Lawrence, A.N. *Claviceps cyperi*, a new cause of severe ergotism in dairy cattle consuming maize silage and teff hay contaminated with ergotised *Cyperus esculentus* (nut sedge) on the Highveld of South Africa. *Onderstepoort J. Vet. Res.* **2005**, *72*, 23–37. [CrossRef]
32. Cerri, M.; Reale, L.; Moretti, C.; Buonaurio, R.; Coppi, A.; Ferri, V.; Foggi, B.; Gigante, D.; Lastrucci, L.; Quaglia, M. *Claviceps arundinis* identification and its role in the die-back syndrome of *Phragmites australis* populations in central Italy. *Plant Biosyst.* **2018**, *152*, 818–824. [CrossRef]
33. Boestfleisch, C.; Drotleff, A.M.; Ternes, W.; Nehring, S.; Pažoutová, S.; Papenbrock, J. The invasive ergot *Claviceps purpurea* var. *spartinae* recently established in the European Wadden Sea on common cord grass is genetically homogeneous and the sclerotia contain high amounts of ergot alkaloids. *Eur. J. Plant Pathol.* **2015**, *141*, 445–461. [CrossRef]
34. van der Linde, E.J.; Pešicová, K.; Pažoutová, S.; Stodůlková, E.; Flieger, M.; Kolařík, M. Ergot species of the *Claviceps purpurea* group from South Africa. *Fungal Biol.* **2016**, *120*, 917–930. [CrossRef] [PubMed]
35. Brady, L. Phylogenetic distribution of parasitism by *Claviceps* species. *Lloydia* **1962**, *25*, 1–36.
36. Franck, B.; Gottschalk, E.M.; Ohnsorge, U.; Hüper, F. Mutterkorn-Farbstoffe, XII. Trennung, Struktur und absolute Konfiguration der diastereomeren Secalonsäuren A, B and C. *Chem. Ber.* **1966**, *99*, 3842–3862. [CrossRef]
37. McClymont Peace, D.; Harwig, J. Screening for ergot particles in grain products by light microscopy. *Food Res. Int.* **1982**, *15*, 147–149. [CrossRef]
38. Maríne Font, A.; Moreno Martin, F.; Costes, C. Study of the pigments of ergot. New method for studying ergot in flours. *Ann. Falsif. Expert. Chim.* **1971**, *64*, 80.
39. Neubauer, L.; Dopstadt, J.; Humpf, H.-U.; Tudzynski, P. Identification and characterization of the ergochrome gene cluster in the plant pathogenic fungus *Claviceps purpurea*. *Fungal Biol. Biotechnol.* **2016**, *3*, 2. [CrossRef] [PubMed]
40. Komarova, E.; Tolkachev, O. The chemistry of peptide ergot alkaloids. Part 1. Classification and chemistry of ergot peptides. *Pharm. Chem. J.* **2001**, *35*, 504–513. [CrossRef]
41. Wäli, P.P.; Wäli, P.R.; Saikkonen, K.; Tuomi, J. Is the pathogenic ergot fungus a conditional defensive mutualist for its host grass? *PLoS ONE* **2013**, *8*, e69249. [CrossRef]
42. Zhang, W.; Krohn, K.; Egold, H.; Draeger, S.; Schulz, B. Diversity of antimicrobial pyrenophorol derivatives from an endophytic fungus, *Phoma* sp. *Eur. J. Org. Chem.* **2008**, 4320–4328. [CrossRef]
43. Pettit, G.R.; Meng, Y.; Herald, D.L.; Graham, K.A.; Pettit, R.K.; Doubek, D.L. Isolation and structure of ruprechstyril from *Ruprechtia tangarana*. *J. Nat. Prod.* **2003**, *66*, 1065–1069. [CrossRef]
44. Menzies, J.; Turkington, T. An overview of the ergot (*Claviceps purpurea*) issue in western Canada: Challenges and solutions. *Can. J. Plant Pathol.* **2015**, *37*, 40–51. [CrossRef]

45. Greatorex, J.; Mantle, P. Experimental ergotism in sheep. *Res. Vet. Sci.* **1973**, *15*, 337–346. [CrossRef]
46. Griffith, R.; Grauwiler, J.; Hodel, C.; Leist, K.; Matter, B. Toxicologic considerations. In *Ergot Alkaloids and Related Compounds*; Berde, B., Schild, H.O., Eds.; Springer: Berlin, Germany, 1978; pp. 805–851.
47. Tor-Agbidye, J.; Blythe, L.; Craig, A. Correlation of endophyte toxins (ergovaline and lolitrem B) with clinical disease: Fescue foot and perennial ryegrass staggers. *Vet. Hum. Toxicol.* **2001**, *43*, 140–146. [PubMed]
48. Merrill, M.; Bohnert, D.; Harmon, D.; Craig, A.; Schrick, F. The ability of a yeast-derived cell wall preparation to minimize the toxic effects of high-ergot alkaloid tall fescue straw in beef cattle. *J. Anim. Sci.* **2007**, *85*, 2596–2605. [CrossRef] [PubMed]
49. Harada, M.; Yano, S.; Watanabe, H.; Yamazaki, M.; Miyaki, K. Phlogistic activity of secalonic acid A. *Chem. Pharm. Bull. (Tokyo)* **1974**, *22*, 1600–1606. [CrossRef]
50. Steyn, P.S. The isolation, structure and absolute configuration of secalonic acid D, the toxic metabolite of *Penicillium oxalicum*. *Tetrahedron* **1970**, *26*, 51–57. [CrossRef]
51. Mayura, K.; Wallace Hayes, A.; Berndt, W.O. Teratogenicity of secalonic acid d in rats. *Toxicology* **1982**, *25*, 311–322. [CrossRef]
52. Hanumegowda, U.M.; Dhulipala, V.C.; Reddy, C.S. Mechanism of secalonic acid D-induced inhibition of transcription factor binding to cyclic AMP response element in the developing murine palate. *Toxicol. Sci.* **2002**, *70*, 55–62. [CrossRef]
53. Zhai, A.; Zhang, Y.; Zhu, X.; Liang, J.; Wang, X.; Lin, Y.; Chen, R. Secalonic acid A reduced colchicine cytotoxicity through suppression of JNK, p38 MAPKs and calcium influx. *Neurochem. Int.* **2011**, *58*, 85–91. [CrossRef]
54. Zhai, A.; Zhu, X.; Wang, X.; Chen, R.; Wang, H. Secalonic acid A protects dopaminergic neurons from 1-methyl-4-phenylpyridinium (MPP+)-induced cell death via the mitochondrial apoptotic pathway. *Eur. J. Pharmacol.* **2013**, *713*, 58–67. [CrossRef]
55. Kurobane, I.; Iwahashi, S.; Fukuda, A. Cytostatic activity of naturally isolated isomers of secalonic acids and their chemically rearranged dimers. *Drugs Exp. Clin. Res.* **1987**, *13*, 339–344. [PubMed]
56. Millot, M.; Tomasi, S.; Studzinska, E.; Rouaud, I.; Boustie, J. Cytotoxic constituents of the lichen *Diploicia canescens*. *J. Nat. Prod.* **2009**, *72*, 2177–2180. [CrossRef] [PubMed]
57. Hu, Y.-P.; Tao, L.-Y.; Wang, F.; Zhang, J.-Y.; Liang, Y.-J.; Fu, L.-W. Secalonic acid D reduced the percentage of side populations by down-regulating the expression of ABCG2. *Biochem. Pharmacol.* **2013**, *85*, 1619–1625. [CrossRef] [PubMed]
58. Franck, B.; Flasch, H. Die Ergochrome (Physiologie, Isolierung, Struktur und Biosynthese). In *Fortschritte der Chemie Organischer Naturstoffe*; Grisebach, H., Kirby, G.W., Herz, W., Eds.; Springer: Berlin, Germany, 1973; pp. 151–206.
59. Reddy, C.; Hayes, A.; Williams, W.; Ciegler, A. Toxicity of secalonic acid D. *J. Toxicol. Environ. Health A* **1979**, *5*, 1159–1169. [CrossRef] [PubMed]
60. Chen, L.; Li, Y.-P.; Li, X.-X.; Lu, Z.-H.; Zheng, Q.-H.; Liu, Q.-Y. Isolation of 4, 4′-bond secalonic acid D from the marine-derived fungus *Penicillium oxalicum* with inhibitory property against hepatocellular carcinoma. *J. Antibiot.* **2019**, *72*, 34. [CrossRef] [PubMed]
61. Gao, X.; Sun, H.; Liu, D.; Zhang, J.; Zhang, J.; Yan, M.; Pan, X. Secalonic acid-F inhibited cell growth more effectively than 5-fluorouracil on hepatocellular carcinoma in vitro and in vivo. *Neoplasma* **2017**, *64*, 344–350. [CrossRef] [PubMed]
62. Kawai, K.; Nakamaru, T.; Maebayashi, Y.; Nozawa, Y.; Yamazaki, M. Inhibition by secalonic acid D of oxidative phosphorylation and Ca2+-induced swelling in mitochondria isolated from rat livers. *Appl. Environ. Microbiol.* **1983**, *46*, 793–796.
63. Pazoutova, S.; Olsovska, J.; Sulc, M.; Chudickova, M.; Flieger, M. *Claviceps nigricans* and *Claviceps grohii*: Their alkaloids and phylogenetic placement. *J. Nat. Prod.* **2008**, *71*, 1085–1088. [CrossRef]
64. Osmundson, T.W.; Eyre, C.A.; Hayden, K.M.; Dhillon, J.; Garbelotto, M.M. Back to basics: An evaluation of NaOH and alternative rapid DNA extraction protocols for DNA barcoding, genotyping, and disease diagnostics from fungal and oomycete samples. *Mol. Ecol. Resour.* **2013**, *13*, 66–74. [CrossRef]
65. Flieger, M.; Band'ouchová, H.; Černý, J.; Chudíčková, M.; Kolařík, M.; Kováčová, V.; Martínková, N.; Novák, P.; Šebesta, O.; Stodůlková, E. Vitamin B2 as a virulence factor in *Pseudogymnoascus destructans* skin infection. *Sci. Rep.* **2016**, *6*, 33200. [CrossRef]

66. Stodůlková, E.; Císařová, I.; Kolařík, M.; Chudíčková, M.; Novák, P.; Man, P.; Kuzma, M.; Pavlů, B.; Černý, J.; Flieger, M. Biologically active metabolites produced by the basidiomycete *Quambalaria cyanescens*. *PLoS ONE* **2015**, *10*, e0118913. [CrossRef] [PubMed]
67. Hammer, Ø.; Harper, D.; Ryan, P. PAST: Paleontological statistics software package for education and data analysis. *Palaeontol. Electron.* **2001**, *4*, 9.
68. Finney, D.J. *Probit Analysis*, 3rd ed.; Cambridge University Press: Cambridge, UK, 1971.

toxins

MDPI

Article

Aflatoxin B_1 Conversion by Black Soldier Fly (*Hermetia illucens*) Larval Enzyme Extracts

Nathan Meijer [1,*], Geert Stoopen [1], H.J. van der Fels-Klerx [1,*], Joop J.A. van Loon [2], John Carney [3,4] and Guido Bosch [5]

1 Wageningen Food Safety Research, Wageningen Campus P.O. Box 230, 6700 AE Wageningen, The Netherlands; geert.stoopen@wur.nl
2 Wageningen University, Department of Plant Sciences, Laboratory of Entomology, Wageningen Campus P.O. Box 16, 6700 AA Wageningen, The Netherlands; joop.vanloon@wur.nl
3 Mars, Incorporated, McLean, VA 22101, USA, john.carney@effem.com
4 JMC Consulting, Portland, OR 972229, USA
5 Wageningen University, Department of Animal Sciences, Animal Nutrition Group, Wageningen Campus P.O. Box 338, 6700 AH Wageningen, The Netherlands; guido.bosch@wur.nl
* Correspondence: nathan.meijer@wur.nl (N.M.); ine.vanderfels@wur.nl (H.J.v.d.F.-K.)

Received: 24 July 2019; Accepted: 10 September 2019; Published: 12 September 2019

Abstract: The larvae of the black soldier fly (*Hermetia illucens* L., BSFL) have received increased industrial interest as a novel protein source for food and feed. Previous research has found that insects, including BSFL, are capable of metabolically converting aflatoxin B_1 (AFB_1), but recovery of total AFB_1 is less than 20% when accounting for its conversion to most known metabolites. The aim of this study was to examine the conversion of AFB_1 by S9 extracts of BSFL reared on substrates with or without AFB_1. Liver S9 of Aroclor-induced rats was used as a reference. To investigate whether cytochrome P450 enzymes are involved in the conversion of AFB_1, the inhibitor piperonyl butoxide (PBO) was tested in a number of treatments. The results showed that approximately 60% of AFB_1 was converted to aflatoxicol and aflatoxin P_1. The remaining 40% of AFB_1 was not converted. Cytochrome P450s were indeed responsible for metabolic conversion of AFB_1 into AFP_1, and a cytoplasmic reductase was most likely responsible for conversion of AFB_1 into aflatoxicol.

Keywords: aflatoxin; mycotoxin; black soldier fly; BSFL; *Hermetia illucens*; S9 fraction; cytochrome P450; metabolic conversion; enzyme induction

Key Contribution: The S9 fraction of black soldier fly larvae (*Hermetia illucens* L., BSFL) contains cytochrome P450s that metabolically convert aflatoxin B_1 (AFB_1) into AFP_1, and a cytoplasmic reductase is responsible for conversion of AFB_1 into aflatoxicol.

1. Introduction

Aflatoxins are a group of mycotoxins that are primarily produced by the molds *Aspergillus flavus* and *Aspergillus parasiticus*. The four major aflatoxins are B_1, B_2, G_1, and G_2, which can be found in various food products such as peanuts and maize [1]. Aflatoxins are carcinogenic to humans (IARC Group 1) and a major economic and health problem globally, but especially in sub-Saharan Africa, Latin America, and Asia, since people and animals are exposed to levels that substantially elevate mortality and morbidity. Aflatoxin B_1 (AFB_1) has generated the most concern due to its toxicity and high contamination levels in food and feed commodities in certain areas such as Africa [2,3]. AFB_1 is converted by animals and humans into a variety of metabolites, such as aflatoxin M_1, Q_1, P_1, and aflatoxicol (AFL) [1,4]. AFB_1 is a "procarcinogen" in the sense that hepatic microsomal cytochrome

P450 (CYP450) enzymes convert AFB_1 to AFB_1-8,9-epoxide (AFBO), which has reactive and electrophilic properties that underlie the toxicity of the compound [5].

Although prevention of contamination of crops by aflatoxigenic molds is paramount, a variety of decontamination strategies have been developed. Postharvest detoxification methods for AFB_1 include physical (heat and irradiation), chemical (acidification, ammoniation, and ozonation), and biological (whole organism or extracts thereof and enzymatic) treatments [6–9]. Although degradation levels of AFB_1 are generally high for enzymatic treatments, treatment times are also high (up to several days), and there is uncertainty regarding the degradation products formed [6]. Since metabolites in treated products may still be toxic, determination of degradation products is a principal requirement for assessing the safety and efficacy of enzymatic detoxification treatments. Detoxification mechanisms are generally classified into three phases: "(I) introduction of reactive and polar groups into substrates through oxidation, reduction, or hydrolysis; (II) conjugation of metabolites with other compounds to create more polar or more easily excretable molecules; and (III) transport and elimination of compounds" [10]. Cytochrome P450 monooxygenase enzymes play a major role in the bioactivation of AFB_1 in phase I metabolism [1,11]. These enzymes can be found in almost all (aerobic) organisms, but different P450 isoforms are species specific [12,13]. Some compounds may act as inhibitors of certain P450s. The best-known example of such an inhibitor is piperonyl butoxide (PBO) [13].

Insects have developed physiological and metabolic strategies to cope with potential toxic compounds, such as mycotoxins. Earlier work on the fruit fly *Drosophila melanogaster* Meigen (Diptera: Drosophilidae) [14–17] and on yellow mealworm (*Tenebrio molitor* L.; Coleoptera: Tenebrionidae; YMW) [18] has shown that some insects are capable of metabolizing AFB_1. More recently, Bosch et al. (2017) [19] found that both black soldier fly larvae (*Hermetia illucens* L., BSFL) and YMW have a high AFB_1 tolerance and that the toxin did not accumulate in these species. Moreover, the amount of AFB_1 lost (from substrates to insects) varied from 83% to 95% for BSFL and 89% to 96% for YMW. However, the YMW formed AFM_1 (present in the excreta) and AFB_1 was detected in YMW when provided with feed containing 0.023 mg/kg of AFB_1 or more. The concentration decreased when the YMW were starved before harvesting, which resulted in the larvae emptying their guts. This suggested that the gut contents contributed significantly to the measured AFB_1 levels in the YMW. Camenzuli et al. (2018) [20] subsequently assessed the effects of a variety of mycotoxins, including AFB_1, on BSFL and lesser mealworm (*Alphitobius diaperinus* Panzer; Coleoptera: Tenebrionidae). The mycotoxin metabolites AFL, aflatoxin P_1, Q_1, and M_1 were taken into consideration in the chemical and bioaccumulation analyses. Mass balance calculations for BSFL suggested recovery of total AFB_1 of less than 20%. Of the other analyzed metabolites, only AFL was detected at 0.2% of the overall mass balance; aflatoxin Q_1, P_1, and M_1 were not detected (<0.001 mg/kg for larvae, <0.005 mg/kg for residual material (spiked feed and gut clean)).

In the corn earworm (*Helicoverpa zea* L.; Lepidoptera: Noctuidae), the toxicity of AFB_1 depends on the CYP-mediated metabolic bioactivation [21]. Niu et al. (2008) [22] reported that dietary phytochemicals (i.e., xanthotoxin, coumarin, or indole-3-carbinol) induced midgut enzymes including CYP321A1 that can degrade AFB_1 into mainly AFP_1 and, to a lesser extent, an undefined metabolite. Feeding AFB_1 without the phytochemical did not increase CYP321A1 transcripts and resulted in reduced growth and development, confirming that phytochemicals induced CYP enzymes that detoxify AFB_1 [23]. Incubation of AFB_1 with a homogenate of the larvae of the navel orangeworm (*Amyelois transitella* Walker; Lepidoptera: Pyralidae) resulted in the formation of mainly AFL and, to a lesser extent, aflatoxin B_{2a} and AFM_1 [24]. This was in line with findings in testes of the fruit fly using a similar in vitro approach [17]. CYP6AB11 from navel orangeworm did not metabolize AFB_1 [25]. Importantly, the in vitro study of Lee and Campbell (2000) [24] reported that PBO did not impact AFL formation by navel orangeworm, which suggested that this metabolite was formed by cytosolic NADPH-dependent reductase. Incubation of AFB_1 with a homogenate of larvae of the codling moth (*Cydia pomonella* L.; Lepidoptera: Tortricidae) did not result in the metabolites AFL, AFB_{2a}, and AFM_1, which may relate either to absence of the metabolic system, different metabolic pathways, or that the system was not activated in the larvae, as these were not exposed to AFB_1 before the study [24]. In honey bees (*Apis mellifera* L.; Hymenoptera: Apidae), there are also indications of P450-mediated metabolic detoxification of AFB_1 [26].

In summary, BSFL have high tolerance to AFB_1, and when AFB_1 is provided in the feed, most of it cannot be recovered in the larvae and residual material. It is not clear whether and, if so, to what extent AFB_1 is metabolically converted. As an alternative to live animals, an enzyme extract can be prepared to assess the potential for metabolic conversion of the species in vitro. In this manner, individual or several metabolic conversion pathways can be isolated and identified. The aim of this study was to examine the conversion of AFB_1 by S9 extracts of BSFL reared on a substrate with AFB_1. The S9 enzyme fraction contains both the membrane-bound as well as the soluble enzymes [27]. Liver S9 of Aroclor-induced rats was used as a reference. To investigate whether cytochrome P450 enzymes specifically are involved in the conversion of AFB_1, PBO was tested in a number of treatments. We conclude that cytochrome P450s were indeed responsible for metabolic conversion of AFB_1 into AFP_1, and that a cytoplasmic reductase was most likely responsible for conversion of AFB_1 into AFL.

2. Results

2.1. *Effects of AFB_1 in Feed on Larval Development*

Live BSFL were subjected to two treatments, each applied in triplicate: one treatment in which the feed was spiked with AFB_1 to a concentration of 0.5 mg/kg, and one control treatment without AFB_1 added to the feed. Per replicate, 100 larvae less than 24 h old were provided with the feed and harvested after 9 days. Survival after these 9 days was high for both the control (average: 99.0) and the AFB_1 treatment (average: 97.3) ($p = 0.007$). Average total biomass obtained was, respectively, 15.2 and 15.0 g ($p = 0.685$).

2.2. *AFB_1 Conversion by S9 Fractions*

Table S1 shows the molar concentrations of AFB_1 and the analyzed metabolites after incubation for all replicates. The results from the treatment with AFB_1 but without S9 (−S9 + AFB_1, t = 2 h) show that only AFB_1 was found at the same concentration as what was spiked, and that no metabolites were formed. In the treatment with S9 but without AFB_1 (+S9 − AFB_1, t = 2 h), no AFB_1 or metabolites were detected. This indicates that the AFB_1 that was present in the larval feed was not converted into the analyzed metabolites by the larvae and did not accumulate.

Figure 1 shows the average molar concentrations (nM) of AFB_1 and the analyzed metabolites for the three types of S9 fractions (rat, BSFL-control, and BSFL-AFB_1) at two different points in time after addition of AFB_1: after directly (t = 0 h) halting enzymatic activity (+S9 + AFB_1, t = 0 h) and after incubation for 2 h (+S9 + AFB_1, t = 2 h). For all three S9 fractions at t = 0 h, only AFB_1 was present. The AFB_1 concentration at t = 0 h was half of the concentration that was spiked at the start due to the addition of 100 μL of acetonitrile to the 100 μL mixture of Regensys A buffer, NADPH, AFB_1, and S9. The results of the BSFL-control and BSFL-AFB_1 S9 fractions that were incubated for 2 h show that part of the AFB_1 was converted into AFP_1 (23.44 nM, $p = 0.847$) and AFL (21.32 nM, $p = 0.824$). The total molar concentrations (AFB_1 + AFP_1 + AFL) of these two treatments were equal to the total molar concentration of AFB_1 in the t = 0 h treatments (BSFL-control: $p = 0.275$; BSFL-AFB_1: $p = 0.211$). This indicates that no metabolic conversion occurred other than the type that was observed (i.e., AFB_1 into AFP_1 and AFL).

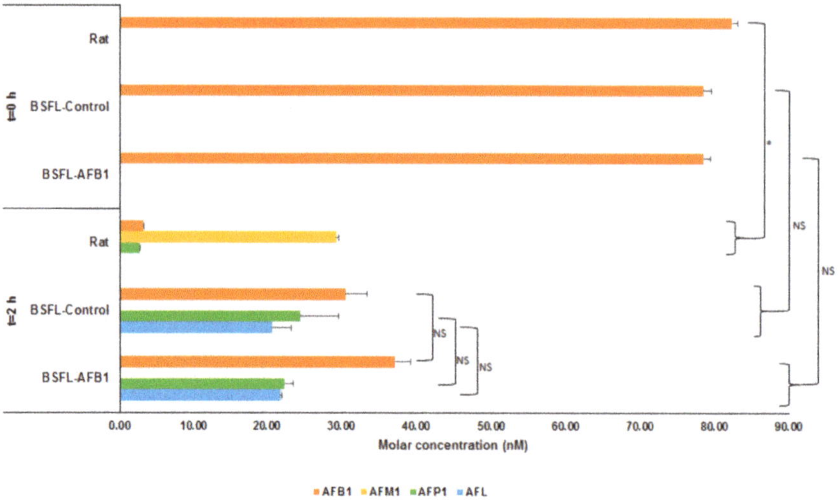

Figure 1. Molar concentrations (nM) of aflatoxin B_1 (AFB_1) and metabolites (AFM_1, AFP_1, and aflatoxicol (AFL)) for incubation of AFB_1 with S9 fractions from rat liver, black soldier fly larvae (*Hermetia illucens* L., BSFL)-control, and BSFL-AFB_1 after directly halting enzymatic activity (t = 0 h) and after 2 h of incubation. Significance of differences is indicated in the figure with * ($p \leq 0.05$) or NS (not significant, $p > 0.05$).

The results of the rat S9 treatments that were incubated for 2 h show that AFM_1 (29.34 nM) and, to a lesser extent, AFP_1 (2.59 nM) had formed. The amount of AFB_1 that was recovered after incubation from the treatment with the rat S9 fraction (3.15 nM) was less than what was recovered from the BSFL treatments (BSFL-AFB_1: 37.23 nM; BSFL-control: 30.57 nM). In addition, the total molar concentration of AFB_1 and analyzed metabolites for the rat S9 treatment after incubation for 2 h (35.17 nM) was less than the total AFB_1 molar concentration for the rat S9 treatment at t = 0 h (82.29 nM). This indicates that some of the spiked AFB_1 was converted by the rat S9 into different metabolites than those that have been analyzed.

2.3. *Effect of PBO on AFB_1 Conversion by S9 Fractions*

Figure 2 shows the average molar concentrations (nM) of AFB_1 and the analyzed metabolites for the two types of S9 fractions (rat and BSFL-AFB_1) after incubation with AFB_1 for 2 h. One treatment contained an S9 fraction (rat or BSFL-AFB_1) and AFB_1 (+S9 + AFB_1, t = 2 h); the second also contained dimethyl sulfoxide (DMSO, (+S9 + AFB_1 + DMSO, t = 2 h); and in the third, PBO (dissolved in DMSO) was added to the S9 fractions and AFB_1 (+S9 + AFB_1 + DMSO + PBO, t = 2h). For the AFB_1 larvae S9 treatments, the differences between the treatment containing DMSO and the treatment without further additives were not significant for each included metabolite (AFB_1 ($p = 0.296$), AFL ($p = 0.758$), AFP_1 ($p = 0.491$)). This indicates that the DMSO in which the PBO was dissolved did not affect the conversion of the BSFL-AFB_1 S9 fraction. Compared with the BSFL treatment without additional additives, the AFP_1 concentration in the PBO treatment was reduced ($p = 0.002$), while the AFL ($p = 0.001$) and AFB_1 ($p = 0.004$) concentrations were elevated. Comparing the rat treatment with PBO to the treatment without additives shows that the conversion into AFP_1 was completely halted and the conversion into AFM_1 was reduced (7.54 nM). The AFB_1 molar concentration was higher in the PBO treatment than in the treatment without additives, but the total molar concentration of the analyzed metabolites in the PBO treatment was equal to the total AFB_1 molar concentration at t = 0 h (+S9 + AFB_1, t = 0 h; $p = 0.129$). This indicates that the PBO halted the conversion of AFB_1 by rat S9 into different metabolites than those that have been analyzed.

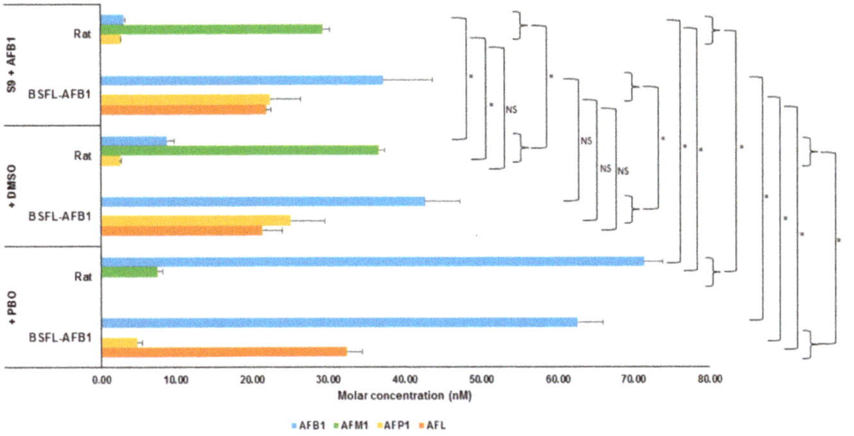

Figure 2. Molar concentrations (nM) of AFB_1 and metabolites (AFM_1, AFP_1, and AFL) for incubation of AFB_1 with S9 fractions from rat liver and BSFL-AFB_1, and with dimethyl sulfoxide (DMSO) or DMSO + cytochrome P450 inhibitor piperonyl butoxide (PBO) added, after 2 h of incubation. Significance of differences is indicated in the figure with * ($p \leq 0.05$) or NS (not significant, $p > 0.05$).

3. Discussion and Conclusions

Body weight and survival of control larvae and larvae exposed to AFB_1 were similar. We therefore conclude that the BSFL were unaffected by the addition of AFB_1 to their feed, which is in line with the findings of Bosch et al. (2017) [19] and Camenzuli et al. (2018) [20].

The study showed that S9 preparations of BSFL converted approximately 60% of the AFB_1 to AFL and AFP_1. The remaining 40% of AFB_1 was not converted into the analyzed metabolites. The amounts of AFL and AFP_1 were more or less equal, and there was no difference in activity of S9 prepared from larvae grown on substrates with or without AFB_1. This suggests that the enzymes involved in the biotransformation of AFB_1 are part of constitutive detoxification systems of the BSFL. Activation of the system in the larvae via pre-exposure—as hypothesized by Lee and Campbell (2000) [24], discussed above—is therefore not required for the system's functioning.

The addition of cytochrome P450 inhibitor PBO partially inhibited the formation of AFP_1 by BSFL S9 extracts, indicating that a P450 enzyme is involved in the conversion from AFB_1 into AFP_1. Conversion to AFL by the BSFL S9 fraction was not inhibited when PBO was added, indicating that it is not catalyzed by P450 enzymes. The total recovery of AFB_1 and metabolites in the BSFL PBO treatment exceeded the total molar concentration of metabolites in the treatment without additives at approximately 122% ($p = 0.001$), but this was within the range of 2 * SD.

Since AFB_1 is converted to AFL by a cytosolic NADPH-dependent reductase [24,28,29], we therefore propose that this conversion to AFL by BSFL occurs via the same pathway. Figure 3 shows selected metabolic conversion pathways known for AFB_1. The black arrows denote metabolic pathways that have been found to be active in BSFL S9 fractions in this study; the grey arrows denote known pathways in other species.

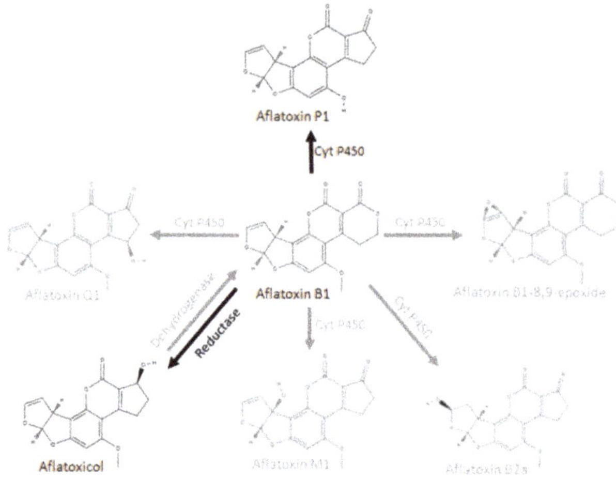

Figure 3. Selected metabolic conversion pathways known for AFB_1 (adapted from Lee and Campbell, 2000 [24] and Dohnal et al., 2014 [5]).

The reaction from AFB_1 to AFL is reversible. The cofactor for the reduction of AFB_1 is NADPH, which was added to the AFB_1 at the start of the trials, together with the Regensys A regenerating system. The cofactor for the dehydrogenation of AFL yielding AFB_1 is NADP, which accumulates when the regeneration of NADPH stops [28]. It cannot be ruled out that BSFL possess this microsomal dehydrogenase, which would revert the reaction and increase the level of AFB_1 again, thereby negating detoxification. This reversion could, for instance, occur in case of an incubation time longer than 2 h or in the absence of an NADPH regenerating system. AFM_1 was not formed by the BSFL S9 fraction in this study. The latter conversion is catalyzed by the cytochrome P450 enzyme CYP1A2 [5]. The absence of the formation of AFM_1 in the BSFL treatment (in this study as well as in Camenzuli et al., 2018 [20]) and its presence in the treatment with rat S9 suggests the absence of this enzyme in BSFL. However, the enzyme may also have been deactivated during preparation of the BSFL S9 fraction.

Compared with the conversion of AFB_1 by live BSFL, as studied by Camenzuli et al. (2018) [20], there are a few major differences in how the AFB_1 was metabolized by the S9 fraction observed in this study. Firstly, no aflatoxin P_1, Q_1, and M_1 could be recovered by Camenzuli et al. (2018) [20], and the amount of AFL was negligible (0.2% of mass balance). In the current study, however, approximately equal proportions of AFL and AFP_1 were recovered. Moreover, while less than 20% of AFB_1 could be recovered in the mass balance of Camenzuli et al. (2018) [20], 100% could be recovered in this study. It is unclear what the exact reasons are for these discrepancies, but the following hypotheses may be considered. Since live larval cells are expected to contain a wider variety of cofactors (other than NADPH, as used in conjunction with the S9 fraction in this study), a larger number of enzymes may be activated. It is possible that enzymes in live larvae first convert the AFB_1 into AFL and AFP_1, which, in turn, are precursors for other compounds. These may, for instance, be reactive metabolites that bind to other proteins. A second option is that the conversion of AFB_1 into AFL and AFP_1 in the S9 fraction is accelerated due to the absence of other cofactors that would catalyze different metabolic pathways. More research on the exact pathways of AFB_1 conversion by live BSFL is recommended in order to identify and quantify degradation products so that the efficacy and safety of reared larvae can be assessed. This could, for instance, be achieved by performing the analyses described in this manuscript with inhibitors of specific cytochrome P450 and/or NADPH-dependent reductase enzymes.

In conclusion, BSFL S9 fractions converted AFB_1 into AFP_1 and AFL. Furthermore, exposing BSFL to AFB_1 did not impact the conversion capacity, suggesting that the enzymes involved are part of a general metabolic system. No other analyzed metabolites were formed. Cytochrome P450s were responsible for metabolic conversion of AFB_1 into AFP_1. A cytoplasmic reductase was most likely responsible for conversion of AFB_1 into AFL.

4. Materials and Methods

The overall methodology for the different treatments is shown schematically in Figure 4. Firstly, BSFL were reared on feed that had been spiked with AFB_1 (0.5 mg/kg). A second batch of larvae was reared on noncontaminated feed as a control. From these two batches of larvae, separate S9 fractions were prepared, and a commercial rat S9 fraction was used for comparison. These S9 fractions were incubated with AFB_1 for 2 h (+S9 + AFB_1, t = 2 h). In addition, an incubation was included in which PBO dissolved in DMSO was added to the mixture of the S9 fraction and AFB_1 (+S9 + AFB_1 + DMSO + PBO, t = 2 h). Four control treatments were used in this study. Firstly, acetonitrile was directly added to an S9 and AFB_1 mixture at t = 0 h in order to halt enzymatic activity (+S9 + AFB_1, t = 0 h). Secondly, one mixture was prepared excluding S9 fractions (−S9 + AFB_1, t = 2 h), and a third control treatment excluded AFB_1 (+S9 − AFB_1, t = 2 h). Finally, a solvent control treatment containing DMSO was used (+S9 + AFB_1 + DMSO, t = 2 h).

Differences between treatments were tested for significance by multiple one-way ANOVA tests ($\alpha = 0.05$) using the Analysis ToolPak add-in for Microsoft Excel 2016 MSO 32-bit (version 16.0.4849.1000, Microsoft Corporation, Redmond, WA, United States of America, 2016). This was done by comparing the molar concentrations of individual (AFB_1, AFM_1, AFP_1, and AFL) and total metabolites between treatments.

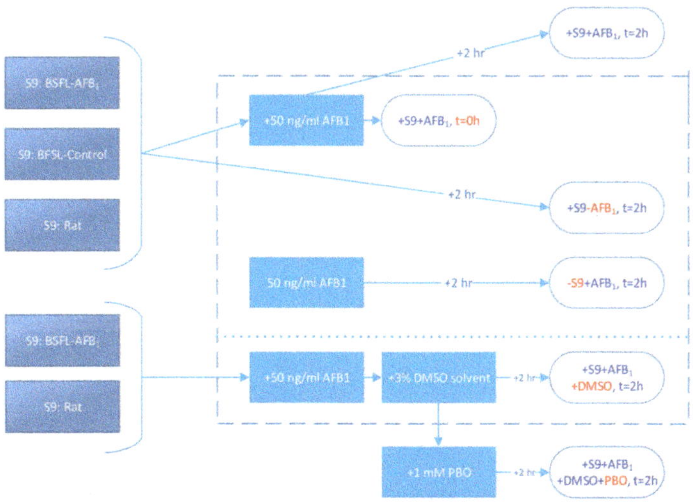

Figure 4. Schematic representation of treatments (control treatments within dotted lines; red letters indicate the difference between that treatment and the + S9 + AFB_1, t = 2 h treatment).

4.1. *Larvae Treatment*

A standard dry wheat-based mash feed (layer meal based) was spiked with AFB_1 (*A. flavus*, 99.6% purity, Sigma-Aldrich, Saint Louis, MO, USA) by an external laboratory (Ducares B.V., Utrecht, The Netherlands) to reach a concentration of 0.5 mg/kg of feed. This was the highest concentration used by Bosch et al. (2017) [19], which had no effect on the mortality and growth of the larvae. The feed used was the same batch that was used by Camenzuli et al. (2018) [20], which had been prepared by Ducares B.V., Utrecht, The Netherlands. A sample of the nonspiked feed was used as a control.

Per dietary treatment, three plastic boxes (17.8 × 11.4 × 6.5 cm) were prepared for each replicate. Each box contained 18 g (±0.1 g) of feed, which was manually mixed with 25 mL (±0.1 mL) of tap water. One hundred larvae less than 24 h old and originating from the BSF colony maintained at the Laboratory of Entomology (Wageningen University, Wageningen, The Netherlands) were added to the box. The box was then closed with a perforated lid. All boxes were kept in a climate cabinet (27 ± 1 °C and 88% ± 1% relative humidity) for 9 days. After 9 days, the larvae were collected and counted. The larvae were cleaned by rinsing with lukewarm tap water, dried with paper, and snap-frozen in liquid nitrogen. Larvae were stored at −80 °C until further analyses.

4.2. Preparation of S9 Fraction

Frozen larvae were ground to a fine powder with a precooled mortar and pestle under addition of liquid nitrogen. The frozen powder was transferred to a precooled polypropylene tube (50 mL Greiner, VWR, Amsterdam, The Netherlands) and 1.5 mL of ice cold buffer (1.15% KCl in 50 mM Tris/HCl pH 7.4) was added per gram of powder (7 g of powder + 10.5 mL of buffer). The sample was mixed thoroughly by tapping on the bench to bring the powder in contact with the buffer. Care was taken that the powder did not thaw before it was mixed with the extraction buffer. After obtaining a homogenous suspension, the material was further extracted by gently inverting the tubes 100 times. The suspensions were centrifuged in a precooled rotor for 25 min at 8960 rcf and 4 °C. The supernatants were collected, pooled, and mixed. Then, 500 µL aliquots were snap-frozen in liquid nitrogen and stored at −80 °C.

The protein concentration was determined using the DC Protein assay (Bio-Rad Laboratories, Veenendaal, The Netherlands) according to the manufacturer's protocol and bovine serum albumin (BSA) was used as a standard. The protein content of the insect S9 fractions was on average 36 mg/mL. The protein content of the rat liver S9 was 38 mg/mL (data provided by the manufacturer).

4.3. S9 Incubations with AFB_1

Samples were prepared on ice and contained 1× Regensys A buffer (Moltox, Boone, USA), 5 mM NADPH, 50 ng/mL AFB_1 (50 µg/kg), and 2.5 mg/mL S9 protein in a final volume of 100 µL. NADPH was prepared freshly in Regensys A buffer. AFB_1 was dissolved in DMSO and dilutions in Regensys buffer were prepared prior to the incubations. The final concentration of DMSO in the assay was 0.03%. The reactions were started by addition of S9 to the mixture and transferring the tubes to 37 °C in an Eppendorf thermomixer. Most samples were incubated for 2 h. t = 0 samples were prepared by adding 100 µL of cold acetonitrile prior to addition of S9.

To study the role of cytochrome P450 enzymes in the conversion of AFB_1, 1 mM of PBO (or 3% DMSO as solvent control) was included in the S9 mixes. Samples were incubated for 2 h and the reactions were stopped by addition of 100 µL of ice cold acetonitrile. Samples were vortexed thoroughly, put on ice for 5 min, and finally stored at −80 °C.

4.4. Chemicals

Regensys A buffer and rat liver S9 (Aroclor-induced rats; lyophilized S9 preparation) were purchased from Trinova Biochem (Gießen, Germany). Regensys A buffer consists of 100 mM phosphate buffer pH 7.4, 33 mM KCl, 8 mM $MgCl_2$, and 5 mM glucose-6-phosphate (NADPH regeneration system). NADPH, AFB_1, AFM_1, DMSO-HybriMax, and PBO were purchased from Sigma-Aldrich (Zwijndrecht, The Netherlands); AFP_1 from TRC (Toronto Research Chemicals, North York, Canada); and AFL from Enzo Life Sciences BVBA, (Brussels, Belgium). Potassium chloride was obtained from Merck (Amsterdam, The Netherlands) and Tris-buffer from Fisher Scientific (Landsmeer, The Netherlands).

4.5. LCMS Analyses

Analyses were performed in largely the same way as in Camenzuli et al. (2018) [20]. Samples were defrosted, vortexed, and centrifuged for 5 min, 14,000 rpm at room temperature. From the supernatant, 190 µL was transferred to an LCMS vial and 10 µL of ^{13}C-labeled internal standard solution was added.

Samples were mixed and 5 μL was analyzed with an LC-MS/MS-based method for the analysis of mycotoxins in feed and food materials. The accredited scope of this method was extended in order to also quantify the AFB_1 and its metabolites in larvae and residual material (excreta and residual feed) of BSFL.

Two MRM transitions were included for each metabolite in the MS/MS method. Details on this and additional MS/MS settings can be found in Tables S2 and S3 of the Supplementary Materials. Each metabolite was identified by its retention time and the peak area ratio between two transitions: the quantifier and the qualifier. Quantification was performed by bracketed calibration (an interval of not more than 10 injections) on the peak area of the quantifier (qn) of calibration solutions in solvent. Concentrations of AFB_1 and metabolites were corrected for matrix effects with the use of their respective ^{13}C-isotope-labeled standards (AFB_1 and AFM_1) or by means of matrix-matched calibration standards (AFP_1 and AFL).

The limit of quantification (LOQ) was defined as the lowest calibrated level which complied with the required QC parameters as mentioned in SANTE/11945/2015. Metabolite-specific LOQs can be found in Table S4 in the Supplementary Materials.

The LC-MS/MS system consisted of an injection and pump system from Waters (Waters, Milford, MA) and an AB Sciex QTRAP 6500 triple quad system equipped with an electrospray ionization (ESI) source operated in positive mode (AB Sciex, Nieuwerkerk a/d IJssel, The Netherlands). For LC separation, a 100 × 2.1 mm ID, 3 μm Restek Ultra Aqueous C18 column (Interscience, Breda, The Netherlands) was used. Details on the LC-MS/MS settings can be found in Table S5 of the Supplementary Materials. The LC eluent gradients were 1 min isocratic at 100% A, followed by a linear gradient to 100% B in 4 min. For complete elution of all matrix coextractants from the column, the final composition at 100% B was kept for 2 min. In 30 s, the initial conditions were restored and then equilibrated for 2 min prior to the next injection.

Supplementary Materials: The following are available online at http://www.mdpi.com/2072-6651/11/9/532/s1. Table S1. Molar concentrations (nmol/L) of aflatoxin B_1 (AFB_1) and analyzed metabolites (aflatoxicol (AFL), aflatoxin P_1 (AFP_1), and aflatoxin M_1 (AFM_1)) after incubation. Results of individual replicates. Table S2. MS/MS parameters. Table S3. MS/MS transitions. Table S4. LOQs of analyzed compounds. Table S5. LC-MS/MS parameters.

Author Contributions: Conceptualization, G.S., H.J.v.d.F.-K., J.J.A.v.L., J.C., and G.B.; Formal analysis, G.S.; Methodology, J.C. and G.B.; Resources, J.J.A.v.L.; Writing—original draft, N.M.; Writing—review and editing, H.J.v.d.F.-K., J.J.A. v.L., and G.B.

Funding: This study was part of the strategic research program of Wageningen UR "Customized Nutrition" and financed by Mars, Inc. (grant no. 1277360201) and Wageningen UR.

Acknowledgments: We want to thank Ruud van Dam (Wageningen Food Safety Research, WFSR) for performing the LCMS analyses, and Lonneke van der Geest (WFSR) for contributing to the design of the experiments.

Conflicts of Interest: This study was part of the strategic research program of Wageningen UR and financed by Wageningen UR, an industrial partner, and the Dutch Ministry of Agriculture, Nature, and Food Quality. The funders had no role in the design of the study; in the collection, analyses, or interpretation of data; in the writing of the manuscript; or in the decision to publish the results. The authors declare no conflicts of interest.

References

1. Do, J.H.; Choi, D.K. Aflatoxins: Detection, toxicity, and biosynthesis. *Biotechnol. Bioproc. E* **2007**, *12*, 585–593. [CrossRef]
2. Wild, C.P.; Miller, J.D.; Groopman, J.D. *Mycotoxin Control in Low-and Middle-Income Countries*; International Agency for Research on Cancer: Lyon, France, 2015.
3. Udomkun, P.; Wiredu, A.N.; Nagle, M.; Bandyopadhyay, R.; Müller, J.; Vanlauwe, B. Mycotoxins in Sub-Saharan Africa: Present situation, socio-economic impact, awareness, and outlook. *Food Control* **2017**, *72*, 110–122. [CrossRef]
4. Shibamoto, T.; Bjeldanes, L.F. *Introduction to Food Toxicology*, 2nd ed.; Academic press: Cambridge, MA, USA, 2009; pp. 1–320.

5. Dohnal, V.; Wu, Q.; Kuča, K. Metabolism of aflatoxins: Key enzymes and interindividual as well as interspecies differences. *Arch. Toxicol.* **2014**, *88*, 1635–1644. [CrossRef] [PubMed]
6. Rushing, B.R.; Selim, M.I. Aflatoxin B1: A review on metabolism, toxicity, occurrence in food, occupational exposure, and detoxification methods. *Food Chem. Toxicol.* **2018**, *124*, 81–100. [CrossRef] [PubMed]
7. Adebo, O.A.; Njobeh, P.B.; Gbashi, S.; Nwinyi, O.C.; Mavumengwana, V. Review on microbial degradation of aflatoxins. *Crit. Rev. Food Sci.* **2017**, *57*, 3208–3217. [CrossRef]
8. Hathout, A.S.; Aly, S.E. Biological detoxification of mycotoxins: A review. *Ann. Microbiol.* **2014**, *64*, 905–919. [CrossRef]
9. Jard, G.; Liboz, T.; Mathieu, F.; Guyonvarc'h, A.; Lebrihi, A. Review of mycotoxin reduction in food and feed: From prevention in the field to detoxification by adsorption or transformation. *Food Addit. Contam. A* **2011**, *28*, 1590–1609. [CrossRef]
10. Birnbaum, S.S.L.; Abbot, P. Insect adaptations toward plant toxins in milkweed-herbivores systems—A review. *Entomol. Exp. Appl.* **2018**, *166*, 357–366. [CrossRef]
11. Bbosa, G.S.; Kitya, D.; Odda, J.; Ogwal-Okeng, J. Aflatoxins metabolism, effects on epigenetic mechanisms and their role in carcinogenesis. *Health* **2013**, *5*, 14–34. [CrossRef]
12. Bergé, R.; Feyereisen, R.; Amichot, M. Cytochrome P450 monooxygenases and insecticide resistance in insects. *Philos. Trans. R. Soc. B Biol. Sci.* **1998**, *353*, 1701–1705. [CrossRef]
13. Scott, J.G. Cytochromes P450 and insecticide resistance. *Insect Biochem. Mol. Biol.* **1999**, *29*, 757–777. [CrossRef]
14. Llewellyn, G.C.; Chinnici, J.P. Variation in sensitivity to aflatoxin B1 among several strains of *Drosophila melanogaster* (Diptera). *J. Invertebr. Pathol.* **1978**, *31*, 37–40. [CrossRef]
15. Gunst, K.; Chinnici, J.P.; Llewellyn, G.C. Effects of aflatoxin B1, aflatoxin B2, aflatoxin G1, and sterigmatocystin on viability, rates of development, and body length in two strains of *Drosophila melanogaster* (Diptera). *J. Invertebr. Pathol.* **1982**, *39*, 388–394. [CrossRef]
16. Delawder, S.; Chinnici, J.P. Degree of aflatoxin B1 sensitivity in Virginia natural populations of *Drosophila melanogaster*. *Va. J. Sci.* **1983**, *34*, 48–57.
17. Foerster, R.E.; Würgler, F.E. In vitro studies on the metabolism of aflatoxin B1 and aldrin in testes of genetically different strains of *Drosophila melanogaster*. *Arch. Toxicol.* **1984**, *56*, 12–17. [CrossRef]
18. Davis, G.R.F.; Schiefer, H.B. Effects of dietary T-2 toxin concentrations fed to larvae of the yellow mealworm at three dietary protein levels. *Comp. Biochem. Physiol. C* **1982**, *73*, 13–16. [CrossRef]
19. Bosch, G.; Van der Fels-Klerx, H.; De Rijk, T.; Oonincx, D. Aflatoxin B1 tolerance and accumulation in black soldier fly larvae (*Hermetia illucens*) and yellow mealworms (*Tenebrio molitor*). *Toxins* **2017**, *9*, 185. [CrossRef]
20. Camenzuli, L.; Van Dam, R.; de Rijk, T.; Andriessen, R.; Van Schelt, J.; der Fels-Klerx, V. Tolerance and excretion of the mycotoxins aflatoxin B1, zearalenone, deoxynivalenol, and ochratoxin A by *Alphitobius diaperinus* and *Hermetia illucens* from contaminated substrates. *Toxins* **2018**, *10*, 91. [CrossRef]
21. Zeng, R.S.L.; Niu, G.; Wen, Z.; Schuler, M.A.; Berenbaum, M.R. Toxicity of aflatoxin B1 to *Helicoverpa zea* and bioactivation by cytochrome P450 monooxygenases. *J. Chem. Ecol.* **2006**, *32*, 1459–1471. [CrossRef]
22. Niu, G.; Wen, Z.; Rupasinghe, S.G.; Zeng, R.S.; Berenbaum, M.R.; Schuler, M.A. Aflatoxin B1 detoxification by CYP321A1 in *Helicoverpa zea*. *Arch. Insect Biochem. Physiol.* **2008**, *69*, 32–45. [CrossRef]
23. Zeng, R.S.; Wen, Z.; Niu, G.; Schuler, M.A.; Berenbaum, M.R. Allelochemical induction of cytochrome P450 monooxygenases and amelioration of xenobiotic toxicity in *Helicoverpa zea*. *J. Chem. Ecol.* **2007**, *33*, 449–461. [CrossRef]
24. Lee, S.U.; Campbell, B.C. In vitro metabolism of aflatoxin B1 by larvae of navel orangeworm, *Amyelois transitella* (Walker) (Insecta, Lepidoptera, Pyralidae) and codling moth, *Cydia pomonella* (L.) (Insecta, Lepidoptera, Tortricidae). *Arch. Insect Biochem. Physiol.* **2000**, *45*, 166–174. [CrossRef]
25. Niu, G.; Rupasinghe, S.G.; Zangerl, A.R.; Siegel, J.P.; Schuler, M.A.; Berenbaum, M.R. A substrate-specific cytochrome P450 monooxygenase, CYP6AB11, from the polyphagous navel orangeworm (*Amyelois transitella*). *Insect Biochem. Mol. Biol.* **2011**, *41*, 244–253. [CrossRef]
26. Niu, G.; Johnson, R.M.; Berenbaum, M.R. Toxicity of mycotoxins to honeybees and its amelioration by propolis. *Apidologie* **2011**, *42*, 79–87. [CrossRef]
27. Duffus, J.H.; Nordberg, M.; Templeton, D.M. Glossary of Terms Used in Toxicology. 2nd Edition. *Pure Appl. Chem.* **2007**, *79*, 1153–1344. [CrossRef]

28. Salhab, A.S.; Edwards, G.S. Comparative in vitro metabolism of AFL by liver preparations from animals and humans. *Cancer Res.* **1977**, *37*, 1016–1021.
29. Eaton, D.L.; Beima, K.M.; Bammler, T.K.; Riley, R.T.; Voss, K.A. *Hepatotoxic Mycotoxins Comprehensive Toxicology*; Elsevier: Amsterdam, The Netherlands, 2010; pp. 527–569.

toxins

Article

Efficacy of Azoxystrobin on Mycotoxins and Related Fungi in Italian Paddy Rice

Paola Giorni [1,*], Umberto Rolla [2], Marco Romani [2], Annalisa Mulazzi [3] and Terenzio Bertuzzi [3]

1 Department of Sustainable Crop Production—DIPROVES, Faculty of Agriculture, Food and Environmental Science, Università Cattolica del Sacro Cuore, via Emilia Parmense 84, 29122 Piacenza, Italy
2 Ente Nazionale Risi, Rice Research Centre, Strada per Ceretto 4, Castello d'Agogna, 27030 Pavia, Italy; u.rolla@enterisi.it (U.R.); m.romani@enterisi.it (M.R.)
3 Department of Animal, Food and Nutrition Science—DIANA, Università Cattolica del Sacro Cuore, Via Emilia Parmense 84, 29122 Piacenza, Italy; annalisa.mulazzi@unicatt.it (A.M.); terenzio.bertuzzi@unicatt.it (T.B.)
* Correspondence: paola.giorni@unicatt.it

Received: 14 May 2019; Accepted: 28 May 2019; Published: 30 May 2019

Abstract: AbstractThe efficacy of azoxystrobin was evaluated in the presence of mycotoxigenic fungi and relative mycotoxins in Italian paddy rice during the growing season in the field. Three experimental fields were considered and the applied experimental design was a strip plot with three replicates; rice samples were collected at four different growing stages. The efficacy of the fungicide treatment on rice fungal population was demonstrated with around 20% less total fungal incidence in sprayed samples compared to untreated ones; the same decrease was noted also in *Fusarium* spp. species but not in *Aspergillus versicolor*. Of the mycotoxins considered, ochratoxin A (OTA) and aflatoxins (AFBs) were never detected, deoxynivalenol (DON) was found in 46% of samples at levels always lower than 100 µg/kg, while sterigmatocystin (STC) occurred in all the paddy rice samples collected after flowering, with a maximum value of 15.5 µg/kg. Treatment with azoxystrobin was not effective in reducing DON contamination, but it had an important and significant effect on STC content, showing a decrease of 67% in the sprayed samples.

Keywords: rice; mycotoxins; sterigmatocystin; STC; deoxynivalenol; DON; growing season; azoxystrobin; fungicide

Key Contribution: This study takes into consideration, for the first time, the effect of fungicide treatment on mycotoxigenic fungi population in Italian paddy rice and on the presence of mycotoxins during the growing season with particular interest to fungicide influence on sterigmatocystin, a relevant emerging mycotoxin.

1. Introduction

Rice (*Oryza sativa* L.) is the staple food for almost half of the world's population [1]; it is cultivated mainly in Asian regions and China is the largest producer. The main rice producer in Europe is Italy, accounting for around 50% of total European production. Rice cultivation is principally in Northern Italy (Piedmont and Lombardy) and is destined for several food uses, baby foods included.

Different diseases can affect rice and, in particular, fungi can be particularly dangerous for plant and grain health [2] during both the growing season and post-harvest [3]. Panicle blast caused by *Pyricularia grisea* [4] and brown spot caused by *Bipolaris oryzae* [5] are the most dangerous diseases for Italian rice crops, occurring frequently and causing production and economic losses [4]. Nowadays, particular attention must also be paid to fungal species which can produce, in favorable environmental and substrate conditions, various mycotoxins that can impact human health. The presence of mycotoxigenic fungi on paddy rice has been indicated in several reports; in particular, *Fusarium* spp., responsible for trichothecenes (expecially deoxynivalenol (DON)) and fumonisins (FBs) [6,7], *Aspergillus flavus*, able to produce aflatoxins (AFs) [8], and *Penicillium* spp. for ochratoxin A (OTA) and citrinin (CIT) [9]. Recently, sterigmatocystin (STC) produced by *Aspergillus versicolor* was also found in rice and resulted the most common mycotoxin in Italian rice [10]. The European Commission fixed strict limits for mycotoxins in cereals; in particular, for rice destined for human consumption limits are present for AFs (2.0 μg/kg), OTA (3.0 μg/kg), and DON (750 μg/kg), making mycotoxin containment very important for product exchanges (EU Regulation 165/2010; EC Regulation 1881/2006; EU Regulation 1006/2015).

Among possible strategies to control mycotoxigenic fungi development in the field and, consequently, mycotoxin production, fungicides can be used. Negative effects have been reported in some cases, such as the reduction of beneficial microorganisms for plant growth due to acidification of the soil [11] or the possible selection of fungicide-resistant fungal strains [12]. Moreover, each toxigenic fungal species responds differently to fungicides because several factors can contribute to their reaction; in particular, weather, active ingredients, plant development stage, and cultivar resistance can play a role [13,14] and can act as stressors in the production of mycotoxins [15]. For example, it has been found that triazole applications can reduce both *F. graminearum* and DON occurrence [16,17], especially if the treatments are carried out before fungal infection [11]. However, in some cases the use of fungicide can increase mycotoxin content; Dors et al. [15] reported that tebuconazole was able to act as an elicitor of stress for mycotoxigenic fungi and, consequently, enhanced the presence of several mycotoxins.

There are few fungicides allowed by Italian Regulations for rice; of these, azoxystrobin is an active ingredient belonging to the strobilurin chemical group and it is one of the most used on Italian rice because of its demonstrated efficacy on several crops and its major role in reducing *Pyricularia grisea* [18] and *Bipolaris oryzae* infections in rice [19] and Fusarium Head Blight (FHB) in wheat [20]. However, its possible effect on mycotoxins is still uncertain since in some studies the use of azoxystrobin in wheat could result in an increase in DON content up to 42% [21,22]; for this reason, this possible effect needs to be evaluated also in rice in order to assist farmers in their selection of fungicides.

The aim of this study was to define the efficacy of azoxystrobin on mycotoxigenic fungal species present in paddy rice during the growing season from flowering to over ripening (1 June–30 September) and determine its possible effect on the production of their relative mycotoxins.

2. Results and Discussion

2.1. *Efficacy of Azoxystrobin on Mycotoxigenic Fungi*

The highest fungal incidence was found at the full ripening stage with more than 70% of the rice kernels infected (Table 1). Fungi seem to increase their incidence throughout the growing season up to ripening, then they significantly decrease if left in field for an additional 14 days obtaining around a 10% reduction for total fungi incidence (Table 1). The same level of reduction was not observed for mycotoxigenic species that reach their maximum incidence at harvest time (full ripening) and maintain their presence even in the case of over ripening. Both for *Fusarium* spp. and *A. versicolor*, the only mycotoxigenic species resulting with a significant presence in field, no differences were found between the full ripening and over-ripening stages (Table 1).

The same was found in a previous study on paddy rice [10] with the only exception of *Fusarium* spp. that seemed to decrease in over ripening in accordance with the total fungi trend; probably, different meteorological conditions registered after full ripening, in particular the almost total absence of rain observed in the area in year 2018, could have influenced *Fusarium* spp. vitality.

As expected, different rice varieties showed different levels of fungal contamination; in particular, Terra CL showed the highest fungal content while CL26 the lowest (Table 1). *Fusarium* spp. exhibited the same trend while *A. versicolor* presence resulted always very low and with no significant differences between rice varieties. However, interestingly, *A. versicolor*, differently from other fungal species, showed a higher incidence in CL26, which was the rice variety least contaminated by other fungal species, and a lower incidence in Terra CL and CL15 varieties which were the most contaminated by other fungal species (Table 1). This was probably due to varying fungal abilities to compete in extreme environmental conditions; the year 2018, in fact, was notable in Italian rice cultivation areas for an almost total absence of rain (total rainfall was only 157.4 mm in the period 1 June–30 September) and extreme temperatures (up to 36 °C). This was undoubtedly favorable for xerophilic species, such as *A. versicolor* [23], in particular on rice varieties where fungal incidence and, as a consequence, fungal competition were lower.

The efficacy of the fungicide treatment on rice fungal population was demonstrated with around 20% less total fungal incidence in sprayed samples than the untreated ones (Table 1). The same decrease was noted also in the *Fusarium* spp. species but not in *A. versicolor* which was unchanged (Table 1). The effect of strobilurins against fungi is well documented, they appear able to enhance rice plant defenses against pathogen attacks [19,24], shown also in wheat against mycotoxigenic *Fusarium* species like *F. graminearum* [20]. The incidence of *A. versicolor* was too low to obtain a significant reduction in treatment with azoxystrobin, although a reduction of 5% was observed.

Table 1. Analysis of variance (ANOVA) of fungal incidence and contamination of sterigmatocystin (STC) and deoxynivalenol (DON) at different sampling times in different rice varieties sprayed or unsprayed with fungicides formulated with azoxystrobyn (250 g/L) in three different experimental fields. Data refer to mean data; all experiments were conducted with three replicates.

	Total Fungi Incidence (%)		Incidence of *Fusarium* spp. (%)		Incidence of *A. versicolor* (%)		STC (µg/kg)		DON (µg/kg)	
Sampling time (A)	**		**		**		**		**	
Flowering (BBCH 69)	4.6	d	1.1	c	0.0	b	0.0	d	0.0	c
Early dough (BBCH 83)	33.3	c	7.8	b	0.1	b	1.3	c	14.4	b
Full Ripening (BBCH 89)	73.2	a	14.1	a	1.2	a	2.8	a	62.1	a
Over ripening (BBCH 92)	61.6	b	14.9	a	1.1	a	1.5	b	35.2	a
Rice variety (B)	**		**		n.s.		**		**	
Sirio CL	48.9	ab	9.2	abc	1.2		0.7	cd	11.8	ab
CLXL 745	37.8	cd	9.0	bcd	1.3		0.6	d	31.7	ab
Mare CL	31.2	de	6.6	cd	0.8		0.5	d	15.2	ab
CL26	26.7	e	5.5	d	1.6		0.8	c	30.8	ab
Terra CL	53.6	a	12.0	a	0.2		1.2	b	22.5	ab
Selenio	41.3	bcd	11.3	ab	0.3		1.7	b	19.1	ab
CL15	45.7	abc	10.5	abc	0.2		1.6	b	63.0	a
Centauro	42.4	bc	7.5	bcd	0.5		1.4	b	11.3	b
Sole CL	47.0	abc	9.9	abc	0.6		2.6	a	34.5	ab
Fungicide (C)	**		**		n.s.		**		n.s.	
Unsprayed	47.6	a	10.5	a	0.61		2.1	a	26.8	
Sprayed	38.7	b	8.4	b	0.58		0.7	b	29.0	
Experimental field (D)	**		**		n.s.		**		*	
A	36.1	b	7.6	c	1.2		0.7	c	22.4	b
B	38.0	b	9.6	b	0.4		1.6	b	20.0	b
C	54.0	a	10.9	a	0.3		1.9	a	40.2	a

Different letters mean significant differences according to Tukey Test; n.s.: not significative; *: $p \leq 0.05$; **: $p \leq 0.01$.

Differences in fungal contamination were found between the three different experimental fields; in particular, experimental field C was the most contaminated with also the highest *Fusarium* spp. incidence. No significant differences were found between experimental fields in the presence of *A. versicolor*.

2.2. Efficacy of Azoxystrobin on Mycotoxin Production

Among the considered mycotoxins considered, OTA and AFs were never detected; DON was found in 46% of the samples at levels always lower than 100 μg/kg, while STC occurred in almost all the paddy rice samples, showing a maximum value of 15.5 μg/kg. These data partially accord with a previous study, carried out on rice samples collected in the same area, that found DON and AFs only sporadically and in low amounts, while STC was always detected, appearing as crucial in rice contamination [10].

Regarding mycotoxin accumulation, it is important to note that both DON and STC follow the same trend of their producing fungi. In particular, DON was highest at full ripening and remained constant up to over ripening as happened for *Fusarium* spp. fungi, while STC was highest at full ripening and significantly decreased in over-ripening, as happened to the presence of *A. versicolor* (Table 1). A similar result for STC was found in a previous research, even if this decrease was not so intensive [10]. This could be due to environmental and substrate conditions that probably reduce fungal ability to produce STC while they have no effect on DON production. Significant differences in mycotoxin contamination were found between rice varieties with Sole CL resulting one of the most contaminated by DON and the one with the highest STC content (Table 1).

The highest DON contamination was found in the rice variety CL15 while the lowest was in the rice variety Centauro (Table 1); none of the rice varieties considered in the study showed a DON contamination above the limits fixed by the European Commission of 1250 μg/Kg for paddy rice (EU Regulation 1881/2006). These results seem to confirm the findings of a previous study where DON was found only in low amounts [10] suggesting that this mycotoxin could be considered a minor risk for Italian paddy rice.

The treatment with azoxystrobin was inefficient in reducing DON contamination; contrarily, DON increased in sprayed samples even if the results were not statistically different (Figure 1). The fungicide had an important and significant effect on STC content, showing a decrease of 67% in the sprayed samples (Table 1). These data partially agree with previous findings on wheat, where the use of strobilurin obtained a good reduction of FHB, but with an uncertain impact on DON reduction [20,25]. The results obtained in STC reduction are very promising because this mycotoxin seems to be the most dangerous for Italian rice production and treatment with azoxystrobin, one of the active ingredients allowed by the Italian government on rice, could be useful for reducing STC contamination in field during the growing season.

Significant differences in mycotoxin contamination were observed between experimental fields ($p \leq 0.01$); in particular, experimental field C was the most contaminated having the highest incidence of total fungi. Moreover, the same experimental field showed the highest STC content (1.9 μg/Kg vs 0.7–1.6 μg/Kg) and the highest DON content (40 μg/Kg vs 20–22 μg/Kg) (Table 1). Differences in mycotoxins contamination between experimental fields were expected since many variables can contribute to their presence such as susceptibility of rice variety, preceding crop, tillage, and pest presence [26,27]. However, even if we tried to keep the differences in agronomic management minimal between experimental fields, environmental factors, such as relative humidity and temperature, can always play a relevant and unpredictable role in both fungal contamination and mycotoxin occurrence.

Considering treatment with azoxystrobin on single rice varieties, important reductions were observed. In particular, Sole showed the highest STC reduction being, respectively, of 62% and 77% in experimental field B and C (Figure 1). The lowest reduction (22%) in STC obtained in sprayed samples was found in the rice variety CLXL745 (Figure 1). Differences in azoxystrobin efficacy between rice varieties were probably due to their different susceptibility to fungicide, as already found in other studies with other active ingredients [28] and on other crops [29,30].

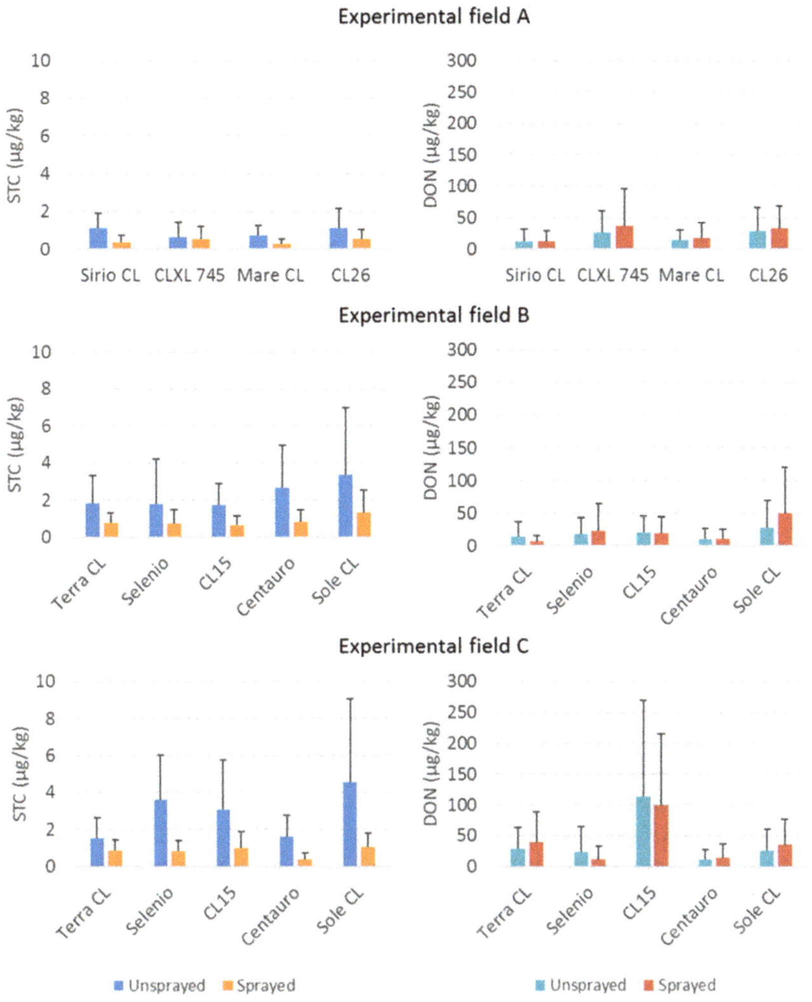

Figure 1. Mean sterigmatocystin (STC) and deoxynivalenol (DON) contamination in the different experimental fields considered in the trial in case of unsprayed and sprayed paddy rice varieties.

3. Conclusions

At first, this study confirmed that *Fusarium* spp. and *A. versicolor* were the most frequently mycotoxigenic species found on Italian paddy rice during the growing season. As a consequence, DON and STC can occur in paddy rice samples at different plant growing stages. Treatment with azoxystrobin as an active ingredient seems to be efficient in reducing total fungi and *Fusarium* spp. incidence and STC contamination, while they have no effect on *A. versicolor* presence and DON level. Rice varieties played an important role for their different and proven susceptibility to fungal diseases and fungicide efficacy.

STC, an emerging mycotoxin that is not routinely checked, has been confirmed as a relevant mycotoxin in paddy rice, confirming a previous survey that collected rice samples of different origin [31]; the contamination level of this mycotoxin could be considered for future EU legislative regulation.

The results obtained showed that the use of azoxystrobin could help farmers to develop a potential method for STC containment in conditions particularly conducive for fungal development and mycotoxin production, being necessarily cautious in their use due to uncertain reduction of the presence of DON.

4. Materials and Methods

4.1. Field Samples

Sampling of rice was conducted at four different growing stages (flowering (BBCH 69), early dough (BBCH 83), ripening (BBCH 89), and over-ripening (BBCH 92, 15 days post-ripening) in 2018 in three experimental fields located close to Mortara (PV) in Lombardy, the main Italian rice production region. Nine rice varieties, both long B and round grain were considered (Table 1). In experimental field A were cultivated four long B grain rice varieties (CLXL 745, CL26, Sirio CL, Mare CL) while five common round grain rice varieties (Sole CL, Selenio, Centauro, Terra CL, CL15) were cultivated in experimental fields B and C. Soil texture and sowing period varied, while the meteorological conditions can be considered similar because of the proximity of the fields (all within 10 km).

4.2. Fungicide Treatment

The applied experimental design was a strip plot with three replicates; each strip (6 m × 100 m), containing rice plants of 1 variety with a sowing density of 150 kg/ha of seeds, was subdivided into three plots considered as replicates. Working at field level, it was not possible to apply a randomized plot design.

In each experimental field, two assays were considered for each rice variety: "unsprayed strip" used as control, where no fungicide was sprayed, and "sprayed strips" where treatment with fungicide was carried out. The distance between "unsprayed" and "sprayed" strips was 20 meters, which was considered sufficient to prevent problems linked to spray drift and possible contamination between the two considered assays.

Commercial formulations with azoxystrobin in the same concentration (250 g/L) were distributed in open field, on the whole width of plots chosen as "sprayed", using a backpack sprayer (mod. SP 126, Oleo-Mac Bagnolo in Piano, Reggio Emilia, Italy) calibrated to spread 250 L/ha of solution. In all the sprayed experimental assays, only 1 fungicide treatment was scheduled when rice plants were at the stage of panicle emergence (BBCH 51-55). We decided to do the fungicide treatment at this plant growing stage because this time is normally chosen also for the scheduled paddy rice treatment against the main pathogens such as *Pyricularia grisea* and *Bipolaris oryzae*.

For each rice variety and experimental field, rice plants were collected from each plot with an X-shape design, then the plants were shelled and the grains obtained considered as representative. For each plot, representing a replicate, 500 g of grains were randomly chosen as sample. Samples were used for mycological analyses and then dried, milled using a cyclone hammer mill (1 mm sieve, Pulverisette, Fritsch GmbH, Idar-Oberstein, Germany), homogenized and kept at 4 °C until chemical analysis.

4.3. Monitoring of Mycotoxigenic Fungi

Fifty kernels were randomly selected from each sample, surface disinfected in 1% sodium hypochlorite for 2 min and in 90% ethyl alcohol for 2 min and then transferred onto Petri dishes containing potato dextrose agar (PDA, Biolife, Milano, Italy). The Petri dishes were incubated at 25 °C (12 h light photoperiod) and after 5–7 days the incidence of kernels infected by fungi was quantified. *Fusarium* spp. and *Penicillium* spp. isolates were identified at Genus level thanks to observations with binocular microscope (40×); only *Aspergillus* spp. isolates were identified at species level observing their morphological characteristics with magnification between 100× and 400× according to Raper and Fennell [32].

4.4. Monitoring of Mycotoxins

The analyses were carried out using the following methods: AFs were determined by HPLC-FLD (liquid chromatography with fluorimeter detector) as reported by Bertuzzi et al. [33]; OTA by HPLC-FLD [34], DON by GC-MS (gas chromatography coupled to mass spectrometer) [35], STC by LC-MS/MS (liquid chromatography coupled to mass spectrometer) [36]. The analyses were recently described in the work of Bertuzzi et al. [10].

4.5. Data Analysis

The data were transformed before statistical analysis; in particular, fungal incidence was arcsine transformed and mycotoxin content was ln transformed [37]. Analysis of variance (ANOVA) was calculated using the generalized linear model (GLM) procedure of the statistical package IBM SPSS Statistics 21 (IBM Corp., Armonk, NY, USA) while significant differences were highlighted using the Tukey test ($p \leq 0.05$) for mean separation.

Author Contributions: The manuscript was written through contributions of all authors. All authors have given approval to the final version of the manuscript. T.B., M.R., and P.G. designed the research. P.G. and A.M. performed the experiment. T.B. and P.G. analyzed the data and wrote the manuscript. U.R., M.R., P.G., and A.M. assisted with the experiment. T.B. and P.G. supervised the research and edited and approved the final manuscript.

Funding: This work supported by Lombardy region, PSR 2014-2020 program, project BABYRICE.

Conflicts of Interest: The authors declare no conflict of interest. The funders had no role in the design of the study; in the collection, analyses, or interpretation of data; in the writing of the manuscript, or in the decision to publish the results.

References

1. Chen, C.F.; Son, N.T.; Chang, L.Y. Monitoring of rice cropping intensity in the upper Mekong Delta, Vietnam using time-series MODIS data. *Adv. Space Res.* **2012**, *49*, 292–301. [CrossRef]
2. Kushiro, M. Historical review of researches on yellow rice and mycotoxigenic fungi adherent to rice in Japan. *Jpn. Soc. Mycotoxicol. (JSM)* **2015**, *65*, 19–23. [CrossRef]
3. Oerke, E.C.; Dehne, H.W. Safeguarding production–losses in major crops and the role of crop protection. *Crop. Prot.* **2004**, *23*, 275–285. [CrossRef]
4. Piotti, E.; Rigano, M.; Rodino, D.; Rodolfi, M.; Castiglione, S.; Picco, A.M.; Sala, F. Genetic structure of *Pyricularia grisea* (Cooke) Sacc. Isolates from Italian paddy fields. *J. Phytopathol.* **2005**, *153*, 80–86. [CrossRef]
5. Bregaglio, S.; Donatelli, M.; Confalonieri, R. Fungal infections of rice, wheat, and grapein Europe in 2030–2050. *Agron. Sustain. Dev.* **2013**, *33*, 767–776. [CrossRef]
6. Kushiro, M.; Nagata, R.; Nakagawa, H.; Nagashima, H. Liquid chromatographic detection of fumonisins in rice seed. *Rep. Natl. Food Res. Inst.* **2008**, *72*, 37–44.
7. Tanaka, K.; Sago, Y.; Zheng, Y.; Nakagawa, H.; Kushiro, M. Mycotoxins in rice. *Int. J. Food Microbiol.* **2007**, *119*, 59–66. [CrossRef] [PubMed]
8. Reddy, K.; Reddy, C.; Muralidharan, K. Detection of Aspergillus spp. and aflatoxin B1 in rice in India. *Food Microbiol.* **2009**, *26*, 27–31. [CrossRef] [PubMed]
9. Wawrzyniak, J.; Waskiewicz, A. Ochratoxin A and citrinin production by Penicillium verrucosum on cereal solid substrates. *Food Addit. Contam. A* **2014**, *31*, 139–148. [CrossRef]
10. Bertuzzi, T.; Romani, M.; Rastelli, S.; Giorni, P. Mycotoxins and related fungi in Italian paddy rice during the growing season and storage. *Toxins* **2019**, *11*, 151. [CrossRef]
11. Oliveira, P.M.; Zannini, E.; Arendt, E.K. Cereal fungal infection, mycotoxins, and lactic acid bacteria mediated bioprotection: From crop farming to cereal products. *Food Microbiol.* **2014**, *37*, 78–95. [CrossRef]
12. Suzuki, F.; Yamaguchi, J.; Koba, A.; Nakajima, T.; Arai, M. Changes in fungicide resistance frequency and population structure of Pyricularia oryzae after discontinuance of MBI-D fungicides. *Plant. Dis.* **2010**, *94*, 329–334. [CrossRef] [PubMed]
13. Dallagnol, L.J.; Navarini, L.; Balardin, R.S.; Gosenheimer, A.; Maffini, A.A. Damage of leaf diseases in irrigated rice crop and efficiency of fungicides control. *R. Bras. Agrociência* **2006**, *12*, 313–318.

14. Chen, Y.; Zhou, M.G. Characterization of Fudarium graminearum isolates resistant to both carbendazim and a new fungicide JS399-19. *Phytopathology* **2009**, *99*, 441–446. [CrossRef]
15. Dors, G.C.; Caldas, S.S.; dos Santos Hackbart, H.C.; Primel, E.G.; Fagundes, C.A.A.; Badiale-Furlong, E. Fungicides and the effects of mycotoxins on milling fractions of irrigated rice. *J. Agr. Food Chem.* **2013**, *61*, 1985–1990. [CrossRef]
16. Jordahl, J.; Meyer, S.; McMullen, M. Results of the 2010 uniform fungicide trial on barley, Fargo, ND. In Proceedings of the 2010 National Fusarium Head Blight Forum, Milwaukee, WI, USA, 7–9 December 2010; pp. 81–83.
17. Ransom, J.; Pederson, J.; Halley, S. Influence of row spacing, seeding rate, fungicide and variety on field and FHB development in spring wheat, durum and barley. In Proceedings of the 2010 National Fusarium Head Blight Forum, Milwaukee, WI, USA, 7–9 December 2010; p. 93.
18. Sundravadana, S.; Kuttalam, S.; Alice, D.; Samiyappan, R. Fungicidal activity of azoxystrobin agaist *Pyricularia grisea* (Cooke) sacc and its controlling activity against rice blasts. *Arch. Phytopathol. Plant Prot.* **2008**, *41*, 608–615. [CrossRef]
19. Debona, D.; Fortunato, A.A.; Araujo, L.; Rodrigues, A.L.C.; Rodrigues, F.A. Rice defense responses to Bipolaris oryzae mediated by a strobilurin fungicide. *Trop. Plant. Pathol.* **2018**, *43*, 389–401. [CrossRef]
20. Feksa, H.R.; Couto, H.T.Z.; do Garozi, R.; Almeida, J.L.; de Gardiano, C.G.; Tessmann, D.J. Pre- and postinfection application of strobilurin-triazole premixes and single fungicides for control of fusarium head blight and deoxynivalenol mycotoxin in wheat. *Crop. Prot.* **2019**, *117*, 128–134. [CrossRef]
21. Mesterházy, Á.; Bartók, T.; Lamper, C. Influence of cultivar resistance, epidemic severity, and *Fusarium* species on the efficacy of fungicide control of Fusarium head blight in wheat and deoxynivalenol (DON) contamination of grain. *Plant. Dis.* **2003**, *87*, 1107–1115. [CrossRef]
22. Mesterházy, Á.; Tóth, B.; Varga, M.; Bartók, B.; Szabó-Hevér, Á.; Farády, L.; Lehoczki-Krsjak, S. Role of fungicides, application of nozzle types, and the resistance level of wheat varieties in the control of Fusarium Head Blight and deoxynivalenol. *Toxins* **2011**, *3*, 1453–1483. [CrossRef]
23. Atalla, M.M.; Hassanein, N.M.; El-Beih, A.A.; Youssef, Y.A. Mycotoxin production in wheat grains by different Aspergilli in relation to different relative humidities and storage periods. *Nahrung* **2003**, *47*, 6–10. [CrossRef]
24. Naik, M.R.; Akila, R.; Thiruvudainambi, S. Management approaches for brown spot of rice caused by Bipolaris oryzae. *J. Farm. Sci.* **2016**, *29*, 370–376.
25. Blandino, M.; Reyneri, A. Effect of fungicide and foliar fertilizer application to winter wheat at anthesis on flag leaf senescence, grain yield, flour bread-making quality and DON contamination. *Eur. J. Agron.* **2009**, *30*, 275–282. [CrossRef]
26. Ferrigo, D.; Raiola, A.; Causin, R. Fusarium toxins in cereals: Occurrence, legislation, factors promoting the appearance and their management. *Molecules* **2016**, *21*, 627. [CrossRef] [PubMed]
27. Camardo Leggieri, M.; Bertuzzi, T.; Pietri, A.; Battilani, P. Mycotoxin occurrence in maize produced in Northern Italy over the years 2009-2011: focus on the role of crop related factors. *Phytopathol. Mediterr.* **2015**, *54*, 212–221.
28. Mani, K.K.; Hollier, C.A.; Groth, D.E. Effect of planting date, fungicide timing and cultivar susceptibility on severity of narrow brown leaf spot and yield of rice. *Crop. Prot.* **2016**, *90*, 186–190. [CrossRef]
29. Morgounov, A.; Akin, B.; Demir, L.; Keser, M.; Kokhmetova, A.; Martynov, S.; Orhan, S.; Ozdemir, F.; Ozseven, I.; Sapakhova, Z.; Yessimbekova, M. Yield gain due to fungicide application in varieties of winter wheat (*Triticum aestivum*) resistant and susceptible to leaf rust. *Crop. Pasture Sci.* **2015**, *66*, 649–659. [CrossRef]
30. Newton, A.C.; Lees, A.K.; Hilton, A.J.; Thomas, W.T.B. Susceptibility of oat cultivars to groat discoloration: causes and remedies. *Plant Breeding* **2003**, *122*, 125–130. [CrossRef]
31. Mol, H.G.J.; MacDonald, S.J.; Anagnostopoulos, C.; Spanjer, M.; Bertuzzi, T.; Pietri, A. European survey on sterigmatocystin in cereals, cereals-based products, beer and nuts. *World Mycotoxin J.* **2016**, *9*, 633–642. [CrossRef]
32. Raper, K.B.; Fennell, D.I. The Genus Aspergillus. Robert, E., Ed.; Krieger Publishing Company Inc.: Malabar, FL, USA, 1965.
33. Bertuzzi, T.; Rastelli, S.; Mulazzi, A.; Pietri, A. Evaluation and improvement of extraction methods for the analysis of aflatoxins B1, B2, G1 and G2 from naturally contaminated maize. *Food Anal. Method.* **2012**, *5*, 512–519. [CrossRef]

34. Bertuzzi, T.; Leggieri, M.C.; Battilani, P.; Pietri, A. Co-occurrence of type A and B trichothecenes and zearalenone in wheat grown in northern Italy over the years 2009–2011. *Food Addit. Contam. B* **2014**, *7*, 273–281. [CrossRef] [PubMed]
35. Rossi, F.; Bertuzzi, T.; Comizzoli, S.; Turconi, G.; Roggi, C.; Pagani, M.; Cravedi, P.; Pietri, A. Preliminary survey on composition and quality of conventional and organic wheat. *Italian J. Food Sci.* **2006**, *4*, 355–366.
36. Bertuzzi, T.; Romani, M.; Rastelli, S.; Mulazzi, A.; Pietri, A. Sterigmatocystin occurrence in paddy and processed rice produced in Italy in the years 2014–2015 and distribution in milled rice fractions. *Toxins* **2017**, *9*, 86. [CrossRef] [PubMed]
37. Clewer, A.G.; Scarisbrick, D.H. *Practical Statistics and Experimental Design for Plant and Crop Science*; John Wiley & Sons Ltd.: Chichester, UK, 2001.

toxins

MDPI

Article

Removal of Small Kernels Reduces the Content of *Fusarium* Mycotoxins in Oat Grain

Guro Brodal *, Heidi Udnes Aamot, Marit Almvik and Ingerd Skow Hofgaard

Norwegian Institute of Bioeconomy Research (NIBIO), P.O.Box 115, N-1431 Ås, Norway; heidi.udnes.aamot@nibio.no (H.U.A.); marit.almvik@nibio.no (M.A.); ingerd.hofgaard@nibio.no (I.S.H.)

* Correspondence: guro.brodal@nibio.no

Received: 30 April 2020; Accepted: 22 May 2020; Published: 23 May 2020

Abstract: Cereal grain contaminated by *Fusarium* mycotoxins is undesirable in food and feed because of the harmful health effects of the mycotoxins in humans and animals. Reduction of mycotoxin content in grain by cleaning and size sorting has mainly been studied in wheat. We investigated whether the removal of small kernels by size sorting could be a method to reduce the content of mycotoxins in oat grain. Samples from 24 Norwegian mycotoxin-contaminated grain lots (14 from 2015 and 10 from 2018) were sorted by a laboratory sieve (sieve size 2.2 mm) into large and small kernel fractions and, in addition to unsorted grain samples, analyzed with LC-MS-MS for quantification of 10 mycotoxins. By removing the small kernel fraction (on average 15% and 21% of the weight of the samples from the two years, respectively), the mean concentrations of HT-2+T-2 toxins were reduced by 56% (from 745 to 328 μg/kg) in the 2015 samples and by 32% (from 178 to 121 μg/kg) in the 2018 samples. Deoxynivalenol (DON) was reduced by 24% (from 191 to 145 μg/kg) in the 2018 samples, and enniatin B (EnnB) by 44% (from 1059 to 594 μg/kg) in the 2015 samples. Despite low levels, our analyses showed a trend towards reduced content of DON, ADON, NIV, EnnA, EnnA1, EnnB1 and BEA after removing the small kernel fraction in samples from 2015. For several of the mycotoxins, the concentrations were considerably higher in the small kernel fraction compared to unsorted grain. Our results demonstrate that the level of mycotoxins in unprocessed oat grain can be reduced by removing small kernels. We assume that our study is the first report on the effect of size sorting on the content of enniatins (Enns), NIV and BEA in oat grains.

Keywords: T-2 toxin; HT-2 toxin; deoxynivalenol (DON); enniatin B (EnnB); size sorting; unprocessed cereals

Key Contribution: Removing small kernels can reduce the mycotoxin content of oat grain lots, and thereby improve the grain quality and increase the number of lots that can be accepted as safe for food and feed.

---

1. Introduction

Several species of the fungal genera *Fusarium* are common pathogens of small grain cereals. *Fusarium* spp. infect and cause damage to the head and grain of cereals, especially under moist conditions. The disease, known as Fusarium Head Blight (FHB), is one of the most important diseases in wheat (*Triticum aestivum*), oats (*Avena sativa*) and barley (*Hordeum vulgare*). During development and maturation of infected heads, *Fusarium* species can produce several mycotoxins which can lead to severe contamination of grain [1]. Mycotoxin-contaminated grains do not necessarily show disease symptoms which makes them difficult to identify. Consumption of grain and grain-based products containing *Fusarium* mycotoxins can cause many harmful health effects in humans and animals, and *Fusarium* toxins are therefore one of the most important quality and safety risks of cereal grain for food and feed [2–4]. In addition, workers at grain elevators and mills may be exposed to mycotoxins by inhalation and skin permeation of grain dust during grain processing [5]. To reduce the risk, the European Union (EU) has set maximum levels for some mycotoxins in cereal grain and cereal-based food products for human consumption, and has recommended guidance values for its content in animal feed [6,7].

The mycotoxin deoxynivalenol (DON) is common and frequently occurs in oat grains [8–11]. Moreover, the HT-2 toxin and T-2 toxin are often found more frequently in oats than in other cereal species, and sometimes at high concentrations [9,10,12–15]. HT-2 and T-2 toxins are closely related (HT-2 is the deacetylated form of T-2), often occur together [12] and their occurrence concentrations are often considered together as a sum of HT-2 and T-2. Throughout this study we use the denomination HT2+T2 for the sum of these toxins. In addition to DON and HT2+T2 toxins, zearalenone (ZEA) and several unregulated mycotoxins such as nivalenol (NIV), enniatin A (EnnA), enniatin A1 (EnnA1), enniatin B (EnnB), enniatin B1 (EnnB1) and beauvericin (BEA) often occur in oat grains [8–11]. In Norway, 3-acetyl-deoxynivalenol (3-ADON) is the dominating acetylated chemotype, although 15-acetyl-deoxynivalenol (15-ADON) has been detected [16].

Besides the importance of oats as a raw material for animal feed concentrate (compound feed), oats grown for human consumption have increased during the last few years due to their beneficial nutritive properties [17]. On the other hand, it has been reported that consumers with a high relative intake of cereals compared to their body weight have a HT2+T2 and a DON exposure that may exceed the Tolerable Daily Intake (TDI) [18]. HT2+T2 toxins are considerably more toxic than DON (TDI 0.02 and 1.0 μg/kg body weight/day, respectively) [19]. The maximum levels for DON and ZEA in unprocessed oat grain for food are 1750 and 100 μg/kg, respectively [6]. However, no regulated maximum levels have been set so far for HT2+T2 in cereals and cereal products, but the European Commission has recommended an indicative level of 1000 μg/kg for HT2+T2 in unprocessed oats [20]. When concentrations of HT2+T2 are detected above this level, the EU member states should perform investigations to identify factors resulting in these levels and investigate the effect of feed and food processing on the presence of these toxins.

In oats, the largest proportion of the mycotoxins is located in the hulls. Thus, de-hulling, i.e., removing hulls (glumes and husk) from the kernels before further processing into oat flakes and other products is an efficient method to reduce the mycotoxin content of oats. Commercial processing of oats has been reported to reduce the content of DON, T2 and HT2 by 80%–95%, with the major loss occurring during de-hulling [21–25]. However, de-hulling is part of the processing of cereal grain. On the other hand, cleaning and size-sorting of raw grain, normally performed as a first step to remove dust, weed seeds, chaff/straw pieces and small, lightweight and damaged kernels before further processing, is accepted according to European legislation, to be carried out on unprocessed grains [6,20]. Several studies have shown that cleaning and sorting of cereal grain can reduce the content of mycotoxins, although variable effects have been reported. Most data are available for reduction of DON in wheat, but also other *Fusarium* toxins, e.g., HT2+T2, NIV and ZEA have been analyzed. The effects of cleaning and sorting by various methods and procedures on the reduction of mycotoxins in wheat, as well as in a few studies in barley and oats, have been reported to vary from no reduction to up to more than an 80% reduction and have even been reported to increase levels in a few cases [3,26–28]. The effect of removing the small grain fractions by size sorting, i.e., after separating the kernels on sieves according to kernel size, varies depending on the sieve sizes used. Despite different degrees of mycotoxin reduction reported by the cleaning and sorting of grains, overall results indicate that these operations may efficiently reduce the mycotoxin levels in highly contaminated cereals before further use/processing.

Data on the effects of removing small grain kernels on the mycotoxin content in oats are limited. The aim of the present study was therefore to investigate to what extent the removal of small kernels can contribute to the reduction of the mycotoxin content in oat grains and thereby improve the quality of the remaining grain. Our hypothesis was that it is feasible/achievable to reduce the mycotoxin content in raw oat grain by size sorting/cleaning out the smaller kernels. Grain from 24 Norwegian oat grain lots (14 from 2015 and 10 from 2018) were sorted into a large and a small kernel fractions by passing the grain through a 2.2 mm laboratory sieve. The large and small kernel samples, in addition to samples of unsorted grain, were analyzed for content of HT2 and T2 (reported together as HT2+T2), DON, ADON (3- and 15-acetyl-deoxynivalenol analyzed together), NIV, EnnA, EnnA1, EnnB, EnnB1, BEA and ZEA. The mycotoxin concentrations in the two grain fractions were compared with the concentrations in the unsorted grain.

2. Results and Discussion

2.1. Mycotoxin Content in the Oat Grain Lots

A visual summary of the concentrations of the ten mycotoxins detected in the 24 oat grain lots (unsorted grain) is shown in Figure 1A,B. Most grain lots contained all the tested mycotoxins. Moderate to high mycotoxin levels in unsorted grain samples were detected for HT2+T2 toxins and EnnB in 2015, and DON in 2018 (Figure 2). Similar contrasting occurrences of HT2+T2 vs. DON in oats have been reported in other studies [9,29,30]. The mycotoxin levels in samples of unsorted grain of the remaining mycotoxins, i.e., ADON, NIV, EnnA, EnnA1, EnnB1, BEA and ZEA were generally low in samples from both years. ZEA was only detected in 2015 samples. Our results are in line with other reports on occurrences of mycotoxins in Norwegian oat grains [9,12,25,31].

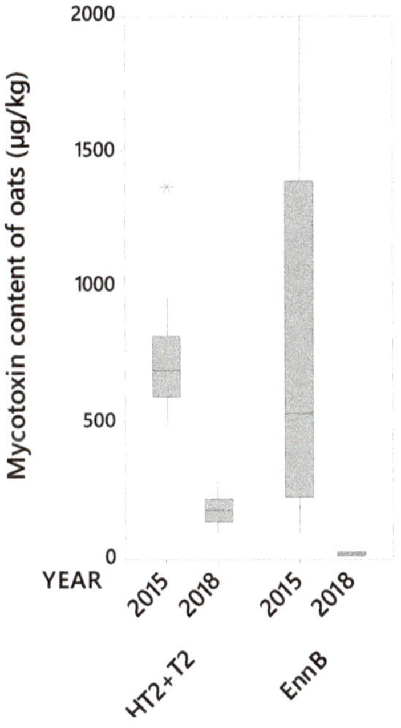

(A)

Figure 1. *Cont.*

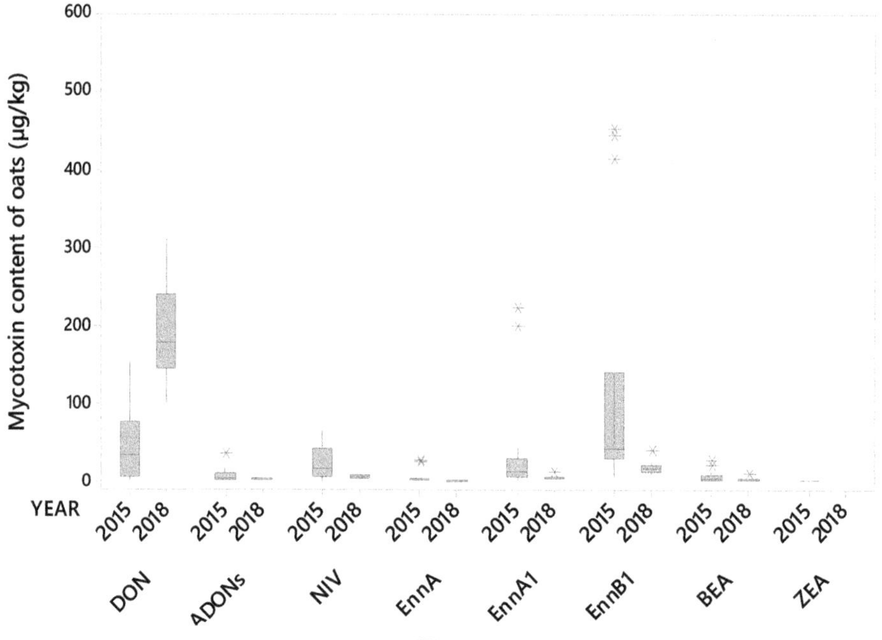

(B)

Figure 1. (**A**) Median, interquartile range, range and outlier (*) for the content (µg/kg) of the mycotoxins HT2+T2 and EnnB (Enniatin B) in 14 oat grain lots from 2015 and 10 oat grain lots from 2018 (unsorted samples). (**B**) Median, interquartile range, and outliers (*) for the content (µg/kg) of the mycotoxins DON (deoxynivalenol), ADON (3- and 15-acetyl-deoxynivalenol), NIV (nivalenol), EnnA (enniatin A), EnnA1 (enniatin A1), EnnB1 (enniatin B1), BEA (beauvericin) and ZEA (zearalenone) in 14 oat grain lots from 2015 and 10 oat grain lots from 2018 (unsorted samples).

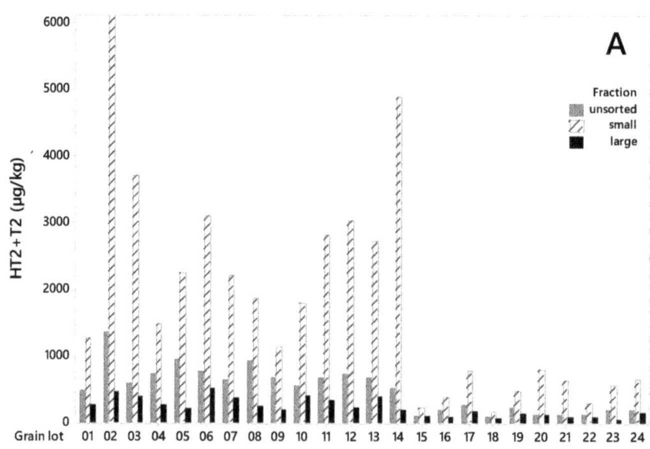

Figure 2. *Cont.*

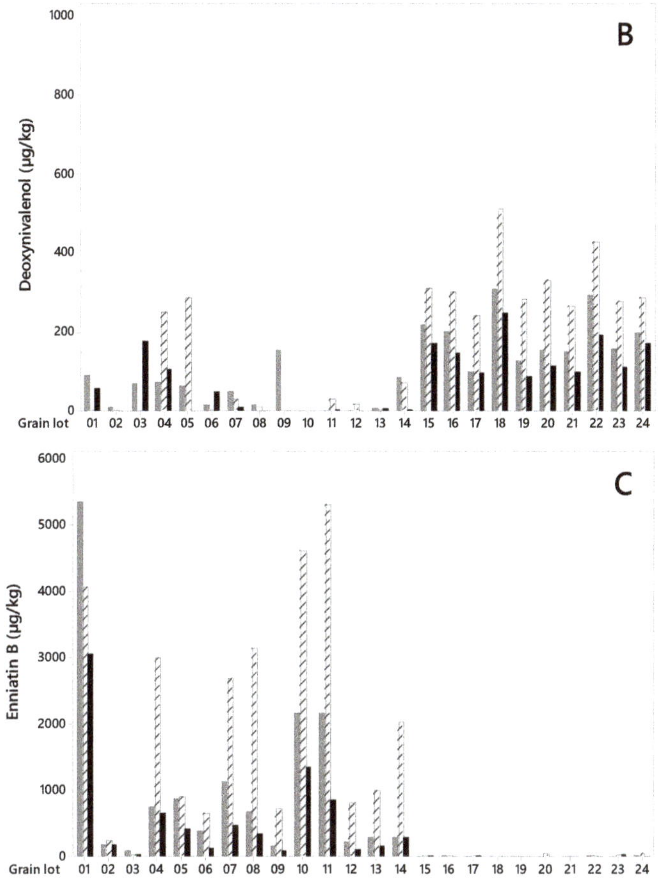

Figure 2. Concentration levels (µg/kg) of HT2+T2 toxins (**A**), deoxynivalenol (**B**) and Enniatin B (**C**) in 24 unsorted oat grain lots and in large and small kernel fractions after size sorting on sieve size 2.2 mm. Lot 1–14 from 2015, lot 15–24 from 2018. Note the different values on the concentration level axes.

2.2. Mycotoxin Content in Unsorted and in Large Kernel Fraction of Oats

2.2.1. HT2+T2

All grain lots contained HT2+T2 toxins (Figure 2A). The levels were considerably higher in the grain from 2015 (lot 1–14) than in the grain from 2018 (lot 15–24). The HT2+T2 concentrations in unsorted grain varied from 486 to 1368 µg/kg (mean 745 µg/kg) among the samples from 2015, and from 92 to 282 µg/kg (mean 178 µg/kg) among the samples from 2018 (Table 1). After sorting, we detected significantly lower HT2+T2 in the large kernel fractions than in the unsorted grain. The concentrations in the large kernel fraction varied from 197 to 522 µg/kg (mean 328 µg/kg) among the samples from 2015, and from 70 to 187 µg/kg (mean 121 µg/kg) among the samples from 2018. In 2015, this corresponds to an average reduction in HT2+T2 concentration of 56% (varying from 24% in lot 10 to 76% in lot 5) in the large kernels compared to the unsorted grain. In 2018, the average reduction in HT2+T2 concentration was 32% (varying from only 2% in lot 15 to 66% in lot 23) (Table 1). The average weight reduction after removal of the small grain fraction was 15% and 21% of the weight of the samples from the two years respectively (Table 2). We did not observe any relationship between the percentage weight reduction and percentage of HT2+T2 reduction (R^2 = 0.00, p = 0.919), or between weight reduction and HT2+T2 levels in unsorted samples (R^2 = 0.04, p = 0.328) when calculated for all 24 grain lots together. However, a significant relationship between percentage weight reduction and HT2+T2 levels was observed (R^2 = 0.47, p = 0.010) for samples from 2015, by omitting the highest contaminated seed lot (No. 2). Only a few studies on the effects of removing small grain kernels on HT2+T2 in oats by size sorting have been found. A Swedish study reported markedly reduced concentrations of HT2+T2 (not quantified) after removing the kernels that passed through a sieve size of 2 mm [32]. A study in Finland, also using a sieve size of 2 mm obtained around a 30%–35% reduction [33], which agrees with our results from 2018 samples and is somewhat lower than what we obtained from the 2015 samples. It was interesting to observe that the effect of removing small kernels was considerably higher in the oats with relatively high HT2+T2 levels (mean 745 µg/kg, 2015 samples) than in oats with lower levels (mean 178 µg/kg, 2018 samples). The extent of toxin reduction increased with toxin levels, and linear regression showed that this relationship was significant (p = 0.000, R^2 = 0.44, Figure 3). Moreover, a few other studies have reported the highest reduction of HT2+T2 in the highest contaminated oats by size sorting and de-hulling [21,32].

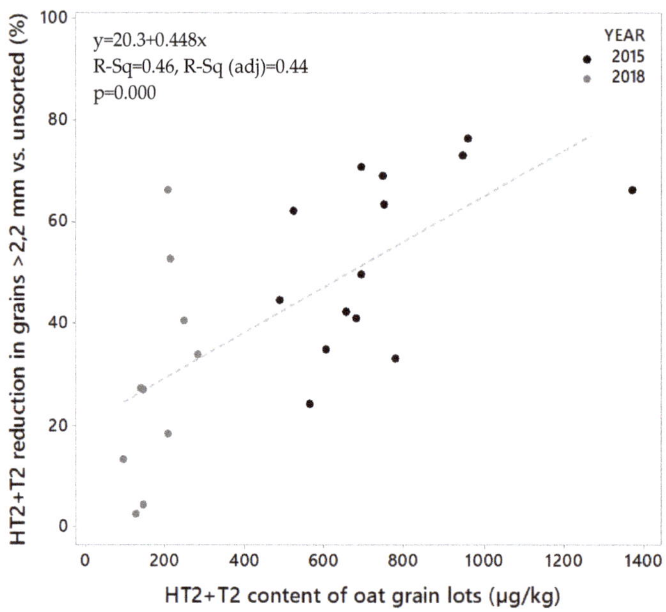

Figure 3. Percentage reduction of HT2+T2 toxins in oat grain samples from 2015 and 2018 in large kernel fraction (after removing small kernel fraction by sieve size = 2.2 mm) vs. concentration level in grain lots (unsorted grain).

Table 1. Mean, minimum (min) and maximum (max) mycotoxin concentrations (μg/kg) in unsorted oat grain samples, and large and small grain fractions after size sorting (2.2 mm sieve) and mean and range in percentage change in toxin concentrations in sorted grain fractions (large or small) compared to unsorted grain.

		2015 (n = 14)				2018 (n = 10)			
Mycotoxin	Grain Category	Mean Toxin Conc. (p-Value) [1]	Min–Max Toxin Conc.	Mean % Change in Toxin Conc. [2]	Range of % Change in Toxin Conc.	Mean Toxin Conc. (p-Value) [1]	Min–Max Toxin Conc.	Mean % Change in Toxin Conc. [2]	Range of % Change in Toxin Conc.
HT2+T2	unsorted	745	486–1368			178	92–282		
	large	328 (0.000)	197–552	−56	−24/−76	121 (0.001)	70–187	−32	−2/−66
	small	2775 (0.000)	1149–6427	+272	+66/+840	510 (0.005)	192–804	+187	+87/+470
DON	unsorted	46	1–153			191	100–309		
	large	30 (0.341)	0–178	n.a. [3]	n.a.	145 (0.000)	89–249	−24	−3/−35
	small	52 (0.811)	0–290	n.a.	n.a.	326 (0.000)	245–514	+71	+42/+145
ADON	unsorted	8	1–35			2.2	1–4		
	large	5 (0.461)	0–30	n.a.	n.a.	1.6 (0.009)	1–4	−27	n.a.
	small	17 (0.435)	0–156	n.a.	n.a.	4.3 (0.000)	3–8	+95	n.a.
NIV	unsorted	23	0–66			6	3–9		
	large	11 (0.035)	0–48	n.a.	n.a.	6 (n.a.)	3–7	n.a.	n.a.
	small	57 (0.164)	0–295	n.a.	n.a.	6 (n.a.)	4–10	n.a.	n.a.
EnnA	unsorted	6	1–27			1	1–2		
	large	4 (0.167)	0–20	n.a.	n.a.	1 (n.a.)	0–2	n.a.	n.a.
	small	16 (0.095)	1–91	n.a.	n.a.	2 (n.a.)	1–4	n.a.	n.a.
EnnA1	unsorted	42	1–221			6	3–11		
	large	24 (0.064)	1–151	n.a.	n.a.	7 (0.588)	2–13	n.a.	n.a.
	small	134 (0.099)	1–896	n.a.	n.a.	12 (0.016)	4–23	+120	−32/+340
EnnB	unsorted	1059	92–5356			15	8–25		
	large	594 (0.018)	48–3064	−44	+2/−63	18 (0.524)	4–43	n.a.	n.a.
	small	2101 (0.008)	37–5319	+98	−60/+568	33 (0.014)	12–67	+120	−10/+500

Table 1. *Cont.*

Mycotoxin	Grain Category	2015 (n = 14) Mean Toxin Conc. (p-Value) [1]	2015 Min–Max Toxin Conc.	2015 Mean % Change in Toxin Conc. [2]	2015 Range of % Change in Toxin Conc.	2018 (n = 10) Mean Toxin Conc. (p-Value) [1]	2018 Min–Max Toxin Conc.	2018 Mean % Change in Toxin Conc. [2]	2018 Range of % Change in Toxin Conc.
EnnB1	unsorted	120	6–452			18	9–38		
	large	62 (0.034)	2–296	n.a.	n.a.	19 (0.708)	5–32	n.a.	n.a.
	small	229 (0.043)	2–1001	n.a.	n.a.	34 (0.022)	13–64	+89	−15/+337
BEA	unsorted	7	1–26			3	1–8		
	large	5 (0.083)	1–22	n.a.	n.a.	3 (n.a.)	1–9	n.a.	n.a.
	small	10 (0.154)	1–48	n.a.	n.a.	4 (n.a.)	1–13	n.a.	n.a.
ZEA	unsorted	1	0–2			n.d. [4]			
	large	2	1–3	n.a.	n.a.	n.d.			
	small	4	2–7	n.a.	n.a.	n.d.			

[1] p-value in paired t-test where the mean toxin levels of the large or small fraction is compared to the level of the unsorted fraction. p-values ≤ 0.05/2 represent a toxin level that is significant different from the unsorted fraction. [2] Percentage change in toxin level in large or small grain fractions compared to the unsorted fraction. Reductions in toxin level compared to the unsorted fraction are shown as negative values and increase as positive values. [3] n.a.—not analysed due to no significant difference and/or low toxin levels. [4] n.d.—not detected.

Table 2. Origin (municipality, field number) and cultivars of oat grain lots from 2015 and 2018, and weight proportions (%) of small and large kernel fractions after size sorting (sieve size 2.2 mm).

Harvest Year	Lot Number	Municipality, Field Number	Cultivar	Weight Proportion (%)	
				Small Kernels	Large Kernels
2015	1	Kongsvinger 1	Belinda	18	82
	2	Kongsvinger 2	Belinda	8	92
	3		Belinda	6	94
	4	Kongsvinger 1	Belinda	24	76
	5		Vinger	27	73
	6		Belinda	15	85
	7		Belinda	22	78
	8		Vinger	33	67
	9		Belinda	22	78
	10	Østre Toten	Dovre	11	89
	11		GN12142	9	91
	12	Hamar	Odal	13	87
	13		Nord09/127	9	91
	14		Poseidon	6	94
	Average weight proportion [1]			15	85
2018	15	Kongsvinger 3	Ringsaker	32	68
	16		GN1311	25	75
	17		Belinda	14	86
	18		Vinger	28	72
	19		Årnes	28	72
	20		Nord13/322	9	91
	21		Gunhild	16	84
	22		GN14182	26	74
	23		GN14209	17	83
	24		GN15154	16	84
	Average weight proportion [1]			21	79

[1] Based on fraction weights of all samples.

As in our study, large differences between samples on the effect on HT2+T2 levels in oats by cleaning/sieving (laboratory-scale grain cleaner, sieve size 1.75 × 20 mm) were reported in a German study [22]. They observed reductions in the range from 0% to 100%, which is even more inconsistent than our data. In a study of barley, the content of HT2 was reduced by 68% and T2 by 81% on average, after around 13% of the sample was removed by using a 2.5 mm sieve [34]. In durum wheat, 54% reduction in the HT2+T2 concentration was observed after a vigorous cleaning procedure (aspiration and two sieves: 5 × 15 mm and 2 × 19 mm) [35]. Concentration levels of HT2+T2 in oats have been reported to be higher in rachis and glumes than in kernels [36]. As small kernels contain a higher proportion of glumes and pericarp than large kernels, removing small kernels will contribute to a reduced mycotoxin content. Our results and other reported data imply that cleaning and size sorting can be useful methods to reduce the concentrations of HT2+T2 in unprocessed grain of oats and other small grain cereals, although the effect will vary among grain lots.

2.2.2. DON

DON was detected in all grain lots (Figure 2B), however its concentration levels were higher in the grain from 2018 (lot 15–24) than in the grain from 2015 (lot 1–14). The concentration levels varied from 100 to 309 µg/kg (mean 191 µg/kg) in unsorted samples from 2018 and from quantification limit (LOQ = 1 µg/kg) to 153 µg/kg (mean 46 µg/kg) in samples from 2015 (Table 1). For the grain harvested in 2018, removing the small kernels resulted in significantly lower DON concentrations in the large kernels (varying from 89 µg/kg to 249 µg/kg, mean 145 µg/kg) compared to the unsorted grain. On average, we detected 24% less DON in the large kernels in 2018 samples, however, the reduction varied from only 3% (lot 17) to up to 35% (lot 22). Despite low DON levels in the 2015 samples, we observed a trend towards a lower mean concentration in large kernel fractions (30 µg/kg) compared to unsorted grain (46 µg/kg) (Table 1). However, the effect of removing the small kernels varied from a reduction to an increase in DON content, and no significant difference in DON levels was detected between the grain fractions.

Limited data exist on the size-sorting effects on DON in oats. A Finnish study observed a 30%–40% reduction in DON concentrations using a 2 mm sieve [33], which is somewhat higher than the 24% reduction we obtained in our 2018 samples. Size sorting of barley in the same study resulted in around a 50% lower content of DON in large grain. Another study in barley reported an 80% reduction of DON after removing the small kernels by using a sieve size of 2.5 mm, however, the effect differed between cultivars [34]. Several studies in wheat, using different sieve sizes, aspiration and cleaning technologies resulting in large variations in the amounts of by-products (e.g., waste, screenings, offals, dockage, pellets etc.) have reported from no and up more than 80% reduction in DON concentrations by cleaning and sorting, but also increased levels have been observed in a few cases [26–28]. For industrial cleaning, an expected reduction rate of 20% has been suggested for DON in wheat [37], which is near the 24% reduction we detected in oats by removing the small kernel fraction in the 2018 materials. Our result supports the previous finding that removing small kernels can reduce the concentration of DON in oats, however as with other small grain cereal species, the effect is likely to vary among grain lots.

2.2.3. Enniatins (Enns) and BEA

The prevalence and concentration levels of Enns and BEA in our grain lots were in accordance with previous studies from Nordic countries where these toxins have been reported as common contaminants of cereals occurring generally at low concentration levels. However, they occur occasionally at high levels, and often EnnB is the most common [8–10,25,31].

All grain lots contained EnnB (Figure 2C). The concentration levels in unsorted samples were considerably higher in most grain lots from 2015 than in grain from 2018, ranging from 92 to 5356 µg/kg (mean 1059 µg/kg), and from 8 to 25 µg/kg (mean 15 µg/kg), for the two years respectively. After removing the small kernel fraction, the EnnB concentrations in large kernel samples from 2015 was significantly lower than in unsorted grain and varied between 48 and 3064 µg/kg (mean 594 µg/kg) (Table 1). On average, this represents 44% less EnnB content than in unsorted grain. However, the reduction varied between 5% (lot 14) and 63% (lot 6), and in lot 2 we recorded an increase of 2%. For samples from 2018, no reduction in the mean EnnB concentrations was detected after size sorting. EnnB1 was detected in all grain lots. In samples from 2015, the concentrations ranged from 6 to 452 µg/kg (mean 120 µg/kg), and a trend towards lower EnnB1 concentrations in large grain (mean 62 µg/kg) compared to unsorted was observed (Table 1). The EnnB1 concentrations in samples from 2018 ranged from 9 to 38 µg/kg (mean 18 µg/kg), with no difference in the content between large and unsorted grain. EnnA and EnnA1 were also detected in all unsorted grain samples, however, the levels were low, especially in samples from 2018 (Table 1). In samples from 2015, a trend towards a lower content of EnnA and EnnA1 in the large grains compared to unsorted grain was observed. BEA occurred at very low levels in all unsorted grain lots, however, a trend towards a reduction was observed after removing the small kernel fraction in samples from 2015 (Table 1). We assume that our study is the first report on the effect of size sorting on the content of Enns and BEA in cereal grains, as we did not find any published data on this. However, a study of Enns in milling fractions of wheat reported that approximately 40% remained in the final wheat flour, compared to whole grain [38].

Enns and BEA have shown cytotoxic, genotoxic and immunomodulating effects, as well as toxic effects on reproductive systems [39,40]. These toxins have been reported to accumulate in animal tissues and eggs [41]. In 2014, the European Food Safety Authority (EFSA) concluded that acute exposure to Enns and BEA do not indicate concern for human health, but chronic exposure might be of concern [42]. However, due to a lack of relevant in vivo toxicity data, a human risk assessment could not be performed. So far, maximum levels for content of these mycotoxins in food and feed have not been established and at present there is no regulatory requirement to consider or reduce the contamination of Enns and BEA in cereal grains. Our results indicate than EnnB can be substantially reduced in oats by removing small kernels, although no consistent effect in relation to concentration levels was found.

2.2.4. NIV, ADON and ZEA

NIV was detected in all but two grain lots from 2015 and in all 10 lots from 2018, however, the overall concentration levels were low (Figure 1B). After removing the small kernel fraction, NIV was detected in all large kernel samples from 2018, but only in 8 of the 14 large kernel samples from 2015. Despite the low levels, a trend towards lower content of NIV in the large grains (mean 11 μg/kg) compared to unsorted grains (mean 23 μg/kg), was observed in samples from 2015 (Table 1). No published data on the effect of sorting and cleaning on the NIV content in oats have been found, however, what is almost an elimination (> 98%) of NIV during oat processing has been reported [21]. In barley, 94% less NIV were reported after removing the small kernels using sieve size 2.5 mm [43]. In wheat, from below a 10% to around an 80% reduction in NIV by cleaning and size sorting has been reported [28]. Based on our limited results and the literature on the effect on NIV in other cereal species, we assume that removal of small kernels can reduce the NIV content in oat grain.

In this study 3- and 15-ADON were analyzed together as ADON. Although 15-ADON is detected in Norway, 3-ADON is the most common chemotype [16]. ADON was detected in all 24 grain lots. However, the overall concentration levels were low (Figure 1B), ranging from 1 (= LOQ) to 35 μg/kg (mean 8 μg/kg) in the samples from 2015, and from 1 to 4 μg/kg (mean 2.2 μg/kg) in the samples from 2018 (Table 1). After removing the small kernel fraction, ADON was still detected in all large kernel samples from 2018 (mean 1.6 μg/kg), and the level was significantly lower than in the unsorted samples. In 2015, ADON could not be detected in five samples after removal of small kernels. Although the average level (5 μg/kg) in the large kernel fraction was lower than in the unsorted grain, this was not statistically significant. A recent Norwegian study on the distribution of mycotoxins in oat grain reported around a 90% reduction of 3-ADON by de-hulling of grain containing relatively high levels of 3-ADON (mean 485 μg/kg) [25]. Based on that study, together with our limited data, it is reasonable to believe that the content of ADON can be reduced by removing small oat kernels.

ZEA was detected at very low levels (close to LOQ = 1 μg/kg) in 12 of the 14 unsorted oat grain samples from 2015, and no ZEA was detected in the 2018 samples (Table 1). Studies in wheat have found ZEA to be mainly concentrated in the outer tissues of the grain, however, the reduction of ZEA content by cleaning and processing has been reported to vary from a few to up to around 40% [43–45]. As no data have been found on the effect of size sorting on the level of ZEA in oats, and because we only detected very low levels in our study, it is not possible to conclude on the effect of size sorting on ZEA in oats.

2.3. *Mycotoxin Content in the Small Kernel Fraction*

Since most mycotoxins are mainly concentrated in the small kernel fractions, in the hulls and in the outer tissues of the grains [21,24,26,44] cleaning, size sorting, de-hulling and further processing will increase the mycotoxin concentrations in the by-products (e.g., screenings, offals, dockage, pellets, bran etc.) [3] In our study, the mean concentration of HT2+T2 in the small kernel fraction was 272% higher for the 2015 samples, and 187% higher in the 2018 samples, compared to the unsorted grain (Table 1). The increase in single samples varied from below 100% to up to 840%, which is the same magnitude that has been measured for HT2+T2 in oat by-products from other size sorting and cleaning studies [21,24,32]. The DON concentrations in our samples were generally low, and despite a mean increase of 71% (ranged from 42% to 145%) in the small grain fraction in samples from 2018, the levels were still moderate (Table 1). A high accumulation (ten-fold) of DON in the offals after cleaning was reported in oats in a Polish study [46]. In our study, the mean concentration of EnnB in the small kernel fraction was 98% and 120% higher in samples from 2015 and 2018, respectively, compared to the unsorted grain (Table 1). However, the concentrations in the small kernel samples varied considerably from a reduction of 60% to an increase of 568%. Higher EnnB1 concentrations were found in the small grain fraction compared to unsorted grain in samples from 2018, representing an increase of 89% (Table 1), whereas in samples from 2015, a trend towards higher mean EnnB1 concentrations in small grains compared to unsorted grains was observed. Except for a study reporting a considerably higher content of EnnB (200% and 375% in shorts and bran respectively) and EnnB1 (around 240% and 300% in shorts and bran respectively) after milling of wheat, no other data have been found on the distribution of Enns in cereal grain fractions [38]. Despite low ADON levels, a significant increase was detected in the small kernel fraction compared to unsorted grain for 2018 samples (Table 1). The by-product fractions are commonly used as raw materials for animal feed. It is important for feed producers to be aware of the risk of extensive increases in the mycotoxin content in by-products. To manage the mycotoxin risk and to decide what to be done with potentially contaminated by-products, proper sampling and analysis are necessary. Based on the contamination level, an evaluation of the economic value of the by-products and the carry-over potential of the mycotoxins, a decision on the inclusion level of feed ingredients can be made [3]. In our study, the highest measured HT2+T2 concentration in the small kernels fraction was 6427 µg/kg (lot No. 2) and 4889 µg/kg (lot No. 14) which would have been of concern if it had been used in feed production.

2.4. Conditions Influencing on the Effect of Grain Size Sorting

We observed variable effects of size sorting on the content of HT2+T2, DON and EnnB among the grain lots (Figure 2). One reason for this variation can be the diversity in cultivars (Table 2) which is likely to differ in resistance to *Fusarium* infections and mycotoxin development. In addition, our grain lots originated from two different years and partly from different locations. The degree of *Fusarium* mycelium growth into the kernels and mycotoxin development varies between *Fusarium* species and are in addition to host plant resistance against infection, influenced by cultivation conditions and local weather during the susceptible stages of the host plant and during grain-filling and maturation stages [36,47,48]. This can result in a different distribution of the different mycotoxins in kernels and therefore likely contribute to the different effects of size sorting among the samples in our study. Moreover, cultivar differences in phenological kernel traits itself, such as kernel size probably also contributed to the variation in size-sorting effects. Grain materials for this study were not selected to allow for an examination of the influence of cultivar or location on the size-sorting effect. One important reason for the variation between different studies in the effect of cleaning and size sorting on the mycotoxin content in grain is in the use of different sorting and cleaning methods/technologies, e.g., different sieve sizes and machinery settings, and some studies have included a pre-cleaning step without or with aspiration with varying fan speeds to remove dust, broken grain and other debris. By removing some of the "waste products" prior to sorting, less effects will be obtained by further cleaning and size sorting. This diversity in method will also result in large differences in volume and weight proportions removed in the pre-processing stages e.g., [21,34,44].

2.5. Grain Weight Reduction by Size Sorting and Mass Balance Calculations

By passing the raw grain samples through a laboratory sieve (sieve size 2.2 mm) and removing the small kernel fraction, the grain weight was in average reduced by 15% and 21% for samples from 2015 and 2018, respectively (Table 2), i.e., a larger proportion passed through the sieve in the samples from 2018 than in the samples from 2015, indicating generally smaller kernels in 2018 than in 2015. However, the weight reduction varied between 6% and 33% among the 14 samples from 2015, and between 9% and 32% among the 10 samples from 2018. No data was found in the literature on the weight reduction by cleaning or size sorting in oats, however, dehulling has been reported to remove around 30% to 40% of the whole grain weight [21,25]. In a study of barley, the weight reduction varied between 6% and 25% among 15 samples of different cultivars when grain passed a sieve size of 2.5 mm [34].

Mass balance calculation of mycotoxin concentrations in unsorted grain and in the sum of the size fractions is an important quality control tool [44]. Mass balance calculated for amounts of HT2+T2

(2015, 2018), DON (2018) and EnnB (2015) in the two fractions from the mycotoxin concentrations and the weight of each fraction, and the sum was compared to the mycotoxin content in the unsorted sample (Table 3). For HT2+T2, the recovery in the sum of the two fractions compared to unsorted grain ranged between 59% and 120% (mean 87%) for 2015 samples and between 75% and 138% (mean 105%) for 2018 samples. For DON, the recovery in the sum of the two fractions ranged between 85% and 117% (mean 96%). The recovery of EnnB in the sum of the two fractions ranged between 51% and 188% (mean 77%). Regression analysis of the mycotoxin amounts in the unsorted grain and the sum amounts in the two fractions (Figure 4) indicated rather a good relationship for DON (R^2 = 0.93, 2018 samples) and EnnB (R^2 = 0.90, 2015 samples), however, some variation in the recovery among the samples were observed for HT2+T2 in samples from both years (R^2 = 0.60 and R^2 = 0.64, for 2015 and 2018 samples respectively). This indicates that the analysis was somewhat inaccurate.

Table 3. Comparison between mycotoxin concentrations (μg/kg) in unsorted grain and the mycotoxin mass balance calculated from the weighted sum of mycotoxins in the large and small kernel fractions and percentage recovery in calculated compared to measured amounts.

Mycotoxin (Harvest Year)	Unsorted Grain (Measured)	Weighted Sum of Large and Small Kernel Fractions (Calculated)	% Recovery (Range)
HT2+T2 (2015)	745	648	87 (59–120)
HT2+T2 (2018)	178	187	105 (75–138)
DON (2018)	191	184	96 (85–117)
EnnB (2015)	1054	820	77 (51–188)

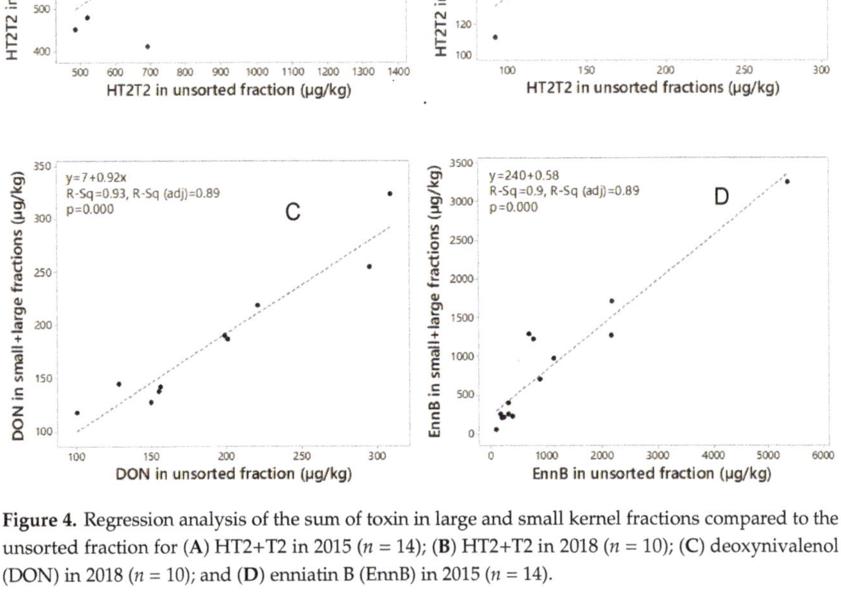

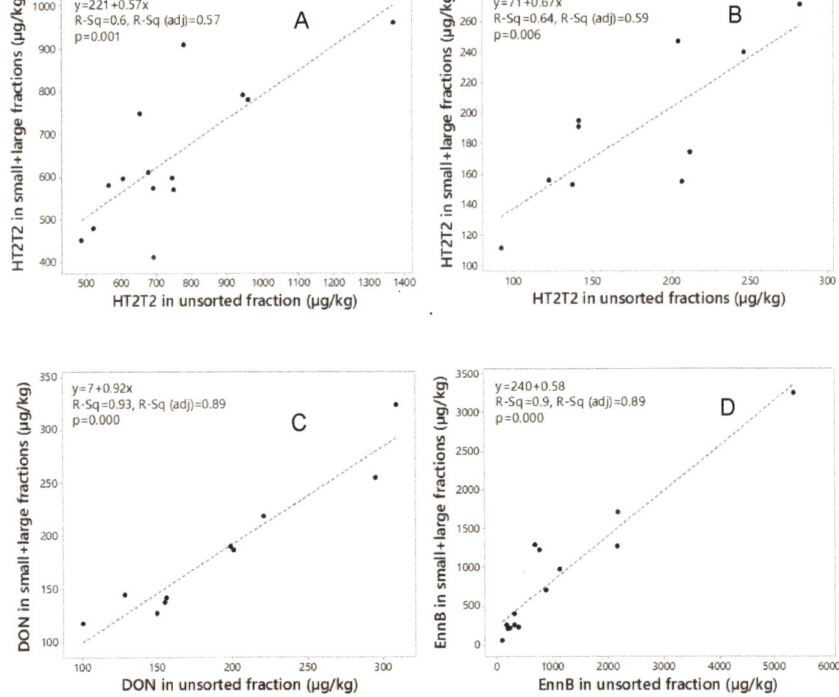

Figure 4. Regression analysis of the sum of toxin in large and small kernel fractions compared to the unsorted fraction for (**A**) HT2+T2 in 2015 (n = 14); (**B**) HT2+T2 in 2018 (n = 10); (**C**) deoxynivalenol (DON) in 2018 (n = 10); and (**D**) enniatin B (EnnB) in 2015 (n = 14).

Reasons for some of the discrepancies between the sum of the two fractions and the amounts in the unsorted sample may be due to inaccuracies in sampling, including sample preparation before analysis, the drawing of a small ground sample (5 g) for analysis, and the recovery of the analysis method itself. Sampling is a major source of error in monitoring mycotoxins in cereal grains. It is difficult to obtain homogenous samples partly due to an uneven distribution of mycotoxins within a grain lot [49]. If a sample is not representative it can cause an over- or under- estimation of mycotoxin contamination, and this might have contributed to the variable effects on the mycotoxin content we obtained by size sorting. The type of grinder as well as the method for dividing can influence on the heterogeneity of mycotoxins in a sample. The grinder and sieve size (1 mm) used in our study gave what was perhaps a higher heterogeneity due to a higher particle size than what is optimal [50]. Moreover, small samples with low mycotoxin levels can cause considerable measurement uncertainty.

3. Conclusions

Our study showed that by removing the small kernel fraction from the grain, representing on average 15% and 21% of the weight of the samples from the two years respectively, the content of *Fusarium* mycotoxins was considerably reduced. The most notable effects were seen on the concentrations of T2+HT2 toxins, which were reduced by 56% and 32% on average for samples from 2015 and 2018 respectively, and EnnB, which was reduced by 44% in grain lots from 2015. We also observed a clear reduction, on average 24%, in the DON concentrations in the 2018 samples. Moreover, despite low levels, our analyses showed a trend towards reduced content of DON, ADON, NIV, EnnA, EnnA1, EnnB1 and BEA after removing the small kernel fraction in samples from 2015.

For HT2+T2, the reduction obtained by sorting increased with the mycotoxin levels of unsorted grain lots. Ours and other studies experienced variable effects on the mycotoxin content by size sorting, however, removing the small kernel fraction in oats can be a useful method to reduce the mycotoxin contamination. Grain lots are still defined as unprocessed after cleaning and size sorting. Thus, by performing these operations, the grain industry may safely utilize a higher number of unprocessed oat grain lots for further processing in the food and feed chain. Knowledge about the different content of mycotoxins in various grain size fractions increases the possibility of better utilization of oat grains for food and feed and can help to identify grain lots at risk. Because of variable effects, it is also important to analyze the mycotoxin content after size sorting. For several of the mycotoxins, the concentrations were considerably higher in the small kernel fraction compared to unsorted grain. We assume that our study is the first report on the effect of size sorting on the content of Enns, NIV and BEA in oat grains.

4. Materials and Methods

4.1. Oat Grain Materials

Samples (approximately 0.5 kg, 14% moisture) from 24 oat grain lots (several cultivars) were obtained from various field experiments in southeast Norway (Table 2). Fourteen lots were harvested in 2015 at four different field locations, and ten were harvested in 2018 at one location. The grain lots were chosen based on preliminary tests showing that they contained HT-2 and T-2 toxins, which were the mycotoxins we were most interested in in this study. A sample of approximately 300g of harvested grain (raw material) of each lot was obtained by deviding on a riffle divider (Rationell Kornservice AS, Esbjerg, Denmark). After slight air cleaning (blowing) at "low speed" to remove dust, weed seeds and trash/straw pieces, each sample was further divided into sub-samples of approximately 100 g (unsorted sample) and 200 g. Each of the 200 g samples was size sorted into a large and small kernel fraction by passing the grain through a laboratory scale grain screening machine (in-house made, sieve size = 2.2 mm) at Kimen Seed Laboratory. The weight of unsorted, large and small kernel samples from each grain lot was recorded. Materials of the two size fractions, in addition to the unsorted sample, were ground on a high-speed rotor mill (ZM 200, Retsch, Haan, Germany) fitted with a 1 mm sieve and stored at −20 °C until analyses.

4.2. Mycotoxin Analyses

All grain samples were analyzed for the content of eleven different mycotoxins by using LC-MS/MS. The sample preparation was done according to the procedure published by Klötzer and Lauber [51] except that only 5 g aliquot of each sample was extracted with 20 mL mixture of acetonitrile and water (80:20 v/v). The analyses of the mycotoxins detected as cations (HT-2, T-2, Enns, BEA and ZEA) in grain samples harvested in 2015 were carried out using a Waters Ultima Pt MS/MS-detector, whereas the analyses of the mycotoxins detected as anions (DON, NIV, sum of 3-acetyl-DON and 15-acetyl-DON) were performed with a Thermo high resolution accurate mass (HRAM) Q-Exactive Orbitrap instrument. The mycotoxin analysis of grain from 2018 was carried out using HRAM Q-Exactive Orbitrap exclusively, using electrospray polarity switching in order to detect all the ionized mycotoxins in one run (Table 4). The toxins were separated on a Thermo Accucore aQ (100 × 2.1 mm i.d., 2.6 μm) column. A linear mobile phase gradient was used, starting with 100% water in 5 mM ammonium acetate reaching 100% methanol in 5 mM ammonium acetate after 9 min. The total run time was 18 min. The injection volume was 5 μL (Waters instrument) or 1 μL (Thermo instrument), the flow 0.3 mL/min and the column temperature was 30 °C. In the negative mode, mycotoxins were detected as acetate-adducts $[M+CH_3COO]^-$ and in the positive mode mycotoxins were detected as ammonium adducts $[M+NH_4]^+$ or hydrogen adducts $[M+H]^+$. The identification criteria were retention time (RT) matched to reference standard, precursor ion accurate m/z mass within 5 ppm accuracy and the presence of at least one targeted product ion with accurate mass within 5 ppm accuracy and produced by fragmentation of the precursor ion. An in-house library of product ion spectra (MS2) for the mycotoxins aided in the identification. Quantification was based on the peak height of the precursor ions. Reference standards of the mycotoxins were purchased from Merck, Darmstadt, Germany. Calibration standards were prepared in the range of 1–1000 μg/kg. Limit of quantification (LOQ) was 1–10 μg/kg. The recovery of HT-2 and T-2 was confirmed to 100% using a certified oat reference material. Recovery of the other toxins was determined from spiked control samples that were prepared with each batch of samples. Recovery was 100% for DON, 3+15-Acetyl-DON and EnnB, 60%–70% for NIV, ZEA, EnnA, EnnA1 and EnnB1, and 45% for BEA. Our method reported the correct levels of HT-2, T-2, DON and ZEA (z-scores lower than 0.35) in oat meal in a proficiency test in 2019 [52].

Table 4. Parameters for the high resolution accurate mass (HRAM) detection of the analytes including retention time, precursor ion, adducts type of precursor and one of the product ions.

Mycotoxin	Retention Time (min)	Precursor Ion (m/z)	Adduct	Product Ions (m/z)
NIV	3.12	371.13476	[M+CH3COO-]	281.10284
DON	3.83	355.13984	[M+CH3COO-]	295.11835
3+15-Acetyl-DON	5.48	397.15041	[M+CH3COO-]	307.11914
HT-2	7.68	442.24354	[M+NH4+]	363.12781
T-2	7.99	484.25411	[M+NH4+]	305.13818
ZEA	8.71	319.15400	[M+H+]	187.07544
Enn B	9.93	657.44331	[M+H+]	196.13345
Enn B1	10.07	671.45896	[M+H+]	654.43317
BEA	10.09	801.44331	[M+H+]	134.09669
Enn A	10.16	685.47461	[M+H+]	210.14906
Enn A1	10.28	699.49026	[M+H+]	228.15967

4.3. Data Analyses

The mean, minimum and maximum toxin concentration was calculated for each toxin for both years using Minitab 18. Percentage reductions of toxins in the large grain fractions and percentage increases in the small grain fractions were calculated compared to concentrations in the unsorted grain. Percentage weight reduction was calculated from the weight of the unsorted sample (= 100%) and the weight of the large and small kernel fractions (sum = 100%). The mean toxin levels in the small or the large grain fractions were compared to the mean toxin level in the unsorted grain fraction using a paired *t*-test in Minitab 18. The confidence level was adjusted according to the Bonferroni method to obtain a simultaneous confidence level of 95%, and the differences between the means were considered as significant when p-values $\leq 0.05/2$. The following relationships were analyzed by linear regression in Minitab 18: (i) the percentage of HT2+T2 reduction vs. the concentration level in the grain lots (unsorted grain), (ii) the sum of toxin concentration (HT2+T2 2015, 2018; DON 2018; EnnB 2015) in the small and the large grain fraction vs. the toxin concentration in the grain lots (unsorted grain), (iii) the percentage weight reduction vs. the percentage HT2+T2 reduction, and (iiii) the percentage of weight reduction vs. the HT2+T2 level in the grain lots. The relationships in (i), (iii) and (iiii) were studied across both years.

Author Contributions: G.B. designed the experiments, supervised the research and wrote the major parts of the manuscript; H.U.A. contributed to the data calculations and to the writing of the manuscript; M.A. analyzed the mycotoxins and contributed to the writing of the manuscript; I.S.H. was project leader, contributed to the data calculations and the writing of the manuscript. All authors have read and agreed to the published version of the manuscript.

Funding: This research was funded by The Agriculture and Food Industry Research Funds—FFL/JA (The Research Council of Norway grant number 254751/E50), Graminor AS, Lantmännen Corporate R&D, Felleskjøpet Agri SA, Felleskjøpet Rogaland Agder, Fiskå Mølle Moss AS, Strand Unikorn AS, Norgesmøllene AS and Kimen Seed Laboratory.

Acknowledgments: Grain lots were provided from field experiments at NIBIO and the Norwegian Agricultural Extension Service. We thank Kari Wahltoft at Kimen Seed Laboratory for cleaning/size sorting and weighing the samples, Ely Gauslaa and Chloè Grieu at NIBIO for grinding samples, Børge Holen for the development of the mycotoxin extraction method and analysis method on Waters LC-MS/MS, Jan Kristian Larsen for mycotoxin extraction of oat grain samples and Torfinn Torp for advice on statistical calculations.

Conflicts of Interest: The authors declare no conflict of interests related to this research. The funders had no role in the design of the study; in the collection, analysis, or interpretation of data; or in the writing of the manuscript and agreed to publish the results.

References

1. Desjardins, A.E. *Fusarium Mycotoxins: Chemistry, Genetics and Biology*; American Phytopathological Society (APS Press): St. Paul, MN, USA, 2006; p. 260.
2. da Rocha, M.E.B.; Freire, F.C.O.; Maia, F.E.F.; Guedes, M.I.F.; Rondina, D. Mycotoxins and their effects on human and animal health. *Food Control* **2014**, *36*, 159–165. [CrossRef]
3. Pinotti, L.; Ottoboni, M.; Giromini, C.; Dell'Orto, V.; Cheli, F. Mycotoxin Contamination in the EU Feed Supply Chain: A Focus on Cereal Byproducts. *Toxins* **2016**, *8*, 45. [CrossRef] [PubMed]
4. Sundheim, L.; Lillegaard, I.T.; Fæste, C.K.; Brantsæter, A.-L.; Brodal, G.; Eriksen, G.S. Deoxynivalenol Exposure in Norway, Risk Assessments for Different Human Age Groups. *Toxins* **2017**, *9*, 46. [CrossRef] [PubMed]
5. Straumfors, A.; Uhlig, S.; Eriksen, G.S.; Heldal, K.K.; Eduard, W.; Krska, R.; Sulyok, M. Mycotoxins and other fungal metabolites in grain dust from Norwegian grain elevators and compound feedmills. *World Mycotoxin J.* **2015**, *8*, 361–373. [CrossRef]
6. European Commission (EC). Commission Regulation (EC) no. 1881/2006 of 19 December 2006 setting maximum levels for certain contaminants in foodstuffs. *Off. J. Eur. Union* **2006**, *L 364*, 5–24.
7. European Commission (EC). Commission Recommendation of 17 August 2006 on the on the presence of deoxynivalenol, zearalenone, ochratoxin A, T-2 and HT-2 and fumonisins in products intended for animal feeding. *Off. J. Eur. Union* **2006**, *L 229*, 7–9.
8. Fredlund, E.; Gidlund, A.; Sulyok, M.; Börjesson, T.; Krska, R.; Olsen, M.; Lindblad, M. Deoxynivalenol and other selected *Fusarium* toxins in Swedish wheat — Occurrence and correlation to specific *Fusarium* species. *Int. J. Food Microbiol.* **2013**, *167*, 284–291. [CrossRef]
9. Hofgaard, I.S.; Aamot, H.U.; Torp, T.; Jestoi, M.; Lattanzio, V.M.T.; Klemsdal, S.S.; Waalwijk, C.; van der Lee, T.; Brodal, G. Associations between *Fusarium* species and mycotoxins in oats and spring wheat from farmers' fields in Norway over a six-year period. *World Mycotoxin J.* **2016**, *9*, 365–378. [CrossRef]
10. Hietaniemi, V.; Rämö, S.; Yli-Mattila, T.; Jestoi, M.; Peltonen, S.; Kartio, M.; Sieviläinen, E.; Koivisto, T.; Parikka, P. Updated survey of *Fusarium* species and toxins in Finnish cereal grains. *Food Addit. Contam. Part A* **2016**, *33*, 831–848. [CrossRef]

11. Tittlemier, S.A.; Blagden, R.; Chan, J.; Roscoe, M.; Pleskach, K. A multi-year survey of mycotoxins and ergosterol in Canadian oats. *Mycotoxin Res.* **2020**, *36*, 103–114. [CrossRef]
12. Langseth, W.; Rundberget, T. The occurrence of HT-2 toxin and other trichothecenes in Norwegian cereals. *Mycopathologia* **1999**, *147*, 157–165. [CrossRef] [PubMed]
13. Edwards, S.G.; Barrier-Guillot, B.; Clasen, P.-E.; Hietaniemi, V.; Pettersson, H. Emerging issues of HT-2 and T-2 toxins in European cereal production. *World Mycotoxin J.* **2009**, *9*, 365–378. [CrossRef]
14. van der Fels-Klerx, H.; Stratakou, I. T-2 toxin and HT-2 toxin in grain and grain-based commodities in Europe: Occurrence, factors affecting occurrence, co-occurrence and toxicological effects. *World Mycotoxin J.* **2010**, *3*, 349–367. [CrossRef]
15. Schöneberg, T.; Jenny, E.; Wettstein, F.E.; Bucheli, T.D.; Mascher, F.; Bertossa, M.; Musa, T.; Seifert, K.; Gräfenhan, T.; Beat Keller, B.; et al. Occurrence of *Fusarium* species and mycotoxins in Swiss oats—Impact of cropping factors. *Eur. J. Agr.* **2018**, *92*, 123–132. [CrossRef]
16. Aamot, H.U.; Ward, T.J.; Brodal, G.; Vrålstad, T.; Larsen, G.B.; Klemsdal, S.S.; Eleamen, A.; Uhlig, S.; Hofgaard, I.S. Genetic and phenotypic diversity within the *Fusarium graminearum* species complex in Norway. *Eur. J. Plant Pathol.* **2015**, *142*, 501–519. [CrossRef]
17. Clemens, R.; van Klinken, B.J.-W. Oats, more than just a whole grain: An introduction. *Br. J. Nutr.* **2014**, *112*, S1–S3. [CrossRef]
18. Ranking of Substances for Monitoring in Foods, Drinks and Dietary Supplements-Based on Risk and Knowledge Gaps. Available online: https://vkm.no/download/18.59c1cc3017057cd177f1653b/1582108692752/Ranking%20of%20substances%20for%20monitoring%20in%20foods,%20drinks%20and%20dietary%20supplements%20-%20based%20on%20risk%20and%20knowledge%20gaps%20revidert2.pdf (accessed on 10 February 2020).
19. EFSA (European Food Safety Authority); Arcella, D.; Gergelova, P.; Innocenti, M.L.; Steinkellner, H. Human and animal dietary exposure to T-2 and HT-2 toxin. *EFSA J.* **2017**, *15*, 4972. [CrossRef]
20. European Commission (EC). Commission Recommendation of 27 March 2013 on the presence of T-2 and HT-2 toxin in cereals and cereal products. *Off. J. Eur. Union* **2013**, *L 91*, 12–15.
21. Scudamore, K.A.; Baillie, H.; Patel, S.; Edwards, S.G. Occurrence and fate of *Fusarium* mycotoxins during commercial processing of oats in the UK. *Food Addit. Contam.* **2007**, *24*, 1374–1385. [CrossRef]
22. Schwake-Anduschus, C.; Langenkämper, G.; Unbehend, G.; Dietrich, R.; Märtlbauer, E.; Münzing, K. Occurrence of *Fusarium* T-2 and HT-2 toxins in oats from cultivar studies in Germany and degradation of toxins during grain cleaning treatment and food processing. *Food Addit. Contam.* **2010**, *27*, 1253–1260. [CrossRef]
23. Yan, W.; Fregeau-Reid, J.; Rioux, S.; Pageau, D.; Xue, A.; Martin, R.; Fedak, G.; de Haan, B.; Lajeunesse, J.; Savard, M. Response of Oat Genotypes to Fusarium Head Blight in Eastern Canada. *Crop Sci.* **2010**, *50*, 134–142. [CrossRef]
24. Pettersson, H.; Brown, C.; Hauk, J.; Meter, J.; Wessels, D. Survey of T-2 and HT-2 toxins by LC-MS/MS in oats and oat products from European oat mills in 2005-2009. *Food Addit. Contam. Part B* **2011**, *4*, 110–115. [CrossRef] [PubMed]
25. Ivanova, L.; Sahlstrøm, S.; Rud, I.; Uhlig, S.; Fæste, C.K.; Eriksen, G.S.; Divon, H.H. Effect of primary processing on the distribution of free and modified *Fusarium* mycotoxins in naturally contaminated oats. *World Mycotoxin J.* **2017**, *10*, 73–88. [CrossRef]
26. Cheli, F.; Pinotti, L.; Rossi, L.; Dell'Orto, V. Effect of milling procedures on mycotoxin distribution in wheat fractions: A review. *LWT Food Sci. Technol.* **2013**, *54*, 307–314. [CrossRef]
27. Peng, W.-X.; Marchal, J.L.M.; van der Poel, A.F.B. Strategies to prevent and reduce mycotoxins for compound feed manufacturing. *Anim. Feed Sci. Technol.* **2018**, *237*, 129–153. [CrossRef]
28. Schaarschmidt, S.; Fauhl-Hassek, C. The Fate of Mycotoxins during the Processing of Wheat for Human Consumption. *Compreh. Rev. Food Sci. Food Saf.* **2018**, *17*, 556–593. [CrossRef]
29. Edwards, S.G. Fusarium mycotoxin content of UK organic and conventional oats. *Food Addit. Contam.* **2009**, *26*, 1063–1069. [CrossRef]
30. Kaukoranta, T.; Hietaniemi, V.; Rämö, S.; Koivisto, T.; Parikka, P. Contrasting responses of T-2, HT-2 and DON mycotoxins and *Fusarium* species in oat to climate, weather, tillage and cereal intensity. *Eur. J. Plant Pathol.* **2019**, *155*, 93–110. [CrossRef]

31. Uhlig, S.; Torp, M.; Heier, B.T. Beauvericin and enniatins A, A1, B and B1 in Norwegian grain: A survey. *Food Chem.* **2006**, *94*, 193–201. [CrossRef]
32. Petterson, H.; Börjesson, T.; Persson, L.; Lerenius, C.; Berg, G.; Gustafsson, G. T-2 and HT-2 toxins in oats grown in Northern Europe. *Cereal. Res. Commun.* **2008**, *26* (Suppl. B), 591–592.
33. Hietaniemi, V.; Rämö, S.; Manninen, P.; Parikka, P.; Hankomäki, J. The effect of cleaning and de-hulling on the trichothecene content inn oats and barley. In Proceedings of the Nordforsk Mould and Mycotoxin Seminar, Uppsala, Sweden, 14–15 April 2009.
34. Perkowski, J.; Kiecana, I.; Kaczmarek, Z. Natural occurrence and distribution of *Fusarium* toxins in contaminated barley cultivars. *Eur. J. Plant Path.* **2003**, *109*, 331–339. [CrossRef]
35. Pascale, M.; Haidukowski, M.; Lattanzio, V.M.T.; Silvestri, M.; Ranieri, R.; Visconti, A. Distribution of T-2 and HT-2 Toxins in Milling Fractions of Durum Wheat. *J. Food. Prot.* **2011**, *74*, 1700–1707. [CrossRef] [PubMed]
36. Opoku, N.; Back, M.A.; Edwards, S.G. Susceptibility of cereal species to *Fusarium langsethiae* under identical field conditions. *Eur. J. Plant Pathol.* **2018**, *150*, 869–879. [CrossRef]
37. Larsen, J.C.; Hunt, J.; Perrin, I.; Ruckenbauer, P. Workshop on trichothecenes with a focus on DON: Summary report. *Toxicol. Lett.* **2004**, *153*, 1–22. [CrossRef]
38. Vaclavikova, M.; Malachova, A.; Veprikova, Z.; Dzuman, Z.; Zachariasova, M.; Hajslova, J. 'Emerging' mycotoxins in cereals processing chains: Changes of enniatins during beer and bread making. *Food Chem.* **2013**, *136*, 750–757. [CrossRef]
39. Fraeyman, S.; Croubels, S.; Devreese, M.; Antonissen, G. Emerging Fusarium and Alternaria Mycotoxins: Occurrence, Toxicity and Toxicokinetics. *Toxins* **2017**, *9*, 228. [CrossRef]
40. Maranghi, F.; Tassinari, R.; Narciso, L.; Tait, S.; La Rocca, C.; Di Felice, G.; Butteroni, C.; Corinti, S.; Barletta, B.; Cordelli, E.; et al. In vivo toxicity and genotoxicity of beauvericin and enniatins. Combined approach to study in vivo toxicity and genotoxicity of mycotoxins beauvericin (BEA) and enniatin B (ENNB). *EFSA Support. Publ.* **2018**, *15*, EN-1406. [CrossRef]
41. Jestoi, M.; Rokka, M.; Järvenpää, E.; Peltonen, K. Determination of *Fusarium* mycotoxins beauvericin and enniatins (A, A1, B, B1) in eggs of laying hens using liquid chromatography–tandem mass spectrometry (LC–MS/MS). *Food Chem.* **2009**, *115*, 1120–1127. [CrossRef]
42. EFSA CONTAM Panel (EFSA Panel on Contaminants in the Food Chain). Scientific Opinion on the risks to human and animal health related to the presence of beauvericin and enniatins in food and feed. *EFSA J.* **2014**, *12*, 3802. [CrossRef]
43. Neuhof, T.; Koch, M.; Rasenko, T.; Nehls, I. Distribution of trichothecenes, zearalenone, and ergosterol in a fractionated wheat harvest lot. *J. Agric. Food Chem.* **2008**, *56*, 7566–7571. [CrossRef]
44. Edwards, S.G.; Dickin, E.T.; MacDonald, S.; Buttler, D.; Hazel, C.M.; Patel, S.; Scudamore, K.A. Distribution of *Fusarium* mycotoxins in UK wheat mill fractions. *Food Addit. Contam.* **2011**, *28*, 1694–1704. [CrossRef]
45. Schwake-Anduschus, C.; Proske, M.; Sciurba, E.; Muenzing, K.; Koch, M.; Maul, R. Distribution of deoxynivalenol, zearalenone, and their respective modified analogues in milling fractions of naturally contaminated wheat grains. *World Mycotoxin J.* **2015**, *8*, 433–443. [CrossRef]
46. Stuper-Szablewska, K.; Szablewski, T.; Buśko, M.; Perkowski, J. Changes in contents of trichothecenes during commercial grain milling. *LWT Food Sci. Technol.* **2016**, *69*, 55–58. [CrossRef]
47. Edwards, S.G.; Kharbikar, L.L.; Dickin, E.T.; MacDonald, S.; Scudamore, K.A. Impact of pre-harvest rainfall on the distribution of fusarium mycotoxins in wheat mill fractions. *Food Control* **2018**, *89*, 150–156. [CrossRef]
48. Ji, F.; Wu, J.; Zhao, H.; Xu, J.; Shi, J. Relationship of Deoxynivalenol Content in Grain, Chaff, and Straw with *Fusarium* Head Blight Severity in Wheat Varieties with Various Levels of Resistance. *Toxins* **2015**, *7*, 728–742. [CrossRef]
49. Cheli, F.; Campagnoli, A.; Pinotti, L.; Fusi, E.; Dell'Orto, V. Sampling feed for mycotoxins: Acquiring knowledge from food. *It. J. Anim. Sci.* **2009**, *8*, 5–22. [CrossRef]
50. Tittlemier, S.A.; Blagden, R.; Chan, J.; McMillan, T.L.; Pleskach, K.; Izydorczyk, M.S. Effects of processing whole oats on the analysis and fate of mycotoxins and ergosterol. *World Mycotoxin J.* **2020**, *13*, 45–56. [CrossRef]

51. Klötzel, M.; Lauber, U.; Humpf, H.-U. A new solid phase extraction clean-up method for the determination of 12 type A- and B-trichothecenes in cereals and cereal-based food by LC-MS/MS. *Mol. Nutr. Food Res.* **2006**, *50*, 261–269. [CrossRef]
52. Elbers, I.J.W.; Pereboom, D.P.K.H.; Mol, J.G.J.; Nijs, W.C.M. Proficiency test for mycotoxins in oat meal. Wageningen Food Safety Research. *WFSR-Rep.* **2019**, 51. [CrossRef]

toxins

MDPI

Article

Development and Validation of a Liquid Chromatography High-Resolution Mass Spectrometry Method for the Simultaneous Determination of Mycotoxins and Phytoestrogens in Plant-Based Fish Feed and Exposed Fish

Amritha Johny [1,*], Christiane Kruse Fæste [1], André S. Bogevik [2], Gerd Marit Berge [3], Jorge M.O. Fernandes [4] and Lada Ivanova [5]

1 Toxinology Research Group, Norwegian Veterinary Institute, 0454 Oslo, Norway; christiane.faste@vetinst.no
2 Nofima—Norwegian Institute of Food, Fisheries and Aquaculture Research, 5141 Fyllingsdalen, Norway; andre.bogevik@Nofima.no
3 Nofima—Norwegian Institute of Food, Fisheries and Aquaculture Research, 6600 Sunndalsøra, Norway; Gerd.Berge@Nofima.no
4 Faculty of Biosciences and Aquaculture, Nord University, 8049 Bodø, Norway; jorge.m.fernandes@nord.no
5 Chemistry Section, Norwegian Veterinary Institute, 0454 Oslo, Norway; lada.ivanova@vetinst.no
* Correspondence: amritha.johny@vetinst.no; Tel.: +47-9026-1691

Received: 11 March 2019; Accepted: 11 April 2019; Published: 13 April 2019

Abstract: New protein sources in fish feed require the assessment of the carry-over potential of contaminants and anti-nutrients from feed ingredients into the fish, and the assessment of possible health risks for consumers. Presently, plant materials including wheat and legumes make up the largest part of aquafeeds, so evaluation of the transfer capabilities of typical toxic metabolites from plant-infesting fungi and of vegetable phytoestrogens into fish products is of great importance. With the aim of facilitating surveillance of relevant mycotoxins and isoflavones, we have developed and validated a multi-analyte LC-HRMS/MS method that can be used to ensure compliance to set maximum levels in feed and fish. The method performance characteristics were determined, showing high specificity for all 25 targeted analytes, which included 19 mycotoxins and three isoflavones and their corresponding aglycons with sufficient to excellent sensitivities and uniform analytical linearity in different matrices. Depending on the availability of matching stable isotope-labelled derivates or similar-structure homologues, calibration curves were generated either by using internal standards or by matrix-matched external standards. Precision and recovery data were in the accepted range, although they varied between the different analytes. This new method was considered as fit-for-purpose and applied for the analysis of customised fish feed containing wheat gluten, soy, or pea protein concentrate as well as salmon and zebrafish fed on diets with these ingredients for a period of up to eight weeks. Only mycotoxin enniatin B, at a level near the limit of detection, and low levels of isoflavones were detected in the feed, demonstrating the effectiveness of maximum level recommendations and modern feed processing technologies in the Norwegian aquaculture industry. Consequently, carry-over into fish muscle was not observed, confirming that fillets from plant-fed salmon were safe for human consumption.

Keywords: Atlantic salmon; zebrafish; liquid chromatography high-resolution mass spectrometry; mycotoxins; phytoestrogens; plant-based feed

Key Contribution: A multi-analyte LC-HRMS/MS method for 25 targeted mycotoxins and phytoestrogens was developed and validated in feed and fish matrices. Mycotoxins above the respective LOD were not detected in feed and dietary exposed fish, whereas phytoestrogens were found in soy and pea protein-based diets but carry-over into fish was not observed.

1. Introduction

Global fish production reached more than 171 million tonnes by 2016, of which 88% were directly used for human consumption and 12% (20 million tonnes) were used for the production of fishmeal and fish oil in aquaculture [1]. Fish and fishery products are an important source of essential nutrients in the human diet, and demand is growing in line with the increasing world population [2]. Aquaculture is the fastest-growing food industry and the intensification of the production depends on the utilisation of other resources for aquafeeds than fishmeal, for which exploitation is reaching an unsustainable level. Therefore, agricultural crops, mainly legumes, cereal grains and oilseeds, have been introduced in steadily increasing amounts into fish feeds, completely or partially replacing marine protein sources [3].

Plant protein sources mainly include soy, pea, lupine, alfalfa, wheat, corn, rape seeds, sunflower seeds, cotton seeds, sesame seeds, mustard oil cake, and white leadtree leaves [4]. Moreover, proteins from insects, microalgae, krill and single-cell proteins have been explored as replacements for fishmeal, but plant proteins are by far the most used ingredients in feed in aquaculture. The considerable changes in the diet composition of farmed fish include ingredients with physicochemical properties that potentially could lead to challenges regarding fish health and welfare, and product quality [5]. However, new processing technologies for plant protein extraction of undesirable components such as fertilisers, pesticides, persistent organic pollutants and heavy metals have allowed the transition from marine to agricultural sources [6]. The growth performance of plant-fed fish has been found to be adequate in short feeding studies [7], but concern about potential negative health effects from natural toxins and anti-nutritional factors including phytoestrogens remains [4,8]. Some anti-nutritional factors are considerably resistant against heat and digestion and have the potential for carry-over into the food chain. Several studies have shown that bioactive compounds may affect physiological functions in animals and humans including negative effects on intestinal health [9]; however, information for fish is limited [4]. The potential transfer of undesirable substances from new sources of aquafeeds might thus lead to potential health risks for consumers of fish products [10]. The assessment of transmissibility requires analytical methods that can be reliably applied for the detection of relevant natural contaminants in agricultural crops, and the considerable prevalence of mycotoxins and phytoestrogens makes them priority target analytes. However, only a few recent studies have surveyed mycotoxin levels in fish feed or farmed fish [11–16], and phytoestrogens are even less investigated [17,18].

There is a risk of mycotoxicosis in farmed fish due to the presence of mycotoxins in plant feed ingredients, but information on effects in fish is limited [11,19]. Mycotoxins comprise a large variety of secondary metabolites produced by fungi such as *Fusarium* spp., *Aspergillus* spp., *Alternaria* spp. and *Pencillium* spp. that infect agricultural crops both in the field and during storage, depending on their preferred growth conditions [20]. The presence of mycotoxins in practically all feed- and foodstuffs worldwide, although at different levels, is critical for nutritional security and safety, and important for animal and human health and welfare [21]. In moderate climate zones, major mycotoxin classes associated with *Fusarium* crop infections are trichothecenes, zearalenones and enniatins. The most important trichothecenes (polycyclic sesquiterpenoids) are A-type HT-2 toxin (HT-2) and T-2 toxin (T-2) and B-type deoxynivalenol (DON), including the acetylated and glucosidated derivatives 3-acetyl-deoxynivalneol (3-ADON), 15-acetyldeoxynivalenol (15-ADON) and deoxynivalenol-3-glucoside (DON-3G), as well as nivalenol (NIV). Furthermore, the mycoestrogen zearalenone (ZEN) shows considerable occurrence and toxicity. The ionophoric enniatins (ENN) B, B1,

A, and A1 are detectable in almost all grain samples and considered an emerging threat [22]. In contrast, toxicity caused by ergot alkaloids such as ergosine, ergonovine, ergotamine, ergocristin, ergocornine and α-ergocryptine in *Claviceps purpurea*-infected cereals has been known as ergotism for centuries. Ergot contamination is a sporadic issue but appears to have increased in recent years. The storage mycotoxin of main concern in Nordic countries is ochratoxin A (OTA), a pentaketidic isocoumarin produced by *Penicillium* or *Aspergillus* sp. In contrast, aflatoxins and fumonisins normally do not occur in Norwegian feed commodities [23]. The European Commission has recommended maximum levels for important mycotoxins in different feed commodities [24]. Fish ingredients and composite fish feed are not specifically mentioned but the guidance levels for DON (5 mg/kg); ZEN (2 mg/kg) and OTA (0.25 mg/kg) also apply to aquaculture. Additionally, an indicative value for the sum of T-2 and HT-2 (250 μg/kg) in compound feed is provided by the EU Commission recommendation [25]. Comparable values have not been established for NIV, enniatins or ergot alkaloids because of the limited occurrence and toxicity data.

Phytoestrogens are plant-derived polyphenolic non-steroidal compounds with structural and functional similarity to animal oestrogens, which can bind to oestrogen receptors and activate oestrogen receptor-dependent pathways in mammals and fish [26]. Thus, they have the potential to disrupt the endocrine system by competing with endogenous hormones. Phytoestrogens can be broadly differentiated into isoflavones, coumestans and lignans, depending on the alkylation pattern in the basic isoflavone molecule structure [27]. Legumes, especially soy, are rich in isoflavones, which occur in plants mainly in glucosidated form, whereas the unconjugated molecules are prevalent after uptake. Important representatives of this substance class are the glucosides daidzin, genistin, glycitin and their respective free counterpart's daidzein, genistein and glycitein [28]. They are also potential substrates for metabolic glucuronidation or sulphatation reactions in the liver and kidneys due to the hydroxyl groups in the molecule and could be excreted as conjugates [29]. Processed soy protein concentrates have an increased aglycon content, which results in improved phytoestrogen absorption from the diet [30]. Exposure of fish to phytoestrogens in feed has been shown to cause reproductive effects and to affect growth and metabolism [31], but the levels in the edible tissue of soy-fed fish and potential human exposure have not been investigated so far.

The assessment of possible health risks from the consumption of fish fed with plant-derived feed requires the development of appropriate analytical methods for the detection of transferred contaminants and bioactive compounds. Mycotoxins are usually analysed by liquid chromatography tandem mass spectrometry (LC-MS/MS) with different multi-toxin methods and in various matrices such as bulk cereals, flour, nuts, food products and hay bales [32–40]. Advanced sampling schemes and extraction protocols have been developed, resulting in improved homogeneity and recovery so that method validation can be performed [41]. Sample preparation often includes single-step solvent extraction using acidic acetonitrile/water mixtures, followed by solid-phase extraction (SPE) or immunoaffinity purification [39]. Matrix effects can be controlled by using matrix-matched calibration and isotope-labelled internal standards (ISTD), which are available for trichothecenes but not for enniatins and ergot alkaloids [32,33,36–38,40]. Notably, fewer LC-MS/MS methods have been described for ergot alkaloids than for *Fusarium* toxins, focussing on rye, feed and seeds as typical matrices [34,37]. In contrast, phytoestrogens are mostly measured in physiological samples including human and animal plasma, milk and urine in connection with monitoring of dietary exposure [42,43]. The LC-MS/MS methods developed for the detection of phytoestrogens in soy and food items use methanol-water extraction and reversed-phase (RP) chromatography [44,45].

Earlier studies have measured several mycotoxins in feed ingredients, aquafeeds and fish fillets [11,13,14,16,46] but ergot alkaloids were not among the analytes. In addition, we have found one report of the occurrence of phytoestrogens in foods of animal origin, including a few fish samples [47]. Considering the potential consumer health risk resulting from the extensive introduction of agricultural crops into fish feed and contaminant carry-over, analytical methods for the reliable detection of natural toxins and bioactive compounds are required. The present study was thus intended to fill this gap by developing a multiplexed LC-MS/MS method for the simultaneous quantification of 25 relevant feed-borne mycotoxins and phytoestrogens in feed and fish.

2. Results and Discussion

2.1. Fish Feed with Fixed Contents of Wheat Gluten, Soy Protein or Pea Protein

Finished feed has to comply with national and international legislation regarding maximum contents of certain contaminants including some mycotoxins [24,25]. In the present study, the fish diets were prepared in a fully equipped feed technology research facility based on materials that are commonly used in Norwegian aquaculture. Since the focus of the fish experiments was the potential transfer of natural contaminants from feed into fish, and not digestibility or feed utilisation, the composition was balanced with regard to plant-based ingredients (Table 1). Constant levels of 15% or 30% wheat gluten, soy protein concentrate or pea protein concentrate were achieved by adjusting the amount of fishmeal, which resulted in slight differences in the total crude protein and total lipid contents between the diets (Table 1). By keeping the ratio of plant-derived ingredients constant, comparability of the analytical results for the targeted metabolites was ensured.

Table 1. Composition of customised salmon and zebrafish feed (FM, fish meal; SPC, soy protein concentrate; PPC, pea protein concentrate).

Diet Composition (g/100 g)	FM (Control)	SPC15	SPC30	WG15	WG30	PPC15	PPC30
Salmon							
Fish meal	63.35	48.35	33.35	48.35	33.35	-	-
Wheat	12.0	12.0	12.0	12.0	12.0	-	-
Soy prot. conc.	-	15.0	30.0	-	-	-	-
Wheat gluten	-	-	-	15.0	30.0	-	-
Fish oil	20.0	20.0	20.0	20.0	20.0	-	-
Additives #	4.65	4.65	4.65	4.65	4.65	-	-
Total protein	45.2	44.6	44.0	46.7	48.1	-	-
Total lipids	26.5	25.1	23.8	25.4	24.3	-	-
Zebrafish							
Fish meal	79.35	64.35	49.35	64.35	49.35	64.35	49.35
Wheat	12.0	12.0	12.0	12.0	12.0	12.0	12.0
Soy prot. conc.	-	15.0	30.0	-	-	-	-
Wheat gluten	-	-	-	15.0	30.0	-	-
Pea prot. conc.	-	-	-	-	-	15.0	30.0
Fish oil	4.0	4.0	4.0	4.0	4.0	4.0	4.0
Additives #	4.65	4.65	4.65	4.65	4.65	4.65	4.65
Total crude protein	56.2	55.6	55.0	57.7	59.1	53.1	49.9
Total lipids	12.0	10.7	9.4	10.9	9.8	11.3	10.7

Additives: Vitamin mix (2%), Mineral mix (0.59%), Monosodiumphosphate-24% P (2%), Yttrium oxide (0.01%), Carophyll Pink-10% (0.05%).

2.2. Exposure of Zebrafish and Salmon to Plant-Derived Aquafeeds

The zebrafish and salmon included in the feeding experiments showed an overall normal growth performance (data not shown). Observable differences in growth rate between diet groups in on-growing salmon in the order of SPC15 > SPC30 > WG15 ≈ FM > WG30 were small but proportional to the feed intake by the same groups. The zebrafish study also included an exposure to PPC15 and PPC30 feed compositions, resulting in a slight growth reduction that had previously also been described for rainbow trout [48]. We considered, however, that the small weight gain differences observed in the present study would not significantly affect the analysis of potentially transmitted contaminants in fish muscle.

2.3. *Characteristics of Targeted Analytes in Method*

The mycotoxins and phytoestrogens included in the multi-analyte LC-HRMS/MS method had considerable differences in their molecular weights and structures (Table S1). Furthermore, there were sizeable differences in compound solubilities, e.g., between the hydrophilic DON, DON-3G, 3-ADON, 15-ADON and NIV and the lipophilic enniatins. These differences, as reflected by the logP (Table S1), became obvious in the order of retention on the reversed-phase LC-column (Figure 1). Molecular structure and logP were obtained from the PubChem database (https://pubchem.ncbi.nlm.nih.gov/). Retention times differed with up to 30 min under the optimised chromatographic conditions of the ammonium acetate/MeOH gradient, while peak widths were small demonstrating good signal resolution. MeOH proved to be the best eluent for combining the different analytes in one LC method. Previous studies have shown that MeOH improves peak shape and sensitivity in the analysis of trichothecenes [32,33,35,37–39] and the same solvent has been used for phytoestrogen chromatography [45].

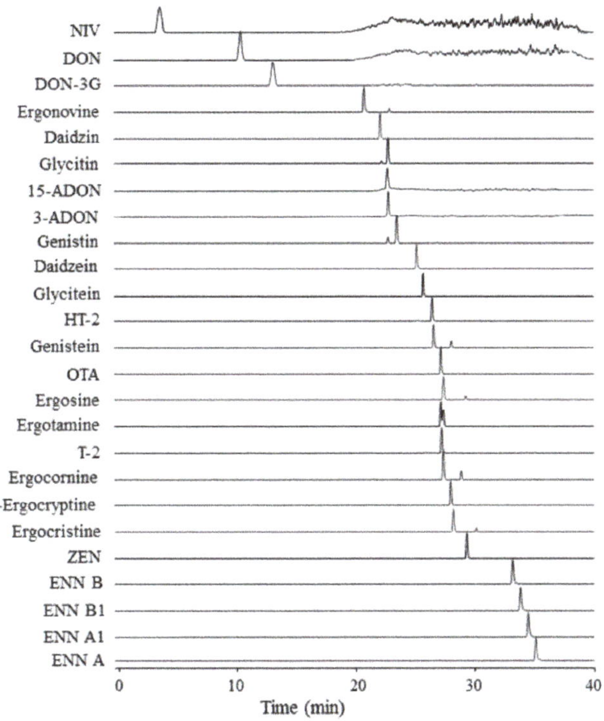

Figure 1. Chromatograms of targeted analysis of 100 µg/L in solvent of the 25 mycotoxins and phytoestrogens included in the multi-analyte LC-HRMS/MS method.

During method development, all compounds were analysed in positive and negative ESI mode for the determination of the highest peak intensities and best target ions, which included proton, ammonium, sodium and acetate adducts (Table 2). The HRMS/MS parameters were adjusted accordingly so that each compound was measured in targeted analysis under optimal conditions.

Table 2. Optimised LC-MS/MS conditions and calibration curve performances (R^2) for target compounds in different matrices.

Compound	Ionisation Mode	Target Ion	RT (min)	Precursor (m/z)	NCE (ev)	Fish Feed (R^2)	Salmon (R^2)	Zebrafish (R^2)	ISTD
DON	ESI neg	$[M+CH_3COO]^-$	12.3	355.1387	17	0.9996	0.9964	0.9996	^{13}C-DON
3-ADON	ESI neg	$[M+CH_3COO]^-$	23.8	397.1493	15	0.9998	0.9975	0.9999	^{13}C-3-ADON
15-ADON	ESI pos	$[M+Na]^+$	23.7	361.1258	15	0.9999	0.9986	0.9969	^{13}C-15-ADON
DON-3G	ESI neg	$[M+CH_3COO]^-$	15.1	517.1916	17	0.9993	0.9935	0.9851	^{13}C-DON-3G
NIV	ESI neg	$[M+CH_3COO]^-$	5.30	371.1337	17	0.9983	0.9901	0.9972	^{13}C-NIV
T-2	ESI pos	$[M+NH_4]^+$	28.0	484.2541	15	0.9995	0.9978	0.9995	^{13}C-T-2
HT-2	ESI neg	$[M+CH_3COO]^-$	26.4	483.2225	15	0.9998	0.9961	0.9998	^{13}C-HT-2
OTA	ESI neg	$[M-H]^-$	27.3	402.0739	32	0.9992	0.9984	0.9998	^{13}C-OTA
ZEN	ESI neg	$[M-H]^-$	29.5	317.1384	50	0.9999	0.9985	0.9998	^{13}C-ZEN
Ergonovine	ESI pos	$[M+H]^+$	21.9	326.1863	50	0.9996	0.9992	0.9999	MetErg
Ergosine	ESI pos	$[M+H]^+$	27.6	548.2868	27	0.9990	0.9979	0.9999	BromCri
Ergotamine	ESI pos	$[M+H]^+$	28.0	582.2711	32	0.9973	0.9985	0.9999	BromCri
Ergocornine	ESI pos	$[M+H]^+$	28.1	562.3024	25	0.9992	0.9973	0.9998	BromCri
α-Ergocryptine	ESI pos	$[M+H]^+$	28.8	576.3180	25	0.9993	0.9980	0.9999	BromCri
Ergoscristine	ESI pos	$[M+H]^+$	29.0	610.3024	27	0.9984	0.9980	0.9999	BromCri
ENN A	ESI pos	$[M+NH_4]^+$	35.1	699.4903	27	0.9943	0.9981	0.9992	-
ENN A1	ESI pos	$[M+NH_4]^+$	34.4	685.4746	27	0.9984	0.9987	0.9991	-
ENN B	ESI pos	$[M+NH_4]^+$	33.1	657.4433	27	0.9986	0.9952	0.9998	-
ENN B1	ESI pos	$[M+NH_4]^+$	33.8	671.4590	27	0.9993	0.9987	0.9993	-
Daidzein	ESI neg	$[M-H]^-$	26.1	253.0506	75	0.9993	0.9980	0.9982	-
Daidzin	ESI neg	$[M+CH_3COO]^-$	23.1	475.1246	10	0.9997	0.9984	0.9998	-
Genistein	ESI neg	$[M-H]^-$	27.3	269.0455	70	0.9997	0.9986	0.9979	-
Genistin	ESI neg	$[M+CH_3COO]^-$	24.4	491.1195	10	0.9994	0.9974	0.9999	-
Glycitein	ESI neg	$[M-H]^-$	26.4	283.0612	35	0.9998	0.9997	0.9989	-
Glycitin	ESI neg	$[M+CH_3COO]^-$	23.6	505.1351	10	0.9994	0.9979	0.9994	-

2.4. Optimisation of Sample Preparation

Appropriate sampling and sample extraction are prerequisites for the reliability of analytical methods [39–41]. Several studies describing sampling strategies for the mitigation of uneven contaminant distribution in different matrices have been published [34]. Sampling plans should aim at achieving pragmatic fit-for-purpose results, providing homogeneity while limiting sample sizes and numbers. In the present experiment, potential distributional heterogeneity was not an issue in the preparation of zebrafish samples since the whole carcasses of three fish were ground and extracted together. In contrast, the salmon fillets were of considerable size and could not be processed in total. Consequently, we attempted to obtain representative samples by punching out tissue at different places in fillet and combining aliquots after grinding (Figure 2a). Additional tissue punches were gathered for proteomic and immunological analyses that were foreseen for subsequent studies (Figure 2b). The composite diets had already a high degree of homogeneity due to the production process. We assumed therefore that the targeted analytes were evenly distributed in samples taken from a few places in the storage bags and ground together.

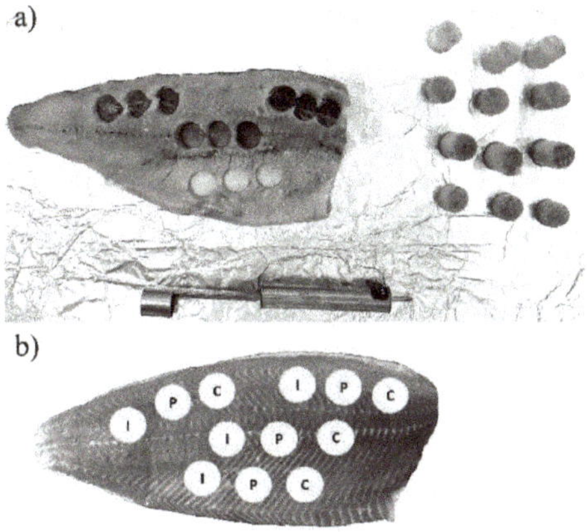

Figure 2. (**a**,**b**) Sampling scheme for homogenous sampling of representative aliquots from a salmon fillet. C: samples used for the chemical analyses in the present study. P and I: samples used for proteomic and immunological analyses in the same project.

Matrix effects impairing analytical method performance can be managed by using clean-up procedures, sample extract dilution, precipitation, filtering, matrix-assisted standard calibration curves and stable-isotope labelled ISTD [34,39]. Clean-up during sample preparation may include passing the extract through immunoaffinity columns or solid-phase extraction (SPE) cartridges, which can be filled with a variety of adsorbents. In the present study, we have not applied clean-up methods during sample preparation to avoid the potential loss of target analytes from surface adhesion. Additionally, the different molecular properties of the 25 compounds would optimally require the use of specific SPE materials. We have therefore attempted to develop a generally applicable sample preparation method by diluting the homogenised material with eight- to tenfold excess of adjusted solvent and using a one-step extraction procedure with subsequent submicron filtering.

Extraction conditions were optimised in a number of preliminary trials by determining recovery rates from spiked matrices with different acidic MeCN/water solvent compositions and, additionally, with a two-step MeCN/water approach [36,40]. However, the two-step extraction produced multiple aqueous and organic layers in the extract, making separation difficult and decreasing analyte recovery. The overall best results for the extraction of the target analytes from feed and fish were achieved with acidic MeCN/water (70:30) (Figure 3), similar to what has been described for other multi-mycotoxin methods [36,37]. This solvent was also suitable for the phytoestrogens that have been extracted with MeOH/water in previous studies [44,45].

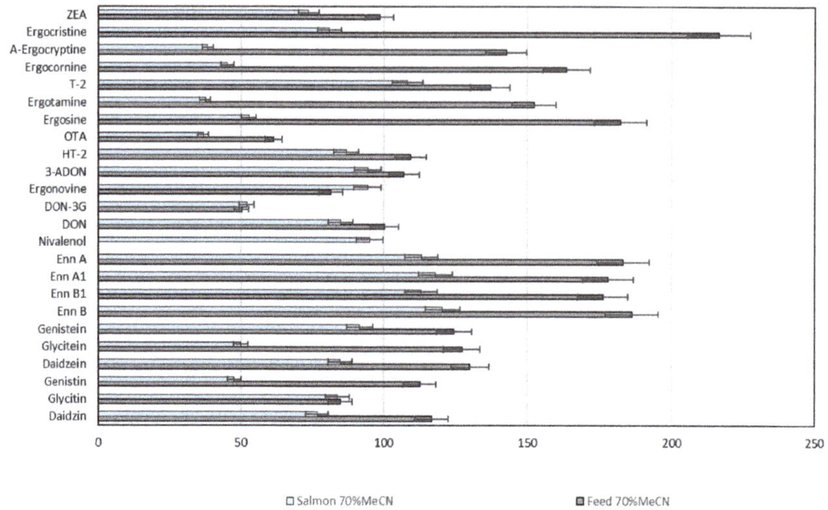

Figure 3. Recovery rates from spiked fish and feed matrices for the mycotoxins and phytoestrogens included in the multi-analyte LC-HRMS/MS method using optimised extraction solvent.

2.5. *Performance of the Multi-Analyte LC-HRMS/MS Method*

The performance characteristics of the new LC-HRMS/MS method for 25 mycotoxins and phytoestrogens were determined with regard to international standardised guidelines [49,50]. The specificity of the method for the selected analytes was excellent due to the high mass accuracy in full scan mode and targeted fragmentation (dd-MS^2) (Figure 1; Table 2). The total run time was slightly increased in comparison to other multi-mycotoxin methods [32,33,35,37–39,41], leading to good chromatographic separation of the analytes. The high resolution of the analysis allowed us to resolve between isomers such as 3-ADON and 15-ADON, which previously has been sometimes a challenge [41].

The 25 analytes were detected with different sensitivities in fish and feed matrices differed considerably between the 25 analytes. The salmon matrix-assisted standard calibration curves showed high sensitivities for the enniatins, ZEN and the phytoestrogens daidzein and genistein, whereas the curve slopes were less steep for the trichothecenes, OTA, ergot alkaloids and remaining phytoestrogens. Interestingly, this order was not identical for solvent, zebrafish and feed matrices, comparable to results reported for other multi-mycotoxin methods that achieved different analyte sensitivities in matrices such as fruit, yoghurt, soya, hazelnut, pepper, wheat, maize, oat, rice, pasta and bread [33,35–38]. The effect of the signal enhancement or suppression by a specific matrix type can be illustrated by the connected SSE% value. Matrix impact is considered as insignificant for SSE 80-120%, while lower values indicate significant signal decrease and higher values signal increase [32,33,35,37–40]. In the present study, SSE varied from 67% to 115% for control fish feed, 58% to 173% for salmon, and 89% to 181% for zebrafish, with ENN A showing the highest signals in the feed and fish matrices (Table 3). Considering all analytes, the feed matrix generally suppressed signals, whereas the fish matrix caused signal enhancement.

Linearity of the standard calibration curves in different matrices was achieved for all analytes in the range 1.0 to 200 µg/L, with the exception of NIV, OTA, DON-3G and 15-ADON that were linear in the range 5.0 to 200 µg/L. The correlation coefficients (Table 2) were $R^2 > 0.98$ for all calibration curves, irrespectively of whether or not stable-isotope labelled ISTD, similar analogue-ISTD or no ISTD were included. Considering the eight times or 10 times sample dilution during matrix extraction, the linear ranges corresponded to 8.0 (40)–1600 μg/kg for feed and salmon and 10 (50)–2000 μg/kg for zebrafish.

The limits of detection (LOD) and quantification (LOQ) in solvent, fish feed, salmon and zebrafish matrices are presented for the undiluted commodities (Table 3). The LOD ranged in solvent from 1 μg/L for ENN A1, B, B1 and genistin to 19 μg/L for NIV, in fish feed from 6 μg/kg for 15-ADON to 85 μg/kg for ENN A, in salmon from 21 μg/kg for glycitein to 144 μg/kg for NIV, and in zebrafish from 8.0 μg/kg for ergonovine and α-ergocryptine to 176 μg/kg for DON-3G. The corresponding LOQ were, as per the definition, 3.3 times higher (Table 3). The values were similar to data shown for comparable multi-mycotoxin methods. LOD ranging from 5.4 to 24 μg/kg for DON, 36 to 50 μg/kg for 15-ADON, 2.8 to 50 μg/kg for NIV, 0.2 to 47 μg/kg for ZEN, 1.0 to 18 μg/kg for T-2, and 0.7 to 12 μg/kg were reported in a number of different matrices [32,35–38]. In contrast, two methods that had been specially developed for the analysis of phytoestrogens in food products had established group LODs of, respectively, 250 μg/kg [44] and 15 μg/kg [45].

The precision of our multi-analyte LC-HRMS/MS method was demonstrated on the one hand by good day-to-day congruency of the solvent and matrix-assisted standard calibration curves. The coefficients of variation (% CV) for all data points in six independent experiments were generally less than 20% in solvent and less than 25% in feed, salmon and zebrafish matrices (data not shown), which was well within the guidance criteria [49]. On the other hand, precision was also assessed by intra-day and inter-day analysis of spiked quality control samples. The total within-laboratory precision was in the range of 1% for ZEN and ENN A to 17% for NIV in the feed matrix and 1% for ergonovine to 41% for NIV in the salmon matrix (Table 3). The precision data were comparable to values reported for other multi-mycotoxin methods in a variety of matrices [32,35,37,38,41]. Published precision data for phytoestrogen analysis in food commodities are scarce. When control samples were analysed using standard calibration in solvent, intra-day and inter-day% CV in the range of 1–13% were reached for a number of analytes [45].

Recovery rates in fish feed ranged from 19% to 161% for all mycotoxins and phytoestrogens in the newly developed method, with the exception of DON-3G, NIV, ergosine, ergotamine, ergocornine and α-ergocryptine that were retrieved less efficiently, and ENN A and ENN A1 that showed enhanced recoveries (Table 3). In the salmon matrix, the analytes were recovered with 69–127% except for a reduced performance for NIV and enhancement for genistein. In the zebrafish matrix, recovery rates of 41–98% were reached, except in DON-3G and NIV, which showed reduced values. The recovery rates established in the present study were similar to those determined with comparable methods ranging from 50% to 150% for a number of mycotoxins [32,35–41]. For phytoestrogens, recoveries between 89% and 107% in spiked solvent have been reported [45]. However, in different food matrices the rates were widely varying and in part very low, which is in strong contrast to our new LC-HRMS/MS method, showing remarkably low interference for phytoestrogen analysis in the three matrices considered (Table 3). Spiking experiments are widely used for the determination of recoveries in the validation of analytical methods, although they only can emulate naturally-contaminated samples to a certain extent. Preferably, the accuracy should be verified with a certified reference material, but this is currently not available for all target analytes and selected matrices of the LC-HRMS/MS method.

Table 3. Performance validation parameters for the multi-analyte LC-HRMS/MS method (*n* = number of analysis for each category; a: solvent; b: fish feed; c: salmon; d: zebrafish).

Compound	*n*	LOD				LOQ				SSE (%)	Total within Laboratory Precision (%)		Recovery ± SD (%)		
		(µg/L)	(µg/kg)			(µg/L)	(µg/kg)								
	(a/b/c/d)	(a)	(b)	(c)	(d)	(a)	(b)	(c)	(d)	(b/c/d)	(b)	(c)	(b)	(c)	(d)
with ISTD															
DON	4/4/3/3	3	23	67	22	9	78	225	74	77/87/133	4	4	90 ± 7	107 ± 13	92 ± 25
3-ADON	4/4/3/3	4	17	57	9	15	56	189	29	98/116/144	3	3	112 ± 17	96 ± 12	78 ± 20
15-ADON	4/3/3/3	5	6	43	63	16	20	142	210	96/161/141	10	3	133 ± 2	107 ± 25	86 ± 14
DON-3G	4/4/3/3	5	36	115	176	18	121	383	588	85/95/119	11	22	19 ± 9	83 ± 20	48 ± 31
NIV	4/4/3/3	19	59	144	76	63	196	479	252	71/65/115	17	41	57 ± 34	69 ± 33	41 ± 24
T-2	4/4/3/3	4	26	53	26	12	88	176	86	97/136/151	3	3	96 ± 17	99 ± 15	90 ± 19
HT-2	4/4/3/3	2	22	70	15	8	73	235	52	89/129/149	2	3	94 ± 18	96 ± 11	98 ± 15
OTA	4/4/3/3	5	41	44	21	18	138	148	68	105/139/150	6	4	75 ± 13	87 ± 23	83 ± 20
ZEN	4/4/3/3	6	11	43	14	22	38	143	47	90/125/125	1	2	109 ± 5	106 ± 18	96 ± 25
Ergonovine	4/4/3/3	6	23	35	8	19	77	115	26	85/130/106	2	1	84 ± 8	98 ± 13	87 ± 30
Ergosine	4/4/3/3	4	35	52	9	12	117	173	32	79/129/138	7	11	69 ± 27	89 ± 31	72 ± 20
Ergotamine	4/4/3/3	2	59	56	10	8	195	188	35	81/134/155	10	9	64 ± 10	84 ± 26	77 ± 18
Ergocornine	4/4/3/3	3	32	59	16	11	108	196	53	93/129/136	11	11	59 ± 16	90 ± 26	70 ± 14
α-Ergocryptine	4/4/3/3	4	15	38	8	14	50	126	28	67/119/137	7	8	53 ± 7	82 ± 21	70 ± 14
Ergoscristine	4/4/3/3	3	30	51	10	10	100	170	32	70/117/135	8	5	77 ± 22	88 ± 24	54 ± 26
without ISTD															
ENN A	4/4/3/3	4	85	49	32	13	284	165	108	115/173/181	1	8	161 ± 14	117 ± 27	81 ± 17
ENN A1	4/4/3/3	1	45	40	33	5	150	133	111	102/122/148	3	11	147 ± 21	110 ± 29	80 ± 16
ENN B	4/4/3/3	1	41	78	17	4	138	260	57	95/132/152	2	10	117 ± 16	107 ± 30	79 ± 17
ENN B1	4/4/3/3	1	29	40	29	5	96	133	96	102/125/147	3	12	134 ± 9	106 ± 35	79 ± 17
Daidzein	4/4/3/3	13	30	50	48	42	100	168	159	86/120/101	4	13	123 ± 9	122 ± 18	93 ± 15
Daidzin	4/4/3/3	3	19	45	15	12	62	152	51	86/113/140	4	16	93 ± 21	93 ± 6	71 ± 13
Genistein	4/4/3/3	11	20	42	52	37	66	141	172	81/120/104	2	13	114 ± 23	127 ± 28	91 ± 18
Genistin	4/4/3/3	1	29	72	11	5	95	241	35	101/143/149	4	12	101 ± 45	88 ± 1	69 ± 14
Glycitein	4/4/3/3	11	18	21	37	36	58	68	124	80/58/89	2	16	127 ± 3	118 ± 24	96 ± 16
Glycitin	4/4/3/3	4	27	51	26	13	90	170	88	94/123/121	4	23	96 ± 14	113 ± 13	97 ± 22

2.6. Mycotoxins and Phytoestrogens in Fish Feed, Zebrafish and Salmon Tissues

The in-house-validated multi-analyte LC-HRMS/MS method was used for the analysis of the customised fish feed and dietary exposed salmon and zebrafish. The feed analysis did not detect any of the targeted mycotoxins, with the exception of ENN B that was found in concentrations close to LOD in WG30 (data not shown). Norwegian aquafeeds ingredients contain generally only low amount of mycotoxins [13,23]. The highest mean contents were found in wheat (DON: 94 μg/kg; T-2+HT-2: 28 μg/kg) and maize (ZEN: 246 μg/kg), which was in compliance with the recommended maximum levels [24,25,51]. Considering that in the present study, the feed contained a maximum of 42% wheat-derived components (WG30) (Table 1), we did not expect sizable levels in the five diets. In contrast, survey data for finished feeds from Central Europe and Asia contained on average 165 μg DON/kg, 188 μg ZEN/kg and 2 μg OTA/kg [11]. Interestingly, our finding of ENN B in WG30 diets is in line with the relatively high prevalence of enniatins in cereals in Northern Europe. ENNs have shown considerable toxicity in in vitro studies and in mice [52]. Carry-over of ENN B and B1 from poultry feed into eggs has been demonstrated [22], but maximum levels for animal feed have not been established yet.

In view of the low mycotoxin content (<LOQ) in the customised feeds in the present study, we consequently did not detect any of the targeted analytes above the respective LOQ in salmon or zebrafish tissues. There were, however, traces of ENN B in several of the WG30-exposed salmon at concentrations close to the LOD, suggesting the carry-over potential of enniatins. A relatively high occurrence of ENNs, especially ENN B, in fish muscle and livers has been previously reported [22,53] and correlates with our data. Transfer of mycotoxins such as DON, T-2 and OTA from low-level contaminated wheat gluten-containing feed into fish fillets has also been demonstrated [13]. In contrast, when salmon was fed with diets containing 2 and 6 mg DON/kg or 0.8 and 2.4 mg OTA/kg for eight weeks, up to 19 μg DON/kg was measured in the muscle, whereas up to 5 μg OTA/kg was detectable in the fish livers [46]. Human exposure following high consumption of salmon fillets with the highest DON concentrations was estimated to amount to only 2% of the established tolerable daily intake (TDI) [46,54]. Consequently, our results in the present study show that the use of plant-based fish feed containing mycotoxins below the recommended maximum levels results in negligible health risks for consumers.

The phytoestrogen analysis of the diets included in the salmon and zebrafish feeding experiments showed dose-dependent levels of all targeted analytes in the soy protein containing feeds (data not shown). Mean concentrations ranged in SPC15 from 21 μg glycitein/kg to 786 μg daidzin/kg and in SPC30 from 40 μg glycitein/kg to 1356 μg daidzin/kg. Glucosidated forms occurred in higher concentrations than the corresponding aglycons, whereas an increase of the free form had been previously observed in extruded protein preparations [30]. In PPC15 and PPC30, 26 and 54 μg glycitein/kg were detected, respectively, confirming results from a screening study on fruits and vegetables [45]. Phytoestrogen levels in food and feed are not regulated so far, and the health risks or benefits of dietary exposure in humans and animals are still under discussion [28,44]. Still, considerable oestrogenic and thyrogenic activities have been determined in vitro in commercial Spanish fish feeds [18], and further evaluation is required. A survey of the phytoestrogen content in food products of animal origin detected the highest concentrations in soy-containing milk products and farmed salmon contained up to 40 μg/kg [47].

In the present experiment, we did not find phytoestrogen concentrations above LOQ in dietary exposed zebrafish or salmon, not even in the respective SPC30 groups. Information on the uptake of isoflavones in fish is not available, but considerable differences in bioavailabilities and biotransformation are reported for warm-blooded vertebrate species [55]. We have recently studied the metabolism of isoflavones in salmon liver microsomes (article in progress) and characterised the major metabolites. Chromatographic peaks corresponding to the retention times and m/z of these metabolites were, however, absent in the muscle of the dietary exposed fish suggesting an efficient detoxification mechanism and excretion of isoflavones without accumulation in the edible parts of fish. Equol, an intestinal metabolite of daidzein, has not been studied in our experiment. Previous studies have suggested that isoflavone metabolisation by the intestinal microbiome varies considerably between producers and non-producers of equol [55]. When gibel carp (*Carassius auratus gibelio*) were exposed to 40–400 mg daidzein/kg in feed, the unchanged compound was recovered with 128 and 261 μg/kg in the fish muscle [56]. In contrast, equol was not found in any of the samples suggesting that fish could lack the necessary gut bacteria. Considering that the highest daidzein level in our experiments was with 0.2 mg/kg in SPC30, about 200-fold smaller than the lowest feed concentration in the gibel carp study, and considering the LOQ of the LC-HRMS/MS method in the fish matrix, the non-detectability of the targeted isoflavones in the salmon fillets was conclusive. However, we intend to investigate the metabolic fate of important isoflavones in fish in depth in a follow-up study.

3. Conclusions

The increasing use of vegetable ingredients in aquafeeds has motivated risk evaluations for mycotoxin exposure of farmed fish, which has resulted in the establishment of recommended maximum levels. Furthermore, the potential consequences of the presence of bioactive compounds such as isoflavones in plant-based feed should be monitored. We have therefore developed and validated a 25-in-1 LC-HRMS/MS method that is suitable for the survey of compliance to feed regulations and for the detection of undesirable compounds in fish fillets. The new method has excellent specificity for all analytes, while there are some differences in sensitivity due to the great diversity of molecular structures. The LOD and LOQ in fish feed, zebrafish and salmon matrices are sufficient to ensure that mycotoxin and phytoestrogen levels are below concentrations that might cause negative health effects. The accuracy of the method, described by precision and recovery of the included analytes, is satisfactory, confirming its applicability for screening and surveillance purposes. The applicability range is limited at present, however, due to the exclusion of aflatoxins. They will be added during the planned extension of the multi-analyte method. In zebrafish and salmon exposed to customised feed containing up to 30% wheat gluten, soy or pea protein concentrate, carry-over of mycotoxins or phytoestrogens could not be detected, confirming that fillets from fish fed commercial plant-based diets are safe for consumption.

4. Materials and Methods

4.1. Chemicals

LC-MS grade acetonitrile (MeCN), methanol (MeOH) and water (Optima, LC/MS grade,) were provided by Fisher Scientific (Loughborough, Leics., UK), and ethanol (EtOH) was obtained from VWR International (Lutterworth, Leics., UK). Acetic acid (CH_3COOH) (>99.8%), formic acid (HCOOH) (>98%) and ammonium acetate (CH_3COONH_4) (>98%) were purchased from Merck KGaA (Darmstadt, Germany).

The mycotoxins deoxynivalenol (DON), 3-actetyl-deoxynivalenol (3-ADON), nivalenol (NIV), T-2 toxin (T-2), HT-2 toxin (HT-2), zearalenone (ZEN), deoxynivalenol-3-glucoside (DON-3G), 15-acetyl-deoxynivalenol (15-ADON), ochratoxin A (OTA), ergosine, α-ergocryptine and ergocristine as well as the stable isotope-labelled analogues U-[^{13}C-15]-NIV, U-[^{13}C-15]-DON, U-[^{13}C-21]-DON-3G, U-[^{13}C-17]-3ADON, U-[^{13}C-17]-15ADON, U-[^{13}C-22]-HT-2, U-[^{13}C-24]-T-2, U-[^{13}C-20]-OTA, U-[^{13}C-18]-ZEN were provided by Romer labs (Tulln, Austria) as solutions in MeCN, ranging from 10 to 100 mg/L. Intermediate standard solutions at 10 mg/L were prepared for DON-3G and 15-ADON by dilution of stock solutions with MeCN. The enniatins A, A1, B, and B1 (ENN A, A1, B, B1), ergonovine, ergotamine, ergocornine, methysergide maleate salt (MetErg) and bromocriptine mesylate (BromCri) were provided as solids by Sigma-Aldrich (St. Louis, MO, USA). Stock solutions in MeOH or MeCN were prepared for ergot alkaloids in the range of 100 to 500 mg/L, and for enniatins with 200 mg/L in MeOH. A combined intermediate standard solution with 10 mg/L was prepared for both enniatins and ergot alkaloids by combining appropriate aliquots of stock standard solutions, evaporating the mixture with a gentle stream of nitrogen and re-dissolving in MeCN/water (50:50). Finally, a combined standard solution containing all mycotoxins (Set A) was prepared by combining aliquots of stock or intermediate standard solutions, evaporating the solvent and re-dissolving in the appropriate volume MeCN/water (50:50) to obtain final concentrations of about 200 μg/L (200.0–200.12 μg/L, depending on the stock solution provided by the manufacturer).

The phytoestrogens daidzin, genistin, glycitin, daidzein, genistein, and glycitein were bought in crystalline form from Sigma-Aldrich (St. Louis, MO, USA), and stock solutions were prepared in MeOH or DMSO (glycitein) ranging from 500 to 1000 mg/L. Individual intermediate standard solutions at a concentration of 5 mg/L were prepared by dilution with MeOH. A combined standard solution (Set B; 200 μg/L) containing all phytoestrogens was prepared by further dilution in MeCN/water (50:50). The finished Set A and Set B solutions were stable at −20 °C for several months and used for the preparation of standard calibration curves.

Additionally, a 25-in-1 multi-analyte mixture was prepared and used in spiking experiments. All analytes were combined with regard to the concentrations of their respective stocks or intermediate standard solutions so that a final concentration of 25 μg/L per analyte was reached after spiking into feed, zebrafish and salmon samples. The multi-analyte mixture was evaporated and re-dissolved in MeCN/water (50:50). It was stable at −20 °C for about a month.

A combined internal standard (ISTD) solution for 15 mycotoxins, containing stable isotope-labelled analogues and the ergot homologues MetErg and BromCri, was prepared in MeCN/water (50:50) to reach final concentrations of 251 μg/L U-[^{13}C-18]-ZEN, 500 μg/L U-[^{13}C-22]-HT-2, 443 μg/L U-[^{13}C-22]-T-2, 506 μg/L U-[^{13}C-15]-DON, 502 μg/L U-[^{13}C-17]-3ADON, 500 μg/L U-[^{13}C-17]-15ADON, 500 μg/L U-[^{13}C-20]-OTA, 530 μg/L U-[^{13}C-15]-NIV, 530 μg/L U-[^{13}C-21]-DON-3G, 624 μg/L BromCri and 500 μg/L MetErg. The different concentrations were chosen with regard to the respective measurement sensitivities in the developed multi-analyte LC-HRMS/MS method. The ISTD solution was stored at −20 °C, adjusted to room temperature (RT) and mixed thoroughly prior to use. It was added in a ratio of 1:5 to the study samples.

4.2. Preparation of Fish Diets

Diets with definite amounts of wheat gluten, soy protein concentrate or pea protein concentrate were produced at Nofima Feed Technology Centre, Fyllingsdalen, Norway. The diets were based on fishmeal (FM) as main protein source, which was replaced by 15% or 30% plant proteins. All diets contained 12% wheat that was required for binding in the extrusion process, in addition to minor inclusion of wheat as carrier for some of the additives used (Table 1). In total seven diets were produced: (1) control feed (FM), (2) 15% soy protein concentrate (SPC15), (3) 30% soy protein concentrate (SPC30), (4) 15% wheat gluten (WG15), (5) 30% wheat gluten (WG30), (6) 15% pea protein concentrate (PPC15), and (7) 30% pea protein concentrate (PPC30). The ingredients used for the preparation of diets included FM Norsildmel AS (Bergen, Norway), SPC from Agilia A/S (Videbæk, Denmark), PPC from AM Nutrition AS (Stavanger, Norway) and WG from Tereos Syral (Marckolsheim, France). All diets had an inclusion of 4% fish oil at extrusion. The feed were produced on a pilot scale twin-screw, co-rotating Wenger TX 52 extruder (Wenger, Sabetha, KS., USA) with a die of 2.5 mm diameter. After extrusion, the diets were dried for 40–70 min in a carousel dryer (Paul Klöckner, Verfahrenstechnik GmbH, Hachenburg, Germany) at 65 °C to a water content of 7–8%. The salmon diets 1 to 5 were, in addition, oil-coated with 16% fish oil after extrusion by vacuum-coating (Dinnissen, Sevenum, Netherlands) to meet the standard dietary inclusion of oil for the fish size studied. The salmon feed had a pellet size of 3.5 mm, while the zebrafish feed were ground and sieved to a pellet size of 0.6–0.8 mm.

4.3. Feeding Studies in Zebrafish and On-Growing Salmon

4.3.1. Zebrafish

Four-month-old zebrafish (*Danio rerio*) (AB strain) with a mean weight of 0.214 g were distributed into 28 tanks (n = 16) and were maintained in a flow-through system with 20 % water exchange per hour (ZebTEC Stand-Alone Toxicology Rack, Techniplast, London, UK) under daily-monitored standard husbandry conditions, including a stable temperature of 28 ± 0.5 °C, pH 7.5, water conductivity of 1500 µS/cm and photoperiod of 12 h light:12 h dark at the Faculty of Biosciences and Aquaculture, Nord University, Bodø, Norway. The feeding study included 336 fish that were distributed into the system's 3.5-litre tanks according to the seven experimental diets. Four replicate groups per diet, each consisting of 12 fish (six per gender) in one tank (and an additional four fish to compensate for potential losses during the study period), were hand-fed twice daily with a total feed amount equal to 2.5% of their body weight over a period of 46 days. The feeding behaviour and health and welfare of the fish were regularly controlled. At the end of the study, the fish were not fed for 24 h prior to sampling. They were separated by gender and euthanised individually by transfer into a tank containing a lethal dose of 200 mg/L tricaine methanesulfonate (MS222) (Sigma-Aldrich, St. Louis, MO, USA), buffered with an equal amount of sodium bicarbonate. The liver, spleen and intestines were carefully dissected under a light microscope and immediately frozen in liquid nitrogen along with the rest of the carcass. All samples were stored at −80 °C for further analyses.

The zebrafish feeding study was conducted in compliance with the guidelines provided by the Norwegian Animal Research Authority (FOTS ID 12581, 27 July 2017) and approved by the Nord University (Norway) ethics committee.

4.3.2. Salmon

One-year-old post-smolt Atlantic salmon (*Salmo salar*; salmo breed strain) with a mean weight of 223 g were randomly distributed into 15 experimental tanks (1 m^3; n = 32) filled with seawater at the Nofima Research Station, Sunndalsøra, Norway. The oil-coated diets 1–5 were given to randomised triplicate tanks by automatic disc feeders. Excess feed was collected once daily for calculation of feed intake. The water temperature was maintained at an average of 10.6 (±0.6) °C. The oxygen level at the tank outlets was higher than 90% at study start and about 80% at the study's end. The water flow in each tank was set to 20 L/min.

The feeding was conducted for nine weeks. At the start of the experiment, 15 fish were sampled, and the muscle, liver and intestine were collected. After five weeks, muscle was sampled from one fish from each tank of the FM, SPC30 and WG30 groups. At the termination of the study, five fish from each tank were collected and weighed. The sampled fish were anaesthetised with 60–80 mg/L MS222, transferred and euthanised with a double dose (120–160 mg/L) MS222. Blood was drawn from the caudal vein using 2.5-mL vacutainers (VACUETTE® 2.5 mL Z serum separator clot activator; Greiner Bio-One, Kremsmünster, Austria) and centrifuged at 2500× *g* for 15 min at 4 °C (Allegra 6R Centrifuge, Beckman, Indianapolis, IN, USA), and sera were stored at −20 °C. The livers and intestines of the fish were removed, and tissue samples were frozen with liquid nitrogen and stored at −80 °C. Fillets were stored at −20 °C. The remaining fish in each tank were weighed in bulk, and their mean weight was calculated, including the sampled fish.

The salmon feeding study was performed in compliance with the national regulations for the use of animals in experiments [57]. The experiment was classified as not requiring a specific license [58] as none of the planned experimental treatments were expected to cause any distress or discomfort for the fish.

4.4. Extraction of Fish Feed, Zebrafish and Salmon Samples

4.4.1. Fish Feed

Fish feed pellets were homogenised with a grinding mill (Retsch, Haan, Germany), and 2.5 g were weighed into 50-mL polypropylene tubes. After the addition of 20 mL extraction solvent, the samples were vortexed for 1 min, extracted on a horizontal shaker (Edmund Bühler, Tübingen, Germany) with 200 min^{-1} at room temperature (RT) for 30 min, and centrifuged with 2000× *g* for 10 min at 4 °C (Beckman Coulter, Brea, CT, USA). The supernatants were transferred into fresh 50-mL tubes and let to settle overnight (ON) at 4 °C. Subsequently, 0.5 mL of the supernatants were centrifuged for 1 min at 20,000× *g* through 0.22 µm nylon filters (Costar Spin-X; Corning, Inc., Corning, NY, USA) and 40 µL of the filtrates were transferred into LCMS vials. Finally, 10 µL ISTD solution were added to each vial. Samples were store refrigerated until analysis by LC-HRMS/MS.

The composition of the extraction solvent was optimised during method development in spiking experiments. Multi-analyte mixture (50 µL) was added to 2.5 g ground feed, which was then kept under a laminar hood for 30 min, allowing the solvent to evaporate. Extractions were performed either in one step with 20 mL acidic (0.1% formic acid (FA)) MeCN/water mixtures of different compositions (50:50; 60:40; 70:30; or 80:20) or in two steps with acidic MeCN/water (I: 80:20; II: 20:80). Based on the best recovery rates for mycotoxins and phytoestrogens, MeCN/water (70:30; 0.1% FA) was selected for all further experiments.

4.4.2. Zebrafish

Three frozen, gutted zebrafish, for each replicate and diet, were thawed and, after separation of the heads, ground to a fine powder with pestle and mortar in liquid nitrogen. The powdered tissue (0.1 g) was weighed and extracted with 1 mL extraction solvent (MeCN/water 70:30; 0.1% FA). The mixture was homogenised by ultra-sonication (Branson, Danbury, CT, USA) for 10 min at 30 °C, centrifuged at 4000× *g* for 10 min at 4 °C (Thermo Scientific, Waltham, MA, USA), and the supernatant was transferred into fresh 5-mL tubes. An aliquot (0.5 mL) was filtered as described before, and 40 µL of the filtrates were transferred into LCMS vials, mixed with 10 µL of the ISTD solution, and analysed by LC-HRMS/MS.

The recoveries of mycotoxins and phytoestrogens from the zebrafish matrix was investigated during method development by different acidic MeCN/water extraction solvents in spiking experiments with multi-analyte mixture.

4.4.3. Salmon

The salmon fillets were half-thawed. Tissue pieces of equal size were sampled from four different areas using a steel puncher (0.5 cm in diameter) (Figure 2). The tissue samples were ground with a pestle and mortar, combined, and 2.5 g were transferred into a 50-mL tube, extracted with 20 mL extraction solvent (MeCN/water 70:30; 0.1% FA) and thoroughly homogenised for 40 s by ultra-turrax (Janke & Kunkel, IKA-Werke, Staufen, Germany). To avoid cross-contamination, the ultra-turrax was washed with water for 20 s between samples from the same fish tank and with water and MeOH for 40 s between samples from different tanks. The samples were vortexed for 30 s and extracted using a horizontal shaker (Edmund Bühler) with 200 min^{-1} at RT for 1 h. Subsequently, they were centrifuged with 2000× *g* for 10 min at 4 °C (Beckman Coulter), and the supernatants were transferred into fresh 50-mL tubes and let to settle overnight at 4 °C. Subsequently, 0.5-mL aliquots were filtered as described before, and 40 µL of the filtrates were transferred into LCMS vials, mixed with 10 µL of the ISTD solution, and analysed by LC-HRMS/MS. The recovery of mycotoxins and phytoestrogens from the salmon matrix was investigated as described for zebrafish.

4.5. *Preparation of Matrix-Assisted Standard Calibration Curves*

Calibration curves in solvent were prepared by evaporating 200 µL Set A solution with nitrogen and re-dissolving with 200 µL Set B, resulting in a standard solution with 200 µg/L for all 25 analytes included in this study. The standard solution was serially diluted with MeCN/water (50:50) to produce calibrants with 200, 100, 50, 10, 5 and 1 µg/L. For the preparation of the matrix-assisted standard calibration curves, 40 µL aliquots of the calibrants were transferred into LCMS vials and 10 µL ISTD solution was added. They were evaporated with nitrogen at 40 °C and re-dissolved in the same volume of blank matrix extract that had been prepared either from control feed or from zebrafish or salmon in the respective FM-control groups by pooling equal volumes of replicates. The calibration standards were transferred into LCMS vials and analysed by LC-HRMS/MS.

4.6. *Development of the Multi-Analyte Liquid Chromatography High-Resolution Mass Spectrometry (LC-HRMS/MS) Method*

Multi-analyte analysis was performed on a Q-Exactive™ Hybrid Quadrupole-Orbitrap HRMS/MS equipped with a heated electrospray ion source (HESI-II) and coupled to a Vanquish UHPLC system (Thermo Scientific). The instrument setup was similar to that described in a previous study [36]; however, there were several modifications and different analytes were included. The HESI-II interface was operated at 300 °C, alternatively in positive and negative mode during one run. The parameters were adjusted as follows: spray voltage 3.2 and 2.5 kV (positive and negative mode, respectively), capillary temperature 280 °C, sheath gas flow rate 35 L/min, auxiliary gas flow rate 10 L/min, and S-lens RF level 55.

The Q-Exactive HRMS/MS was operated in full scan (FS) mode with the inclusion of targeted fragmentation (data-dependent MS/MS: dd-MS^2). For full scans, the mass ranges were set to *m/z* 90–900 and 200–900 in negative and positive mode, respectively. FS data were acquired at a mass resolution of 70,000 full width half-maximum (FWHM) at *m/z* 200, while mass resolution was set to 17,500 FWHM at *m/z* 200 during dd-MS2. The automated gain control (AGC) target was set to 5×10^5 ions for a maximum injection time (IT) of 250 ms in the FS mode, whereas for dd-MS^2 mode the AGC target was 1×10^5 and the IT was 100 ms. The inclusion list for the targeted analysis contained the *m/z*, retention times (RT), and normalised collision energies (NCE) (Table 2). NCE values were determined by direct infusion of standard solutions in the mobile phase (MeCN/water (50:50), containing 5 mM ammonium acetate and 0.1% acetic acid) by using a syringe pump at a flow rate of 5 µL/min. The quadrupole mass filter was operated with an isolation window of *m/z* 3. External mass calibration of the Q-Exactive HRMS/MS was performed every three days over the mass range *m/z* 90–2000, in accordance with the manufacturer's instructions. The identification of the 25 mycotoxins and phytoestrogens included in the multi-analyte method was supported by the determination of specific retention times, fragmentation patterns and accurate masses, which were obtained using a mass accuracy window of ±5 ppm with respect to the theoretical accurate masses (Table S1). Chromatographic separation was achieved at 30 °C on a 150 × 2.1 mm Kinetex reversed-phase F5 column (2.6 µm, 100Å; Phenomenex, Torrance, CA, USA) with a 0.5 µm × 0.004″ ID, HPLC KrudKatcher Ultra Column In-Line filter. The flow rate of the mobile phase was 0.25 mL/min, and the injection volume was 1 µL. Eluent A was water and eluent B was MeOH (both containing 5 mM ammonium acetate and 0.1% acetic acid). Since the solubility of ammonium acetate in MeOH is limited, it was first dissolved in 25 mL water before MeOH was added. The total run time was 43 min, and gradient elution was employed starting at 3% B for 1 min, linearly increasing to 15% B in 15 min, to 79% B in 10 min, and finally, to 100% B in 13 min. After washing the column for 2 min with 100% B, the mobile phase was returned to the initial conditions and the column was eluted isocratically for 2.5 min. The column was regularly washed with 70% methanol to prevent cross-contamination. Calibration standards and samples were analysed in randomised order and intercepted with blank solvent samples to minimise analytical bias from sample positions and to reduce sample-to-sample carry-over.

4.7. Validation of the Multi-Analyte LC-HRMS/MS Method

The method was validated with regard to the guidelines established by the International Organization for Standardization [49,50]. The analytical selectivity was determined by the combination of LC retention time and high-resolution mass detection including dd-MS^2 product ion qualifying of the different analytes. Measured peak areas were used for quantification. Sensitivity for the different analytes was expressed, by the slope of the respective six-point standard calibration curves (mean of three to four independent experiments) that were calculated by linear regression analysis in both solvent (MeCN 50:50) and the different matrices. The linear range was defined as the concentration interval, in which the regression coefficient R^2 was ≥ 0.96. Although internal standard calibrations were used for 15 of the analytes for the compensation of matrix interferences, potential suppression and enhancement (SSE%) of signals from the co-eluting matrix were estimated for all analytes as the ratio of the slope of the matrix-assisted standard calibration curve to the calibration curve in MeCN/water (50:50). If SSE values were above or below 100%, signal enhancement or suppression by the matrix could be assumed.

Considering the negligible noise in the extracted high-resolution mass chromatograms, the limits of detection (LOD) and limits of quantification (LOQ) of the 25 analytes were calculated based on the standard deviation of the y-intercept of the respective calibration curves and their corresponding slopes (m) as $LOD = 3 \times \frac{SD}{m}$, $LOQ = 10 \times \frac{SD}{m}$ [59]. The accuracy of the method was assessed by determining recovery by spiking experiments and precision in terms of total within laboratory precision (RSi_R) considering intra- and interday variabilities together [60]. Furthermore, coefficients of variation (% CV) were determined for all concentration points in the solvent and matrix-assisted standard calibration curves. Recovery rates were calculated for all analytes as the mean of three to four experiments at a spiking level of 25 µg/L. In a few cases, where the matrix-assisted standard curves in feed or fish matrices did not pass through the origin but showed a positive signal on the ordinate due to background noise, this was corrected by virtually moving the curve with parallel shift on the abscissa. The corresponding concentration difference was added to the spike concentration used in the recovery experiments according to $\text{Recovery}_{(\text{spike corrected})}$ = (measured concentration − blank)/(spiked concentration + concentration difference to origin).

Measured results for fish feed and fish study samples were converted from concentrations (µg/L) into content in the respective matrix (µg/kg) by using the factors 0.1 for zebrafish and 0.125 for salmon and feed.

4.8. Data Analysis

The Q-Exactive was calibrated using Xcalibur software, version 2.2 (Thermo Scientific). The molecular formulas and exact masses of the target analytes were calculated using the built-in Qualbrowser of the Xcalibur 2.2 software, which was also applied for signal quantification. Microsoft Excel (Version 2016, Microsoft Corporation, Redmond, WA, USA) was used for basic statistics (e.g., calculation of mean, minimum and maximum values, regression and relative standard deviation).

Supplementary Materials: The following are available online at http://www.mdpi.com/2072-6651/11/4/222/s1, Table S1: Molecular characteristics of target analytes.

Author Contributions: Conceptualization, C.K.F. and L.I.; methodology, L.I.; software, A.J. and L.I.; validation, A.J.; formal analysis, A.J.; investigation, A.J.; resources, A.S.B., G.M.B. and L.I.; data curation, A.J.; writing—original draft preparation, A.J.; writing—review and editing, C.K.F., G.M.B., A.S.B., J.F. and L.I.; supervision, C.K.F., L.I and J.M.O.F.; project administration, C.K.F; funding acquisition, C.K.F. and J.M.O.F.

Funding: This work was supported by the Norwegian Research Council (RCN) as part of the projects SAFEFISH (RCN 254822), EPIGREEN (RCN 267944) and Amritha Johny's PhD scholarship grant.

Acknowledgments: We express our sincere gratitude to Anusha K. S. Dhanasiri at the Faculty of Biosciences and Aquaculture, Nord University, Bodø, Norway, for her substantial help with the zebrafish exposure study. We also would like to thank the technical staff at Nofima's Research Station for Sustainable Aquaculture, Sunndalsøra, Norway, for their valuable assistance in the salmon exposure study. Furthermore, we are thankful to Silvio Uhlig in the Chemistry Section at the Norwegian Veterinary Institute, Oslo, Norway, for supporting the instrumental analyses performed in this study.

Conflicts of Interest: The authors declare no conflict of interest. The funders had no role in the design of the study; in the collection, analyses, or interpretation of data; in the writing of the manuscript, or in the decision to publish the result.

References

1. FAO. *The State of World Fisheries and Aquaculture 2018-Meeting the Sustainable Development Goals*; FAO: Rome, Italy, 2018.
2. Froehlich, H.E.; Runge, C.A.; Gentry, R.R.; Gaines, S.D.; Halpern, B.S. Comparative terrestrial feed and land use of an aquaculture-dominant world. *Proc. Natl. Acad. Sci. USA* **2018**, *115*, 5295. [CrossRef] [PubMed]
3. Kraugerud, O.F.; Jørgensen, H.Y.; Svihus, B. Physical properties of extruded fish feed with inclusion of different plant (legumes, oilseeds, or cereals) meals. *Anim. Feed Sci. Technol.* **2011**, *163*, 244–254. [CrossRef]
4. Francis, G.; Makkar, H.P.S.; Becker, K. Antinutritional factors present in plant-derived alternate fish feed ingredients and their effects in fish. *Aquaculture* **2001**, *199*, 197–227. [CrossRef]
5. Hardy, R.W. Utilization of plant proteins in fish diets: Effects of global demand and supplies of fishmeal. *Aquacult. Res.* **2010**, *41*, 770–776. [CrossRef]
6. Morken, T.; Kraugerud, O.F.; Sørensen, M.; Storebakken, T.; Hillestad, M.; Christiansen, R.; Øverland, M. Effects of feed processing conditions and acid salts on nutrient digestibility and physical quality of soy-based diets for Atlantic salmon (*Salmo salar*). *Aquacult. Nutr.* **2012**, *18*, 21–34. [CrossRef]
7. Opstvedt, J.; Aksnes, A.; Hope, B.; Pike, I.H. Efficiency of feed utilization in Atlantic salmon (*Salmo salar* L.) fed diets with increasing substitution of fish meal with vegetable proteins. *Aquaculture* **2003**, *221*, 365–379. [CrossRef]
8. Krogdahl, Å.; Penn, M.; Thorsen, J.; Refstie, S.; Bakke, A.M. Important antinutrients in plant feedstuffs for aquaculture: An update on recent findings regarding responses in salmonids. *Aquacult. Res.* **2010**, *41*, 333–344. [CrossRef]
9. Bora, P. Anti-nutritional factors in foods and their effects. *J. Acad. Ind. Res.* **2014**, *3*, 285–290.
10. Andersen, L.F.; Andreassen, Å.K.; Elvevoll, E.O.; Hemre, G.I.; Hjeltnes, B.; Hofshagen, M.; Iversen, P.O.; Krogdahl, Å.; Källqvist, T.; Rafoss, T. *Research Needs and Data Gaps of Importance for Food Safety and Protection of Biodiversity*; VKM Report 2005–2015; Scientific Steering Committee of the Norwegian Scientific Committee for Food Safety: Skøyen, Norway, 2016.
11. Gonçalves, R.A.; Naehrer, K.; Santos, G.A. Occurrence of mycotoxins in commercial aquafeeds in Asia and Europe: A real risk to aquaculture? *Rev. Aquacult.* **2016**, *10*, 263–280. [CrossRef]
12. Greco, M.; Pardo, A.; Pose, G. Mycotoxigenic fungi and natural co-occurrence of mycotoxins in rainbow trout (*Oncorhynchus mykiss*) feeds. *Toxins* **2015**, *7*, 4595–4609. [CrossRef]
13. Nácher-Mestre, J.; Ibáñez, M.; Serrano, R.; Pérez-Sánchez, J.; Hernández, F. Qualitative screening of undesirable compounds from feeds to fish by liquid chromatography coupled to mass spectrometry. *J. Agric. Food. Chem.* **2013**, *61*, 2077–2087. [CrossRef]
14. Pietsch, C.; Kersten, S.; Burkhardt-Holm, P.; Valenta, H.; Dänicke, S. Occurrence of deoxynivalenol and zearalenone in commercial fish feed: An initial study. *Toxins* **2013**, *5*, 184–192. [CrossRef]
15. Sele, V.; Sanden, M.; Berntssen, M.; Lunestad, B.T.; Espe, M.; Lie, K.K.; Amlund, H.; Lundebye, A.-K.; Hemre, G.I.; Waagbø, R. *Program for Overvåking av Fiskefôr*; Havforskningen Instituttet: Bergen, Norway, 2018.
16. Woźny, M.; Obremski, K.; Jakimiuk, E.; Gusiatin, M.; Brzuzan, P. Zearalenone contamination in rainbow trout farms in north-eastern Poland. *Aquaculture* **2013**, *416–417*, 209–211. [CrossRef]
17. Matsumoto, T.; Kobayashi, M.; Moriwaki, T.; Kawai, S.i.; Watabe, S. Survey of estrogenic activity in fish feed by yeast estrogen-screen assay. *Comp. Biochem. Physiol. C* **2004**, *139*, 147–152. [CrossRef] [PubMed]
18. Quesada-García, A.; Valdehita, A.; Fernández-Cruz, M.L.; Leal, E.; Sánchez, E.; Martín-Belinchón, M.; Cerdá-Reverter, J.M.; Navas, J.M. Assessment of estrogenic and thyrogenic activities in fish feeds. *Aquaculture* **2012**, *338–341*, 172–180. [CrossRef]
19. Matejova, I.; Svobodova, Z.; Vakula, J.; Mares, J.; Modra, H. Impact of Mycotoxins on Aquaculture Fish Species: A Review. *J. World Aquacult. Soc.* **2017**, *48*, 186–200. [CrossRef]

20. Sweeney, M.J.; Dobson, A.D. Mycotoxin production by Aspergillus, Fusarium and Penicillium species. *Int. J. Food Microbiol.* **1998**, *43*, 141–158. [CrossRef]
21. Da Rocha, M.E.B.; Freire, F.d.C.O.; Maia, F.E.F.; Guedes, M.I.F.; Rondina, D. Mycotoxins and their effects on human and animal health. *Food Control* **2014**, *36*, 159–165. [CrossRef]
22. Jestoi, M.; Rokka, M.; Järvenpää, E.; Peltonen, K. Determination of Fusarium mycotoxins beauvericin and enniatins (A, A1, B, B1) in eggs of laying hens using liquid chromatography–tandem mass spectrometry (LC–MS/MS). *Food Chem.* **2009**, *115*, 1120–1127. [CrossRef]
23. Bernhoft, A.; Eriksen, G.S.; Sundheim, L.; Berntssen, M.; Brantsæter, A.L.; Brodal, G.; Fæste, C.K.; Hofgaard, I.S.; Rafoss, T.; Sivertsen, T.; et al. *Risk Assessment of Mycotoxins in Cereal Grain in Norway. Opinion of the Scientific Steering Committee of the Norwegian Scientific Committee for Food Safety*; VKM Report: Oslo, Norway, 2013.
24. Commission, E. Commission Recommendation NO 2006/576/EC of 17 August 2006 on the Presence of Deoxynivalenol, Zearalenone, Ochratoxin A, T-2 and HT-2 and Fumonisins in Products Intended for animal Feeding. 2006. Available online: https://eur-lex.europa.eu/legal-content/EN/TXT/PDF/?uri=CELEX:32006H0576&from=EN (accessed on 1 March 2019).
25. Commission, E. Commission Recommendation NO 2013/165/EU of 27 March 2013 on the Presence of T-2 and HT-2 Toxin in Cereals and Cereal Products. *Off. J. Eur. Union* **2013**, *L91/12*. Available online: https://eur-lex.europa.eu/legalcontent/EN/TXT/PDF/?uri=CELEX:32013H0165&from=EN (accessed on 1 March 2019).
26. Pinto, P.I.S.; Estêvão, M.D.; Andrade, A.; Santos, S.; Power, D.M. Tissue responsiveness to estradiol and genistein in the sea bass liver and scale. *J. Steroid Biochem. Mol. Biol.* **2016**, *158*, 127–137. [CrossRef]
27. Kurzer, M.S.; Xu, X. Dietary phytoestrogens. *Annu. Rev. Nutr.* **1997**, *17*, 353–381. [CrossRef]
28. Rietjens, I.M.C.M.; Louisse, J.; Beekmann, K. The potential health effects of dietary phytoestrogens. *Br. J. Pharmacol.* **2017**, *174*, 1263–1280. [CrossRef]
29. Ng, Y.; Hanson, S.; Malison, J.A.; Wentworth, B.; Barry, T.P. Genistein and other isoflavones found in soybeans inhibit oestrogen metabolism in salmonid fish. *Aquaculture* **2006**, *254*, 658–665. [CrossRef]
30. Pandjaitan, N.; Hettiarachchy, N.; Ju, Z.Y. Enrichment of genistein in soy protein concentrate with b-glucosidase. *J. Food Sci.* **2000**, *65*, 403–407. [CrossRef]
31. Cleveland, B.M. In vitro and in vivo effects of phytoestrogens on protein turnover in rainbow trout (*Oncorhynchus mykiss*) white muscle. *Comp. Biochem. Physiol. Part C Toxicol. Pharmacol.* **2014**, *165*, 9–16. [CrossRef]
32. Andrade, P.D.; Dantas, R.R.; Moura-Alves, T.L.d.S.d.; Caldas, E.D. Determination of multi-mycotoxins in cereals and of total fumonisins in maize products using isotope labeled internal standard and liquid chromatography/tandem mass spectrometry with positive ionization. *J. Chromatogr. A* **2017**, *1490*, 138–147. [CrossRef]
33. Beltrán, E.; Ibáñez, M.; Sancho, J.V.; Hernández, F. Determination of mycotoxins in different food commodities by ultra-high-pressure liquid chromatography coupled to triple quadrupole mass spectrometry. *Rapid Commun. Mass Spectrom.* **2009**, *23*, 1801–1809. [CrossRef]
34. Berthiller, F.; Brera, C.; Iha, M.H.; Krska, R.; Lattanzio, V.M.T.; MacDonald, S.; Malone, R.J.; Maragos, C.; Solfrizzo, M.; Stranska-Zachariasova, M.; et al. Developments in mycotoxin analysis: An update for 2015–2016. *World Mycotoxin J.* **2017**, *10*, 5–29. [CrossRef]
35. De Santis, B.; Debegnach, F.; Gregori, E.; Russo, S.; Marchegiani, F.; Moracci, G.; Brera, C. Development of a LC-MS/MS method for the multi-mycotoxin determination in composite cereal-based samples. *Toxins* **2017**, *9*, 169. [CrossRef]
36. Ivanova, L.; Sahlstrøm, S.; Rud, I.; Uhlig, S.; Fæste, C.K.; Eriksen, G.S.; Divon, H.H. Effect of primary processing on the distribution of free and modified *Fusarium* mycotoxins in naturally contaminated oats. *World Mycotoxin J.* **2017**, *10*, 73–88. [CrossRef]
37. Malachová, A.; Sulyok, M.; Beltrán, E.; Berthiller, F.; Krska, R. Optimization and validation of a quantitative liquid chromatography–tandem mass spectrometric method covering 295 bacterial and fungal metabolites including all regulated mycotoxins in four model food matrices. *J. Chromatogr. A* **2014**, *1362*, 145–156. [CrossRef]

38. Sulyok, M.; Krska, R.; Schuhmacher, R. A liquid chromatography/tandem mass spectrometric multi-mycotoxin method for the quantification of 87 analytes and its application to semi-quantitative screening of moldy food samples. *Anal. Bioanal. Chem.* **2007**, *389*, 1505–1523. [CrossRef]
39. Sun, W.; Han, Z.; Aerts, J.; Nie, D.; Jin, M.; Shi, W.; Zhao, Z.; De Saeger, S.; Zhao, Y.; Wu, A. A reliable liquid chromatography–tandem mass spectrometry method for simultaneous determination of multiple mycotoxins in fresh fish and dried seafoods. *J. Chromatogr. A* **2015**, *1387*, 42–48. [CrossRef]
40. Varga, E.; Glauner, T.; Köppen, R.; Mayer, K.; Sulyok, M.; Schuhmacher, R.; Krska, R.; Berthiller, F. Stable isotope dilution assay for the accurate determination of mycotoxins in maize by UHPLC-MS/MS. *Anal. Bioanal. Chem.* **2012**, *402*, 2675–2686. [CrossRef]
41. Ciasca, B.; Pascale, M.; Altieri, V.G.; Longobardi, F.; Suman, M.; Catellani, D.; Lattanzio, V.M.T. In-house validation and small-scale collaborative study to evaluate analytical performances of multimycotoxin screening methods based on liquid chromatography–high-resolution mass spectrometry: Case study on Fusarium toxins in wheat. *J. Mass Spectrom.* **2018**, *53*, 743–752. [CrossRef]
42. Lampe, J.W. Isoflavonoid and lignan phytoestrogens as dietary biomarkers. *J. Nutr.* **2003**, *133*, 956S–964S. [CrossRef]
43. Wielogórska, E.; Elliott, C.T.; Danaher, M.; Chevallier, O.; Connolly, L. Validation of an ultra high performance liquid chromatography–tandem mass spectrometry method for detection and quantitation of 19 endocrine disruptors in milk. *Food Control* **2015**, *48*, 48–55. [CrossRef]
44. Horn-Ross, P.L.; Barnes, S.; Lee, M.; Coward, L.; Mandel, J.E.; Koo, J.; John, E.M.; Smith, M. Assessing phytoestrogen exposure in epidemiologic studies: Development of a database (United States). *Cancer Causes Control* **2000**, *11*, 289–298. [CrossRef]
45. Kuhnle, G.G.C.; Dell'Aquila, C.; Low, Y.-L.; Kussmaul, M.; Bingham, S.A. Extraction and quantification of phytoestrogens in foods using automated solid-phase extraction and LC/MS/MS. *Anal. Chem.* **2007**, *79*, 9234–9239. [CrossRef]
46. Bernhoft, A.; Høgåsen, H.R.; Rosenlund, G.; Ivanova, L.; Berntssen, M.H.G.; Alexander, J.; Eriksen, G.S.; Fæste, C.K. Tissue distribution and elimination of deoxynivalenol and ochratoxin A in dietary-exposed Atlantic salmon (*Salmo salar*). *Food Addit. Contam. A* **2017**, *34*, 1211–1224. [CrossRef]
47. Kuhnle, G.G.C.; Dell'Aquila, C.; Aspinall, S.M.; Runswick, S.A.; Mulligan, A.A.; Bingham, S.A. Phytoestrogen content of foods of animal origin: Dairy products, eggs, meat, fish, and seafood. *J. Agric. Food. Chem.* **2008**, *56*, 10099–10104. [CrossRef] [PubMed]
48. Gomes, E.F.; Corraze, G.; Kaushik, S. Effects of dietary incorporation of a co-extruded plant protein (rapeseed and peas) on growth, nutrient utilization and muscle fatty acid composition of rainbow trout (*Oncorhynchus mykiss*). *Aquaculture* **1993**, *113*, 339–353. [CrossRef]
49. Commission, E. Guidance Document on Identification of Mycotoxins in Food and Feed. SANTE/12089. 2016. Available online: https://ec.europa.eu/food/sites/food/files/safety/docs/cs_contaminants_sampling_guid-doc-ident-mycotoxins.pdf (accessed on 6 March 2019).
50. International Organization for Standardization. Guide to Method Validation for Quantitative Analysis in Chemical Testing Laboratories. ISO/IEC 17025. 5 September 2018. Available online: https://www.iso.org/files/live/sites/isoorg/files/store/en/PUB100424.pdf (accessed on 6 March 2019).
51. Norwegian Food Safety Authority. *Anbefalte Grenseverdier for sopp og Mykotoksiner in Fôrvarer*; Norwegian Food Safety Authority: Oslo, Norway, 2018.
52. Maranghi, F.; Tassinari, R.; Narciso, L.; Tait, S.; Rocca, C.L.; Felice, G.D.; Butteroni, C.; Corinti, S.; Barletta, B.; Cordelli, E.; et al. In vivo toxicity and genotoxicity of beauvericin and enniatins. Combined approach to study in vivo toxicity and genotoxicity of mycotoxins beauvericin (BEA) and enniatin B (ENNB). *EFSA Support. Publ.* **2018**, *15*, 1406E. [CrossRef]
53. Tolosa, J.; Font, G.; Mañes, J.; Ferrer, E. Natural Occurrence of Emerging Fusarium Mycotoxins in Feed and Fish from Aquaculture. *J. Agric. Food. Chem.* **2014**, *62*, 12462–12470. [CrossRef]
54. Vitenskapskomiteen for Mat og Miljø. *Risk Assessment of Mycotoxins in Cereal Grain in Norway*; VKM Report: Oslo, Norway, 2013.
55. Miura, A.; Sugiyama, C.; Sakakibara, H.; Simoi, K.; Goda, T. Bioavailability of isoflavones from soy products in equol producers and non-producers in Japanese women. *J. Nutr. Intermed. Metabol.* **2016**, *6*, 41–47. [CrossRef]

56. Li, Y.; Yu, H.; Xue, M.; Zhang, Y.; Mai, K.; Hu, H.; Liu, J. A tolerance and safety assessment of daidzein in a female fish (*Carassius auratus gibelio*). *Aquacult. Res.* **2016**, *47*, 1191–1201. [CrossRef]
57. Lovdata. *Regulations on the Use of Animals in Experiments, FOR-2015-06-18-761*; Ministry of Agriculture and Food: Oslo, Norway, 2015.
58. The European Parliament and Commission. Directive 2010/63/EU of the European Parliament and of the Council of 22 September 2010 on the protection of animals used for scientific purposes. *Off. J. Eur. Union* **2010**, *L276*, 33–79.
59. Shrivastava, A.; Gupta, V. Methods for the determination of limit of detection and limit of quantitation of the analytical methods. *Chron. Young Sci.* **2011**, *2*, 21–25. [CrossRef]
60. Horwitz, W. Protocol for the design, conduct and interpretation of method-performance studies: Revised 1994 (Technical Report). *Pure Appl. Chem.* **2009**, *67*, 331–343. [CrossRef]

toxins

MDPI

Perspective

Aflatoxin Binders in Foods for Human Consumption—Can This be Promoted Safely and Ethically?

Sara Ahlberg [1,2,*], Delia Randolph [1], Sheila Okoth [3] and Johanna Lindahl [4,5,6]

1 Department of Biosciences, International Livestock Research Institute, P.O. Box 30709, Nairobi 00100, Kenya
2 Department of Food and Environmental Sciences, University of Helsinki, P.O. Box 66, FI-00014 Helsinki, Finland
3 School of Biological Sciences, University of Nairobi, P. O. Box 30197, Nairobi 00100, Kenya
4 International Livestock Research Institute, 298 Kim Ma Street, Ba Dinh District, Hanoi, Vietnam
5 Department of Medical Biochemistry and Microbiology, Uppsala University, P.O. Box 582, 75123 Uppsala, Sweden
6 Department of Clinical Sciences, Swedish University of Agricultural Sciences, P.O. Box 7054, 75007 Uppsala, Sweden
* Correspondence: sarahellinahlberg@gmail.com

Received: 2 June 2019; Accepted: 12 July 2019; Published: 14 July 2019

Abstract: Aflatoxins continue to be a food safety problem globally, especially in developing regions. A significant amount of effort and resources have been invested in an attempt to control aflatoxins. However, these efforts have not substantially decreased the prevalence nor the dietary exposure to aflatoxins in developing countries. One approach to aflatoxin control is the use of binding agents in foods, and lactic acid bacteria (LAB) have been studied extensively for this purpose. However, when assessing the results comprehensively and reviewing the practicality and ethics of use, risks are evident, and concerns arise. In conclusion, our review suggests that there are too many issues with using LAB for aflatoxin binding for it to be safely promoted. Arguably, using binders in human food might even worsen food safety in the longer term.

Keywords: Aflatoxins; binding; food safety; biocontrol; food discipline

Key Contribution: Aflatoxin control by binders in human foods as a food safety measure raises concerns and risks not previously discussed. These issues have to be taken into consideration in research planning targeting improved food safety.

---

1. Aflatoxins in Developing Country Food Chains with a Special Focus on Kenya

Mycotoxins, including the important fumonisins, trichothecene toxins, zearalenone, and especially aflatoxins, have caused great concern in African and especially Kenyan markets over the last four decades. These mycotoxins are widespread, contaminating cereals, potatoes, bananas, cotton, and other plants. Additional mycotoxins, such as ochratoxins and patulin, are found in coffee, apples, and citrus fruits [1].

Aflatoxins are an important group of mycotoxins because there is strong evidence of their severe health impacts, causing liver cancer, especially among hepatitis B–positive people [2–4]. Extended exposure is implicated in immunodeficiency, immunosuppression, stunting, kwashiorkor, and interference with the metabolism of micronutrients in children [4]. High prevalence of aflatoxins in staples and consequently chronic exposure is common in regions where control and monitoring systems are poor and regulations are not enforced. Many studies find aflatoxins are present in high levels in both feed and food chains in Africa, exposing consumers to aflatoxins, especially through staple foods [5].

Aflatoxins are produced by toxin-producing fungi *Aspergillus*, but fungal growth does not necessarily entail toxin production. Naturally occurring, there are non-toxic and toxic strains that produce aflatoxins at different levels [6]. Fungal growth and aflatoxin production are driven by climatic conditions. Any pre-harvest contamination of maize with *Aspergillus* fungi can lead to the accumulation of considerable aflatoxin levels when post-harvest conditions are adverse. However, post-harvest preventive measures against fungal contamination are more common than pre-harvest measures [7].

Acute aflatoxicosis is caused by consumption of large amounts of aflatoxins. This has occurred repeatedly in Kenya and other countries resulting in outbreaks with hundreds of human and thousands of animal deaths in the worst cases [8–10]. These widely reported cases have led to increased public concern and stimulated research efforts, policy changes, and investments into the research of suitable and effective mitigation interventions, and increased awareness of safety measures. However, these efforts have not been shown to decrease either the prevalence nor the dietary exposure to aflatoxins [9].

Kenya, a hot-spot of aflatoxins, has frequent, high, and not consistently improving prevalence of aflatoxins in staples and animal feeds. Aflatoxin studies report high proportions of cereals and feeds contaminated to some extent, and many samples exceed the allowable limits [8,11–14]. Likewise, fumonisins are found in almost all crops, often in co-occurrence with aflatoxins [8,15–22]. In consequence of the crop and feed contamination, almost all cattle milk is contaminated with aflatoxins [8,11–13,22–24].

Compared with other common foodborne hazards, aflatoxins are unusual because they can be formed only as a result of fungal infestation, usually at the farm level. This is exacerbated and spread by poor storage conditions. Once the aflatoxins are introduced, products are contaminated, and, if not removed from the chain at the control point when detected, they move further along the food chain and through processing. Heat treatments used in food production cannot eliminate the formed aflatoxins. Aflatoxins and other mycotoxins are invisible and can be detected only with modern analytical methods. However, if visible *Aspergillus* mould is present, this is an indicator of risk. The lack of control and monitoring in developing regions enables the supply of contaminated crops to reach the consumers.

Exposure to aflatoxins can be assessed through blood samples detecting albumin adducts or through detection of metabolites in milk or urine. Surveys report a wide range of exposure levels, from nondetectable to very high. Aflatoxin levels reported from Kenya during the 2010 outbreak were the highest ever reported (even up to 1200 pm/mg albumin) [5,10,25–27]. An indirect assessment of human exposure is the contamination level in food products.

Poverty is associated with poor availability and quality of foods, and this is also associated with aflatoxin exposure levels. Higher aflatoxin exposure levels were associated with the lowest socio-economic conditions in a study in Kenya, although all the women sampled were exposed [28]. In Africa, many small-holder farmers are women, who farm mostly for household consumption and informal markets and lack resources to avoid aflatoxin exposure.

Many mitigation methods have been suggested, from farm- to consumer-level interventions. Wild and Gong [29] have listed reasons for failures in aflatoxin control strategies. This list, which is relevant still a decade later, includes

- The perceived value of interventions may be low and a main reason for this could be the broken food chains where farmers, producers, and supply chain actors are working in isolation from each other, their efforts are not clearly rewarded, and (probably even more importantly) negligence is not sanctioned;
- Toxins are invisible and tasteless, making them difficult for both producers and consumers to assess;
- Control is required along the food chain in several points, and currently, the ability to cover the food chains throughout by food inspectors is poor in developing regions;
- The highest exposure may be in informal markets where regulations and control do not reach;

- Aflatoxins are a multidisciplinary problem of agriculture, public health, and economics.

Staple foods in Africa are the most contaminated with aflatoxins and other mycotoxins. Promotion of healthy diets and diversification of food sources in the diet, e.g., increased diversity of legumes and vegetables, could be one significant way to decrease the levels of exposure. However, most people in Africa cannot afford diverse diets. Nonetheless, diversification of nutrient sources should be promoted, not only from the contamination exposure point of view, but also from agricultural and environmental diversity and nutritional perspective. Focus on staples and fungus-resistant maize can further decrease the promotion of diversity in diets and in agriculture, promoting further monocropping leading to decreased biodiversity levels, which are declining globally in alarming levels.

2. Binding of Aflatoxins as a Biocontrol Method

Novel approaches and new intervention methods focusing strongly on finding solutions to aflatoxin contamination have been called for. Risk mitigation and food safety improving measures have attracted funding resources, leaving other issues and problems, including other mycotoxins, behind. For example, aflatoxin research has benefited from a level of donor support disproportionate to the health burden it causes. According to the World Health Organisation and World Bank, aflatoxins are a relatively minor contributor to the overall health burden of foodborne disease [30,31], but the WHO report only includes the burden from hepatocellular carcinomas.

A specific approach to aflatoxin control is the use of aflatoxin-binding agents in foods. The principle is as follows: aflatoxins, which have contaminated foods, can be bound to an agent to mitigate the aflatoxin-induced health risks after consumption. Binders include bacteria cells, yeasts, proteins, and clays; the latter have been especially analysed for use in animal feeds. The hypothesis is that the binding agent and the bound toxin would pass through the gastrointestinal tract without, or at least with less, uptake and thus less damage caused by the toxins. Binding with lactic acid bacteria (LAB) is discussed below. Some other organic binding agents analysed have been yeasts [32,33].

Evidence of the binding ability of aflatoxins with LAB cells has been shown through a number of studies in laboratory conditions, some with 100% binding efficiency [32,34,35]. Binding is speculated to be an instant phenomenon [32,36–39], but also binding levels have been observed to increase over time [32,36,37,39–43].

Contrary to observed instant binding, some studies have reported no immediate binding at all [43,44]. Govaris [45] also noted several contradictions among the studies since the 1980s. Conflicting results have also been reported from storage studies. While Ahlberg [46] observed both increased binding over time and release of aflatoxins back to the matrix during 21-day trial, Barukčić [47] and Govaris [45] reported binding levels to remain the same even for 21 days. Sokoutifar [44] recorded large amounts of aflatoxins bound to LAB strains up to 30 days at 21 and 37 °C. In practice, however, such high temperature conditions cannot be attained due to food integrity and safety risks.

While some authors reported increasing binding efficiency of LAB with increased aflatoxin concentration, others have reported decreasing effects or no difference or even both [34,41,45,46]. Binding has been shown to be dependent also on the concentration of the LAB cells [34,35,48].

Viability of bacteria strains has been considered a significant factor in binding. However, both viable and non-viable LAB strains have performed better in binding over the other in different studies, and no difference between the two has also been found [36,37,42,48–50]. These results have not brought clarity to the binding mechanisms, whether the binding effect is due to physical binding or influenced by the components produced by the bacteria.

Other factors affecting binding efficiency have been reported to occur in different food matrices such as milk or yoghurt, possibly explained by the compounds in the matrix [40,45], lower pH [45], or even higher pH [37,48]. In conclusion, external conditions seem to strongly affect the binding ability of aflatoxins by LAB.

One factor to consider in the binding analysis is the stability of the bound complex. Even simple washing can release 20–70% of the initially categorized bound aflatoxins back to detectable forms [32,34,36,37,39,51,52]. The stability of the formed bond is an important factor to assess the suitability of binding agents in food systems to reduce the harmful effects of aflatoxins.

As LAB are commonly used in dairy fermentation, the binding efficiencies of milk components have been studied. The milk protein casein is often speculated to be a binding agent in milk, the cheese making process being an indicator for this phenomenon due to the separation of whey and casein fractions. Aflatoxin binding has been concluded both to increase and decrease during cheese making [53]. In some of the binding studies, the controls without LAB cells show very low binding and reduction in aflatoxin shares (2–5%) compared with the binders [43,44]. These findings do not support the binding of milk components or casein to aflatoxins to be anything significant.

One of the first studies in binding concluded LAB removed as much as 80% of aflatoxins during cooking [17], which probably resulted a flourishing of interest in this research sector. Scientific evidence shows good potential in binding methods if certain criteria for evaluation are selected. However, when considering binding from wider perspective, serious concerns and problems arise, which have not been discussed or critically reviewed within these applications.

3. Challenges with Interpreting the Results of Binding Aflatoxins with LAB

Binding mechanisms and efficiency factors for LAB are not clearly understood and are considered still speculative in publications on binding. There seems to be no predictable factor affecting the binding efficiency and stability, resulting in the unpredictability and uncontrollability of the binding process. Optimal conditions for controlled and predictable binding have not been found. One factor can enhance binding shares in one study, but the same factor decreases the binding shares in another study. For example, the level of aflatoxin concentration is speculated to be one major factor in binding efficiency. It is especially important to bear this in mind because, as aflatoxins are contaminants, the levels and prevalence are unpredictable and vary significantly between batches, commodities, regions, and seasons. The approach to increase the safety of foods with aflatoxin binding with LAB cannot depend on the uncontrollable contamination level.

The binding analyses follow fairly simple procedures. Binders and LAB are mixed and possibly incubated in a liquid media (milk, broth, PBS, etc.) with aflatoxins. The mixture is then centrifuged, and the pellet is considered containing the bound aflatoxins attached to the LAB, as the free, unbound aflatoxins are considered remaining in the supernatant, the liquid media. It is possible that in this method the aflatoxins can be "trapped": physically pulled down by the other components of the binding analysis matrix to the pellet during centrifugation. This is even more likely when fermentation is taking place: LAB produce exopolysaccharides, high in molecular weight and large in structure constructing extracellular polymeric substances (EPSs) with proteins. These are partly responsible for the thickening of the product during fermentation. As any high molecular component will be pelletized during centrifugation, so are the fermenting products, which then can easily trap the aflatoxins and further falsely be detected as "bound".

For food safety purposes, both the binding efficiency and the stability of the formed bond are relevant. A weak formed bond releasing the aflatoxin would not have mitigation potential, despite the initial binding efficiency. If the binding phenomenon is only temporary, the suitability as a food safety method will not be relevant due to the uncontrollable conditions and risks induced. Several studies have reported how different levels of aflatoxins are released from formed aflatoxin and LAB complex under different conditions [32,34,36,37,39,51,52].

One major flaw in aflatoxin binding studies is the over-optimistic rhetoric used in the studies and conclusions. A number of studies observed binding in laboratory conditions with limited replications yet concluded it to be a suitable method of improving food safety. These conclusions contradict standard approaches to food safety measures, guidance, and regulations development, which would not support use of additives on the basis of inconclusive evidence. The phrase "aflatoxins could be removed" is often used in aflatoxin-binding studies, but in practice, the aflatoxins are still present in the food at the original levels, whether bound or not.

The analysis of binding of aflatoxins by LAB raises a question about the suitability of the methods. Aflatoxin contamination methods for screening contamination levels from foods uses the same analyses as the binding methods. These results of aflatoxin screening in different studies can sometimes show even higher aflatoxin contamination levels for the fermented food and milk products, which are incompatible with bound aflatoxins [23]. To further speculate, in principle, if the binding of aflatoxins to LAB, to milk components, or other food components occurs, all the analysed levels of aflatoxins from foods would be higher in reality than the given results indicate. Alternatively, it could be implied that the analysis methods for food contamination levels are not appropriate for the binding trials.

4. Big Picture—Safe Food for All

Promotion of aflatoxin binding at the consumer level of the food chain can signal to the producers and operators that the production of unsafe foods is acceptable as the problem could be solved later on. Such new principles can be extremely difficult to reverse later on, especially in poorly regulated markets. The awareness, knowledge, and practice of safety measures about mycotoxins and aflatoxins among farmers [7], producers, and consumers is limited [12,24,54], and promoting a method with uncertainties could easily create new misunderstandings and misperceptions of the causalities behind the contamination patterns and induced health risks.

Development of binders has taken a highly technological approach with little consideration to ethical, political, consumer acceptability, or legal implications. Yet using binders raises serious concerns and questions about risk, trade-offs, and entitlements that have not been discussed, let alone addressed. Without thoroughly understanding these aspects, it is likely that even if LAB is found to be technologically effective, it may not be adopted, or that if adopted, it could have unintended negative consequences.

Today, poor consumers patronising informal market chains cannot enjoy the same fundamental right to safe food as the wealthy consumers in formal markets in high income countries. In developing countries, market regulations, although inadequately implemented, mainly cover the formal markets, leaving informal markets unregulated [23,55]. In Kenya, among branded products sold in formal markets, lowest priced maize was 25% less likely to meet regulatory requirements for aflatoxins than the highest priced products [56]. Some indicators show that the situation might be worse in informal markets, but no systematic comparison has been done between the maize products sold in formal and informal markets in Kenya [56]. Aflatoxin exposure from milk among low-income consumers in urban Nairobi is higher than among mid-income consumers due to the higher aflatoxin levels in products sold in low-income areas and the higher milk consumption [23].

One effect of promoting fermentation with LAB to reduce aflatoxins in the informal sector could be the development of double standards in the food safety and food production systems. In principle, promoting different standards and procedures in different markets will create problems later in the upgrading and formalisation of traditional markets.

While aflatoxins are present in large parts of the world, high exposure levels in humans are mainly a problem in developing regions, and worst among poor purchasers. These people have often less access to information, and their understanding about the options, alternatives, and the relationship between actions at the beginning of the production chain and the consumption level may be lacking. Consumers in informal markets have limited access to the regulated markets without full market structure change.

Promotion of the use of aflatoxin binders in foods could potentially create new layers of problems. These have not received attention because the solution has been developed from a perspective of scientific functionality. Aflatoxins are by far the most studied mycotoxins [57], and when other mycotoxins start to gain more publicity, aflatoxin binding may appear inadequate as a solution. The role of social sciences should be promoted to create collaboration and multidisciplinary academic knowledge to develop new and suitable ways to work against aflatoxins and increase food safety [9].

Notably aflatoxin binding research has approached the issue from a one-component "silver bullet" solution instead of focusing on comprehensive food safety solutions at the farm and value chain level mitigating all the mycotoxins. Other mycotoxins are prevalent and occur together with aflatoxins. The binding solution is a rather simplified solution for a complex problem formed due to several factors and enchased by insufficient practices.

5. Ethical Assessment to Improve Food Safety with Binders in Human Foods

"Humans have a right to food free from mycotoxins that could cause significant health risk".

Declaration by the United Nations Environment Programme (UNEP) and the World Health Organization (WHO) International Programme on Chemical Safety (IPCS) [58]

An aflatoxin binding approach to foods inevitably requires testing and efficient analytical methods at consumer level. This is challenging for a number of reasons. First of all, promoting aflatoxin binding at the consumer level assumes people will deliberately be exposed to aflatoxins from contaminated foods and food products to assess the effectiveness, accepting something many citizens feel to be unacceptable. Second, aflatoxins are more of a problem in poorly regulated countries than in developed regions, especially among the poorest consumers.

Aflatoxins are one of the most regulated contaminants with allowable legal limits in commodities [59,60]. The role of the European Union in trading has pushed EU limits to be followed and adopted in regions with limited resources, creating a situation where limits are strict but resources are scarce to implement, monitor, and control the set limits. Also, the Codex Alimentarius has recommended limits for mycotoxins and aflatoxins, which can be adopted to national legislation [61]. The limits, whether reasonable and realistic from economic and trade perspective, are set to harmonize the safe food production systems to ensure the safety of the products.

The application of binders in human foods is in conflict with the principle of developed food safety regulations, set allowable limits, and regulation implementation and compliance by the operators. Even an emergency application can add new problems to the fragile and developing food safety systems. Officially approving a binder application in foods would be politically ambiguous. It is highly unlikely that developed regions, with strong regulatory systems, would allow aflatoxin binders at the consumer level as it is strongly against the principles of the current food regulatory systems. Implementing such binders legally only in developing regions with poor regulatory systems would raise concerns in terms of promoted double standards.

Clay supplements and LAB have been tested in human trials aimed to be used during an emergency aflatoxins outbreak situations [62,63]. In already poorly regulated regions, it would be challenging to keep the promotion of daily food safety measures and good practices separated from promoting a temporary solution or a quick-fix. It raises the concern at what threshold level would such an emergency outbreak be announced for the binding application in human foods to be "legal" or allowed. For example, in Kenya, many foods continuously contain aflatoxins above the allowable limits. Would high aflatoxin prevalence above legal limits permit the usage of binders in a specific time and region? Instead of supplementing binders to people in an aflatoxin emergency situation to encourage them to eat the contaminated, potentially high-risk maize, it would be more ethical to provide the replacement of safe maize for consumption.

6. Who Can Choose What to Eat?

A food safety method to control harmful contaminants should be robust, reliable, and functional in all conditions the contaminants are present. Also, to be suitable for the purpose, the methods needs to be available, feasible, understandable, and acceptable to the end users.

As the European Union is the largest economy in the world and a major trading partner for many countries, the EU legislation and standards are relevant globally. The EU has strict standards to ensure food safety and comprehensive regulation of practices to ensure the safety and quality of the products. It should be highlighted that set standards and limits alone cannot create food safety, but the comprehensive food industry system from farm practices, through processing to consumers, all controlled and monitored by relevant institutions, can create a chain of controlled and traceable practices. This element of comprehensive approach is lacking in poorly regulated and in informal markets.

Where the legislation is set and executed throughout the practices in food production to protect consumers, unsafe products rarely enter the market chains and can be recalled if necessary. The binding application idea is also related to the food security status, but can the science and research community promote it in regions where people who have no institutional food safety protection, allowing them to consume foods that in regulated regions would be categorised unsafe and not fit for consumption? These are fundamental issues that should be discussed before any binding applications are taken to further testing. Figure 1 illustrates the separation between informal and formal markets and the most likely binder application channel and consequences.

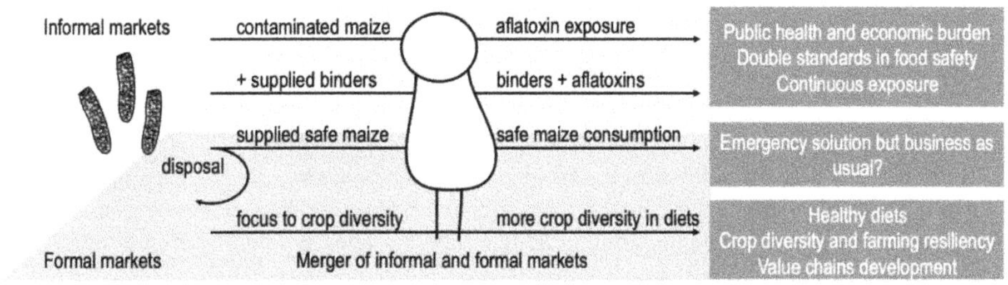

Figure 1. The most likely application chain for binder method applied in informal markets focusing strongly to the consumer actually taking the risk. Implementation of binding method in formal markets would be highly unlikely as the approach conflicts strongly against the regulatory allowable limits set to the aflatoxins. Informal and formal markets currently are not equal and should be merged into formal markets to enable the same food safety standards, economic growth, and new value chains in one coherent food production system.

Consumers and end-users have very little influence on aflatoxin levels. Would consumers accept contaminated foods and milk for consumption with binding methods compared with better management at the farm- and supply chain–level to prevent the contamination altogether? Would poor and less-informed consumers be more approving toward the binding methods than informed, knowledgeable consumers who have more resources to understand the production chains and the consequences of the practices?

Judging from past trends, it is unlikely that the food safety standards and measures will be lightened. Consumers are increasingly conscious, information is ever more readily available, and consumers are demanding safer, high-quality foods produced sustainably, ethically, and fairly. Enabling and promoting the development of different food standards and measures in informal market sectors or poorly regulated regions is a very questionable approach to food safety, and the acceptability of binding applications should be brought to wider discussions from laboratories and the research community.

One of the most important questions in the binding applications should be, would you take it?

7. Suggestions for Way Forward

Using LAB to bind aflatoxins in foods may pose greater short- and long-term risks than benefits. Most important aspects are related to regulations, acceptability, and the creation of double standards when harmonized systems and merged markets are needed. Use of binding agents in foods contradicts all the existing principles and regulations set to ensure food safety. If such a method is promoted, the efforts to combat the aflatoxin problem at farm level and throughout the value chain, to eliminate and reduce the contaminants, could be compromised.

Aflatoxin control is not simple and needs a comprehensive approach covering food safety and economic development to address overall good farming and food production practices. Currently, food safety promotion through binders is discussed as an isolated factor, a magic bullet, to solve the problem. Over-reliance on technological solutions and inadequate attention to legal, ethical, political, and behavioural aspects of technologies as well as unintended consequences reduces the likelihood that agricultural innovations will have beneficial health and development outcomes. Now is the time to start addressing these neglected and important aspects of aflatoxin control.

Aflatoxin problems are prevalent especially in staples, and promoting diverse diets could reduce the exposure, especially from maize. Basically, all measures come with a cost, but creating new systems to promote increasing diversity in diets would directly contribute to diversity in crops in farming, creating resilience against climate change and unpredictable conditions. Promoting new value chains for staples and for a larger variety of plant and animal source foods can create new income sources for farmers while contributing to improved diets and decreased aflatoxin intake, directly contributing to a decreased public health burden from unsafe foods and unhealthy diets. When people become richer, they naturally diversify their diets, and aflatoxin exposure reduces. So, the promotion of development through economic and agricultural policy may be an indirect way of ending the scourge of aflatoxin [64]. Other public health approaches such as hepatitis B vaccination also have potential. Finally, the authorities' role to ensure the food safety in poorly regulated regions covering both informal and formal markets, but also promoting the merge of the two, should be strengthened significantly.

In final conclusion, there are too many issues with the aflatoxin binding methodology and results for it to be promoted. This review also highlights that binders for humans may be counter-productive for food safety.

Author Contributions: Conceptualization, S.A.; D.R.; S.O. and J.L.; Writing—original draft preparation, S.A.; Writing—review and editing, S.A.; D.R.; S.O. and J.L; Visualization, S.A.

Funding: This perspective received no external funding.

Conflicts of Interest: The authors declare no conflict of interest.

References

1. Kirk, P.M.; Cannon, P.F.; Minter, D.W.; Stalpers, J.A. *Dictionary of the Fungi*, 10th ed.; Ainsworth & Bisby's; CABI Europe UK: Wallingford, UK, 2008; ISBN 9780851998268.
2. *Improving Public Health through Mycotoxin Control*; IARC Scientific Publication; Pitt, J.I.; Wild, C.P.; Baan, R.A.; Gelderblom, W.C.A.; Miller, J.D.; Riley, R.T.; Wu, F. (Eds.) International Agency for Research on Cancer: Lyon, France, 2012.
3. WHO; IARC. *Some Naturally Occurring Substances: Food Items and Constituents, Heterocyclic Aromatic Amines and Mycotoxins. IARC Monographs on the Evaluation of Carcinogenic Risks to Humans*; IARCPress: Lyon, France, 2002; Volume 82.
4. Wu, F.; Groopman, J.D.; Pestka, J.J. Public Health Impacts of Foodborne Mycotoxins. *Annu. Rev. Food Sci. Technol.* **2014**, *5*, 351–372. [CrossRef] [PubMed]
5. Okoth, S. *Improving the Evidence Base on Aflatoxin Contamination and Exposure in Africa*; CTA Working Paper, 16/13; CTA: Wageningen, The Netherlands, 2016.
6. Okoth, S.; Nyongesa, B.; Ayugi, V.; Kan'gethe, E.; Korhonen, H.; Joutsjoki, V. Toxigenic Potential of Aspergillus Species Occurring on Maize Kernels from Two Agro-Ecological Zones in Kenya. *Toxins* **2012**, *4*, 991–1007. [CrossRef] [PubMed]
7. Kiama, T.; Lindahl, J.; Sirma, A.J.; Senerwa, D.; Waithanji, E.; Ochungo, P.; Poole, E.; Kang'ethe, E.; Grace, D. Kenya Dairy Farmer Perception of Moulds and Mycotoxins and Implications for Exposure to Aflatoxins: A Gendered Analysis. *Afr. J. Foodagric. Nutr. Dev.* **2016**, *16*, 11106–11125. [CrossRef]
8. Joutsjoki, V.; Ramo, S.; Murithi, G.; Mungatu, J.K.; Korhonen, H.J.; Ouko, E.O.; Kang'ethe, E.K.; Sirma, A.J.; Lindfors, E.; Nduhiu, G.J.; et al. Occurrence of Mycotoxins in Food, Feed, and Milk in Two Counties from Different Agro-Ecological Zones and with Historical Outbreak of Aflatoxins and Fumonisins Poisonings in Kenya. *Food Qual. Saf.* **2017**, *1*, 161–170.

9. Stepman, F. Scaling-up the Impact of Aflatoxin Research in Africa. The Role of Social Sciences. *Toxins* **2018**, *10*, 136. [CrossRef] [PubMed]
10. Azziz-Baumgartner, E.; Lindblade, K.; Gieseker, K.; Rogers, H.S.; Kieszak, S.; Njapau, H.; Schleicher, R.; McCoy, L.F.; Misore, A.; DeCock, K.; et al. Case–Control Study of an Acute Aflatoxicosis Outbreak, Kenya, 2004. *Environ. Health Perspect.* **2005**, *113*, 1779–1783. [CrossRef] [PubMed]
11. Kang'ethe, E.K.; M'Ibui, G.M.; Randolph, T.F.; Lang'At, A.K. Prevalence of Aflatoxin M1 and B1 in Milk and Animal Feeds from Urban Smallholder Dairy Production in Dagoretti Division, Nairobi, Kenya. *East. Afr. Med. J.* **2007**, *84* (Suppl. 11), 83–86.
12. Kang'ethe, E.; Lang'a, K. Aflatoxin B1 and M1 Contamination of Animal Feeds and Milk from Urban Centers in Kenya. *Afr. Health Sci.* **2009**, *9*, 218–226.
13. Obade, M.; Andang'o, P.; Obonyo, C.; Lusweti, F. Exposure of Children 4 to 6 Months of Age to Aflatoxin in Kisumu County, Kenya. *Afr. J. Food Agric. Nutr. Dev.* **2015**, *15*, 9949–9963.
14. Senerwa, D.; Sirma, A.J.; Mtimet, N.; Kang'ethe, E.K.; Grace, D.; Lindahl, J.F. Prevalence of Aflatoxin in Feeds and Cow Milk from Five Counties in Kenya. *Afr. J. Foodagric. Nutr. Dev.* **2016**, *16*, 11004–11021. [CrossRef]
15. Adekoya, I.; Njobeh, P.; Obadina, A.; Chilaka, C.; Okoth, S.; De Boevre, M.; De Saeger, S. Awareness and Prevalence of Mycotoxin Contamination in Selected Nigerian Fermented Foods. *Toxins* **2017**, *9*, 363. [CrossRef] [PubMed]
16. Adekoya, I.; Obadina, A.; Phoku, J.; De Boevre, M.; De Saeger, S.; Njobeh, P. Fungal and Mycotoxin Contamination of Fermented Foods from Selected South African Markets. *Food Control* **2018**, *90*, 295–303. [CrossRef]
17. Kpodo, K.; Sørensen, A.K.; Jakobsen, M. The Occurrence of Mycotoxins in Fermented Maize Products. *Food Chem.* **1996**, *56*, 147–153. [CrossRef]
18. Bankole, S.A.; Adebanjo, A. Mycotoxins in Food in West Africa: Current Situation and Possibilities of Controlling It. *Afr. J. Biotechnol.* **2003**, *2*, 254–263.
19. Kumi, J.; Mitchell, N.; Asare, G.; Dotse, E.; Kwaa, F.; Phillips, T.; Ankrah, N.-A. Aflatoxins and Fumonisins Contamination of Home-Made Food (Weanimix) from Cereal-Legume Blends for Children. *Ghana Med. J.* **2014**, *48*, 121. [CrossRef] [PubMed]
20. Agbetiameh, D.; Ortega-Beltran, A.; Awuah, R.T.; Atehnkeng, J.; Cotty, P.J.; Bandyopadhyay, R. Prevalence of Aflatoxin Contamination in Maize and Groundnut in Ghana: Population Structure, Distribution, and Toxigenicity of the Causal Agents. *Plant Dis.* **2017**, *102*, 764–772. [CrossRef] [PubMed]
21. Chilaka, C.A.; De Boevre, M.; Atanda, O.O.; De Saeger, S. Prevalence of Fusarium Mycotoxins in Cassava and Yam Products from Some Selected Nigerian Markets. *Food Control* **2018**, *84*, 226–231. [CrossRef]
22. Kang'ethe, E.K.; Gatwiri, M.; Sirma, A.J.; Ouko, E.O.; Mburugu-Musoti, C.K.; Kitala, P.M.; Nduhiu, G.J.; Nderitu, J.G.; Mungatu, J.K.; Hietaniemi, V.; et al. Exposure of Kenyan Population to Aflatoxins in Foods with Special Reference to Nandi and Makueni Counties. *Food Qual. Saf.* **2017**, *1*, 131–137. [CrossRef]
23. Ahlberg, S.; Grace, D.; Kiarie, G.; Kirino, Y.; Lindahl, J. A Risk Assessment of Aflatoxin M1 Exposure in Low and Mid-Income Dairy Consumers in Kenya. *Toxins* **2018**, *10*, 348. [CrossRef]
24. Kirino, Y.; Makita, K.; Grace, D.; Lindahl, J. Survey of Informal Milk Retailers in Nairobi, Kenya and Prevalence of Aflatoxin M1 in Marketed Milk. *Afr. J. Foodagric. Nutr. Dev.* **2016**, *16*, 11022–11038. [CrossRef]
25. IFPRI. *Aflatoxins—Finding Solutions for Improved Food Safety*; IFPRI: Washington, DC, USA, 2013.
26. Shephard, G.S. Risk Assessment of Aflatoxins in Food in Africa. *Food Addit. Contam. Part A* **2008**, *25*, 1246–1256. [CrossRef] [PubMed]
27. Yard, E.E.; Daniel, J.H.; Lewis, L.S.; Rybak, M.E.; Paliakov, E.M.; Kim, A.A.; Montgomery, J.M.; Bunnell, R.; Abudo, M.U.; Akhwale, W.; et al. Human Aflatoxin Exposure in Kenya, 2007: A Cross-Sectional Study. *Food Addit. Contam. Part A Chem. Anal. Control. Expo. Risk Assess.* **2013**, *30*, 1322–1331. [CrossRef] [PubMed]
28. Leroy, J.L.; Wang, J.-S.; Jones, K. Serum Aflatoxin B 1 -Lysine Adduct Level in Adult Women from Eastern Province in Kenya Depends on Household Socio-Economic Status: A Cross Sectional Study. *Soc. Sci. Med.* **2015**, *146*, 104–110. [CrossRef] [PubMed]
29. Wild, C.P.; Gong, Y.Y. Mycotoxins and Human Disease: A Largely Ignored Global Health Issue. *Carcinogenesis* **2010**, *31*, 71–82. [CrossRef] [PubMed]
30. Havelaar, A.H.; Kirk, M.D.; Torgerson, P.R.; Gibb, H.J.; Hald, T.; Lake, R.J.; Praet, N.; Bellinger, D.C.; de Silva, N.R.; Gargouri, N.; et al. World Health Organization Global Estimates and Regional Comparisons of the Burden of Foodborne Disease in 2010. *PLoS Med.* **2015**, *12*, e1001923. [CrossRef]

31. The Global Food Safety Partnership (GFSP). *Food Safety in Africa: Past Endeavors and Future Directions*; GFSP: Washington, DC, USA, 2019.
32. Corassin, C.H.; Bovo, F.; Rosim, R.E.; Oliveira, C.A.F. Efficiency of Saccharomyces Cerevisiae and Lactic Acid Bacteria Strains to Bind Aflatoxin M 1 in UHT Skim Milk. *Food Control* **2013**, *31*, 80–83. [CrossRef]
33. Gonçalves, B.L.; Gonçalves, J.L.; Rosim, R.E.; Cappato, L.P.; Cruz, A.G.; Oliveira, C.A.F.; Corassin, C.H. Effects of Different Sources of Saccharomyces Cerevisiae Biomass on Milk Production, Composition, and Aflatoxin M 1 Excretion in Milk from Dairy Cows Fed Aflatoxin B 1. *J. Dairy Sci.* **2017**, *7*, 5701–5708. [CrossRef]
34. Ismail, A.; Levin, R.E.; Riaz, M.; Akhtar, S.; Gong, Y.Y.; de Oliveira, C.A.F. Effect of Different Microbial Concentrations on Binding of Aflatoxin M 1 and Stability Testing. *Food Control* **2017**, *73*, 492–496. [CrossRef]
35. Taheur, F.B.; Fedhila, K.; Chaieb, K.; Kouidhi, B.; Bakhrouf, A.; Abrunhosa, L. Adsorption of Aflatoxin B1, Zearalenone and Ochratoxin A by Microorganisms Isolated from Kefir Grains. *Int. J. Food Microbiol.* **2017**, *251*, 1–7. [CrossRef]
36. Bovo, F.; Corassin, C.H.; Rosim, R.E.; de Oliveira, C.A.F. Efficiency of Lactic Acid Bacteria Strains for Decontamination of Aflatoxin M1 in Phosphate Buffer Saline Solution and in Skimmed Milk. *Food Bioprocess Technol.* **2013**, *6*, 2230–2234. [CrossRef]
37. Elsanhoty, R.M.; Salam, S.A.; Ramadan, M.F.; Badr, F.H. Detoxification of Aflatoxin M1 in Yoghurt Using Probiotics and Lactic Acid Bacteria. *Food Control* **2014**, *43*, 129–134. [CrossRef]
38. Haskard, C.A.; El-Nezami, H.S.; Kankaanpaa, P.E.; Salminen, S.; Ahokas, J.T. Surface Binding of Aflatoxin B1 by Lactic Acid Bacteria. *Appl. Environ. Microbiol.* **2001**, *67*, 3086–3091. [CrossRef] [PubMed]
39. Serrano-Niño, J.C.; Cavazos-Garduño, A.; Hernandez-Mendoza, A.; Applegate, B.; Ferruzzi, M.G.; San Martin-González, M.F.; García, H.S. Assessment of Probiotic Strains Ability to Reduce the Bioaccessibility of Aflatoxin M1 in Artificially Contaminated Milk Using an in Vitro Digestive Model. *Food Control* **2013**, *31*, 202–207. [CrossRef]
40. El Khoury, A.; Atoui, A.; Yaghi, J. Analysis of Aflatoxin M1 in Milk and Yogurt and AFM1 Reduction by Lactic Acid Bacteria Used in Lebanese Industry. *Food Control* **2011**, *22*, 1695–1699. [CrossRef]
41. Adibpour, N.; Soleimanian-Zad, S.; Sarabi-Jamab, M.; Tajalli, F. Effect of Storage Time and Concentration of Aflatoxin M1 on Toxin Binding Capacity of L. Acidophilus in Fermented Milk Product. *J. Agric. Sci. Technol.* **2016**, *18*, 1209–1220.
42. Jebali, R.; Abbès, S.; Salah-Abbès, J.B.; Younes, R.B.; Haous, Z.; Oueslati, R. Ability of Lactobacillus Plantarum MON03 to Mitigate Aflatoxins (B1 and M1) Immunotoxicities in Mice. *J. Immunotoxicol.* **2015**, *12*, 290–299. [CrossRef] [PubMed]
43. Shigute, T.; Washe, A.P. Reduction of Aflatoxin M1 Levels during Ethiopian Traditional Fermented Milk (Ergo) Production. *J. Food Qual.* **2018**, *2018*, 4570238. [CrossRef]
44. Sokoutifar, R.; Razavilar, V.; Anvar, A.A.; Shoeiby, S. Degraded Aflatoxin M1 in Artificially Contaminated Fermented Milk Using Lactobacillus Acidophilus and Lactobacillus Plantarum Affected by Some Bio-physical Factors. *J. Food Saf.* **2018**, *38*, e12544. [CrossRef]
45. Govaris, A.; Roussi, V.; Koidis, P.A.; Botsoglou, N.A. Distribution and Stability of Aflatoxin M1 during Production and Storage of Yoghurt. *Food Addit. Contam.* **2002**, *19*, 1043–1050. [CrossRef]
46. Ahlberg, S.; Kärki, P.; Kolmonen, M.; Korhonen, H.; Joutsjoki, V. Aflatoxin M1 Binding by Lactic Acid Bacteria in Milk (submitted).
47. Barukčić, I.; Bilandžić, N.; Markov, K.; Jakopović, K.L.; Božanić, R. Reduction in Aflatoxin M1 Concentration during Production and Storage of Selected Fermented Milks. *Int. J. Dairy Technol.* **2018**, *71*, 734–740. [CrossRef]
48. Sarlak, Z.; Rouhi, M.; Mohammadi, R.; Khaksar, R.; Mortazavian, A.M.; Sohrabvandi, S.; Garavand, F. Probiotic Biological Strategies to Decontaminate Aflatoxin M1in a Traditional Iranian Fermented Milk Drink (Doogh). *Food Control* **2017**, *71*, 152–159. [CrossRef]
49. Pierides, M.; El-Nezami, H.; Peltonen, K.; Salminen, S.; Ahokas, J. Ability of Dairy Strains of Lactic Acid Bacteria to Bind Aflatoxin M1 in a Food Model. *J. Food Prot.* **2000**, *63*, 645–650. [CrossRef] [PubMed]
50. El-Nezami, H.; Kankaanpää, P.; Salminen, S.; Ahokas, J. Physicochemical Alterations Enhance the Ability of Dairy Strains of Lactic Acid Bacteria to Remove Aflatoxin from Contaminated Media. *J. Food Prot.* **1998**, *61*, 466–468. [CrossRef] [PubMed]
51. Assaf, J.C.; Atoui, A.; Khoury, A.E.; Chokr, A.; Louka, N. A Comparative Study of Procedures for Binding of Aflatoxin M1 to Lactobacillus Rhamnosus GG. *Braz. J. Microbiol.* **2017**, *49*, 120–127. [CrossRef] [PubMed]

52. Kuharić, Ž.; Jakopović, Ž.; Čanak, I.; Frece, J.; Bošnir, J.; Pavlek, Ž.; Ivešić, M.; Markov, K. Removing Aflatoxin M1 from Milk with Native Lactic Acid Bacteria, Centrifugation, and Filtration. *Arch. Ind. Hyg. Toxicol.* **2018**, *69*, 334–339. [CrossRef] [PubMed]
53. Campagnollo, F.B.; Ganev, K.C.; Khaneghah, A.M.; Portela, J.B.; Cruz, A.G.; Granato, D.; Corassin, C.H.; Oliveira, C.A.F.; Sant'Ana, A.S. The Occurrence and Effect of Unit Operations for Dairy Products Processing on the Fate of Aflatoxin M1: A Review. *Food Control* **2016**, *68*, 310–329. [CrossRef]
54. Afum, C.; Cudjoe, L.; Hills, J.; Hunt, R.; Padilla, L.; Elmore, S.; Afriyie, A.; Opare-Sem, O.; Phillips, T.; Jolly, P. Association between Aflatoxin M1 and Liver Disease in HBV/HCV Infected Persons in Ghana. *Int. J. Environ. Res. Public Health* **2016**, *13*, 377. [CrossRef] [PubMed]
55. Lindahl, J.F.; Kagera, I.N.; Grace, D. Aflatoxin M 1 Levels in Different Marketed Milk Products in Nairobi, Kenya. *Mycotoxin Res.* **2018**, *34*, 289–295. [CrossRef]
56. Hoffmann, V.; Moser, C. You Get What You Pay for: The Link between Price and Food Safety in Kenya. *Agric. Econ.* **2017**, *48*, 449–458. [CrossRef]
57. Klingelhöfer, D.; Zhu, Y.; Braun, M.; Bendels, M.H.K.; Brüggmann, D.; Groneberg, D.A. Aflatoxin—Publication Analysis of a Global Health Threat. *Food Control* **2018**, *89*, 280–290. [CrossRef]
58. IARC; WHO. IARC Monographs on the Evaluation of Carcinogenic Risks to Humans. Available online: https://monographs.iarc.fr/list-of-classifications-volumes/ (accessed on 13 July 2019).
59. Sirma, A.J.; Lindahl, J.F.; Makita, K.; Senerwa, D.; Mtimet, N.; Kang'ethe, E.K.; Grace, D. The Impacts of Aflatoxin Standards on Health and Nutrition in Sub-Saharan Africa: The Case of Kenya. *Glob. Food Sec.* **2018**, *18*, 57–61. [CrossRef]
60. FAO. *Worldwide Regulations for Mycotoxins in Food and Feed in 2003*; FAO: Rome, Italy, 2004.
61. Codex Alimentarius (Ed.) *Codex Standard 193-1995*; FAO/WHO, 2010; Available online: http://www.fao.org/fao-who-codexalimentarius/codex-texts/list-standards/en/ (accessed on 13 July 2019).
62. Awuor, A.O.; Yard, E.; Daniel, J.H.; Martin, C.; Bii, C.; Romoser, A.; Oyugi, E.; Elmore, S.; Amwayi, S.; Vulule, J.; et al. Evaluation of the Efficacy, Acceptability and Palatability of Calcium Montmorillonite Clay Used to Reduce Aflatoxin B1 Dietary Exposure in a Crossover Study in Kenya. *Food Addit. Contam. Part A* **2017**, *34*, 93–102. [CrossRef] [PubMed]
63. Nduti, N.; McMillan, A.; Seney, S.; Sumarah, M.; Njeru, P.; Mwaniki, M.; Reid, G. Investigating Probiotic Yoghurt to Reduce an Aflatoxin B1 Biomarker among School Children in Eastern Kenya: Preliminary Study. *Int. Dairy J.* **2016**, *63*, 124–129. [CrossRef]
64. Egner, P.; Wang, J.B.; Zhu, Y.R.; Jacobson, L.P.; Ng, D.; Munoz, A.; Kensler, T.W. Prevention of Liver Cancer in Qidong, China: Lessons from Aflatoxin Biomarker Studies. *Prog. Chem.* **2013**, *25*, 1454–1461.

toxins

MDPI

Review

Fumonisins: Impact on Agriculture, Food, and Human Health and their Management Strategies

Madhu Kamle [1], Dipendra K. Mahato [2], Sheetal Devi [3], Kyung Eun Lee [4], Sang G. Kang [4,5,*] and Pradeep Kumar [1,*]

1 Department of Forestry, North Eastern Regional Institute of Science and Technology, Nirjuli-791109, Arunachal Pradesh, India; madhu.kamle18@gmail.com

2 School of Exercise and Nutrition Sciences, Deakin University, 221 Burwood Hwy, Burwood VIC 3125, Australia; kumar.dipendra2@gmail.com

3 SAB Miller India Ltd., Sonipat, Haryana 131001, India; sheetaldeshwal1993@gmail.com

4 Molecular Genetics Laboratory, Department of Biotechnology, Yeungnam University, 280 Daehak-Ro, Gyeongsan, Gyeongbuk 38541, Korea; keun126@ynu.ac.kr

5 Stemforce, 302 Institute of Industrial Technology, Yeungnam University, Gyeongsan, Gyeongbuk 38541, Korea

* Correspondence: kangsg@yu.ac.kr (S.G.K.); pkbiotech@gmail.com (P.K.)

Received: 4 May 2019; Accepted: 4 June 2019; Published: 7 June 2019

Abstract: The fumonisins producing fungi, *Fusarium* spp., are ubiquitous in nature and contaminate several food matrices that pose detrimental health hazards on humans as well as on animals. This has necessitated profound research for the control and management of the toxins to guarantee better health of consumers. This review highlights the chemistry and biosynthesis process of the fumonisins, their occurrence, effect on agriculture and food, along with their associated health issues. In addition, the focus has been put on the detection and management of fumonisins to ensure safe and healthy food. The main focus of the review is to provide insights to the readers regarding their health-associated food consumption and possible outbreaks. Furthermore, the consumers' knowledge and an attempt will ensure food safety and security and the farmers' knowledge for healthy agricultural practices, processing, and management, important to reduce the mycotoxin outbreaks due to fumonisins.

Keywords: Fumonisins; *Fusarium* spp.; food contamination; health issues; secondary metabolites

Key Contribution: This review gives insight into the occurrence of fumonisins, their outbreak and effects on human health, and agriculture and food along with their management strategies.

1. Introduction

Fumonisins are secondary metabolites produced in cereals by pathogenic fungi, namely *Fusarium verticillioides*, *Fusarium proliferatum*, and related species [1]. Moreover, *Aspergillus nigri* also produces fumonisins in the crop plants of peanut, maize, and grape [2–6]. The maize and maize-based products are most commonly infected with fumonisins besides their presence in several other grains (rice, wheat, barley, maize, rye, oat, and millet) and grain products (tortillas, corn flask, chips) [7,8] which have major influences on health. More than 15 fumonisin homologues have been known and characterized as fumonisin A, B, C, and P [9,10]. Further among fumonisin B, FB1, FB2, and FB3 are most abundant with FB1 being the most toxic form that can co-exists with other forms of fumonisin, i.e., FB2 and FB3 [11]. These (FB1, FB2, and FB3) forms are the main food contaminants. FB1 consists of a diester with propane-1,2,3-tricarboxylic acid (TCA) and 2-amino-12,16-dimethyl-3,5,10,14,15-pentahydroxyleicosane where hydroxyl (OH-) groups at the C-14 and C-15 positions involved with the carboxyl groups (-COOH) of TCA to form an ester. On the other hand, FB2 and FB3 are actually the C-5 and C-10 dehydroxy analogues of FB1 [12].

The toxins are linked with several health issues like cancer of the esophagus as evident from different regions of the world. Fumonisins are a very sensitive issue all around the world, which occur in Europe (51%) and Asia (85%) [13]. The occurrence of fumonisins with other related toxins in feed and food is reported in various countries like Argentina [14], Brazil [15], China [16], Italy [17], Portugal [18], Spain [19], Tanzania [20], and Thailand [21]. They are also reported to have toxic effects on the liver and nephron in all the tested animals [22]. In addition, FB1 is implicated with the incidences of hepatocarcinoma, stimulation and suppression of the immune system, defects in the neural-tube, nephrotoxicity, as well as other ailments. It is prominent as a promoter of hepatocarcinoma [23] where its synergistic interactions with aflatoxin B1 (AFB1) has been exhibited in animal models (rainbow trout and rats) for two stages, i.e., initiation and promotion of cancer [24–26]. The international agency for Research on Cancer (IARC) characterized FB1 as a group 2B possible carcinogen for human. Besides this, it can cause toxicity in several animals like rats, mice, and rabbits [27]. Further, a temporary maximum tolerable daily intake for fumonisins has been set as 2 μg/kg bw/day based on the lack of any observed adverse effects for nephrotoxicity in male rats by the joint Food and Agriculture Organization (FAO) and World Health Organization (WHO) [28].

2. Major Source of Fumonisin

Fumonisins are mainly produced by *F. verticillioides* and *F. proliferatum* and other *Fusarium* spp. The genus *Fusarium*, belonging to the family Nectriaceae, can be found as saprophytes in soil and plants worldwide [29]. *Fusarium* spp. colonize to the rhizospheres of plants and then subsequently enter into the plant system. Furthermore, *F. verticillioides* and *F. proliferatum* are known to be the most common pathogens of maize (*Zea mays*) [30]. Not only the crops, but also many popular ornamental plants (e.g., aster begonia, carnation, chrysanthemum, gladiolus, etc.) are frequently attacked by different *Fusarium* species, viz., *F. oxysporum*, *F. foetens*, *F. hostae*, and *F. redolens* at various stages of production [31].

Fusarium, on the other hand, infects orchids in both pathogenic and non-pathogenic forms. The non-pathogenic forms are either decomposers [32] or in mutual relation where they help in the germination of seeds and the color development of seedlings [33]. The non-pathogenic forms also help to mitigate the infection of *Fusarium* wilt on various crops [34]. Soils responsible for suppressing *Fusarium* wilt are found to be dominant in the *Fusarium* spp. like *F. oxysporum* and *F. solani* which are of agricultural importance [35,36]. The *Fusarium* species infect maize and produce fumonisins mainly at the pre-harvesting stage. Furthermore, fumonisin production has been observed during the post-harvest period; however, under adverse conditions of storage [37]. Dietary exposure of fumonisins can lead to several harmful outcomes in both farm and experimental laboratory animals. For example, these toxins are responsible for leukoencephalomalacia in horses [38], pulmonary edema syndrome in pigs [39], hepatotoxicity and nephrotoxicity in rats [40], and apoptosis in many other types of cells [41].

3. Chemistry and Biosynthesis of Fumonisin

Fumonisins (FBs) consist of two methyls (–CH_3), one amine (-NH_2), one to four hydroxyl (-OH^-), and two tricarboxylic ester groups located at different positions along with the linear polyketide-derived backbone. The biosynthesis step comprises the addition of two molecules of tricarballylic esters and one alanine-derived amine to a C-18 polyketide backbone [42]. FBs structural identity has been established, which are similar to sphingosine and are an integral part of cell signaling, growth, and communication [43]. It was believed that fumonisin formation could be controlled by disrupting the biosynthesis of sphingolipids [44]. The biosynthesis process of the toxin has been initiated to illustrate these cellular mechanisms and to design modified analogs [45,46]; however, to date, single total synthesis has been achieved by Pereira et al. [47]. There are intra-specific differences in the biosynthesis of fumonosins depending on the environmental conditions, e.g., temperature, the wavelength of light, humidity, and media composition for both the *Fusarium* spp. *F. verticillioides* and *F. proliferatum* [48].

Even the responses of strains were found to be different when the plant extracts were added from common hosts of *F. proliferatum* [49].

4. Genes Responsible for Fumonisin Production

Exploring the biosynthesis of trichothecene and fumonisin has revealed the gene cluster fumonisin biosynthetic gene (FUM in *Fusarium* and *Aspergillus*) which is responsible for the production of fumonisins, two transport proteins, and a transcription factor [50]. The expression of these genes is co-regulated and related to the FUM genes expression as well; however, it is influenced by ecological conditions [51,52]. The production of fumonisin is dependent on FUM1 which further expresses an enzyme complex known as polyketide synthase that catalyzes the initial step for fumonisin biosynthesis [53]. Furthermore, a positive correlation has been identified between the proportion of FUM1 transcripts being estimated by real-time RT-PCR and the proportion of fumonisins biosynthesized by the *F. verticillioides* and *F. proliferatum* species [54]. FUM19 lies at a distance of 35 kb downstream of the FUM1 gene that expresses an ATP-binding cassette responsible for exporting extracellular fumonisins [51]. Further, the expression of an aminotransferase by FUM8 functions to maintain the biologically active and mature FB1 molecule [55].

A. niger genome has a *Fusarium* FUM cluster homologue consisting of eleven homologues of the *Fusarium* genes namely fum1 (polyketide synthase), fum3, fum6, and fum15 (hydroxylase), fum7 (dehydrogenase), fum8 (aminotransferase), fum10 (acyl-CoA synthase), fum13 (carbonyl reductase), fum14 (condensation-domain protein), fum19 (ABC transporter), and fum21 (transcription factor) genes [56,57]. The FUM cluster in the *A. niger*, also known to have a dehydrogenase gene (sdr1), which is of a short-chain length, is absent in the *Fusarium* FUM cluster and its role in the process of fumonisin biosynthesis is unknown [56,57]. Further, the *Fusarium* FUM2 gene is also absent from the *A. niger* FUM cluster which causes hydroxylation at the C-10 backbone position of fumonisin [58]. The absence of a FUM2 homologue in the *A. niger* cluster has been seen to be consistent with other studies as well revealing that *A. niger* produces fumonisins (FB2, FB4, and FB6) only when it lacks a hydroxyl at C-10 [59–61]. In addition to these, genes like FUG1 and FST1 have been also confirmed to have an important role in fumonisin biosynthesis in *F. verticillioides* besides their role in maize kernel colonization [62,63]. Furthermore, Niehaus et al. [64] have identified 21 polyketide synthase (PKS) in the genome of the *F. proliferatum* where PKS3 and PKS11 are predicted to be linked with the biosynthesis of fumonisin.

5. Occurrence in Food

The contamination of foods by fumonisin depends on agroclimatic conditions (Table 1). The most commonly infected groups in food are the cereals (rice, wheat, barley, maize, rye, oat, and millet). The FB1 has been reported to contaminate numerous food products like asparagus and garlic [65], barley foods [66], beers [67], dried figs [68], and milk [69]. Maize (*Zea mays* L.) and maize-based products are one of the most commonly infected foods by FB1 [70]. Maize is used for manufacturing several products like tortillas and tortilla chips, corn flakes and corn starch, popcorn, grits, flour, and oils. However, the contamination by FB1 and FB2 is decreased by 59% during the manufacturing of tortilla chips from maize flour, while 60% for flour and 50% for grits and snack products due to the heat treatment by extrusion [71]. Further, several other products like cornflakes [72], the Portuguese maize bread [73], tea (black and herbal), along with some medicinal plants [74] have also been contaminated by fumonisins.

Table 1. Occurrence of Fumonisin B1 and FB2 in cereals and cereal-based foods around the world.

Country	Food Matrix	FB1 (Range, µg/kg)	FB2 (Range, µg/kg)	Detection Technique	Reference
UK	Corn	200–6000	-	TLC	[75]
The Netherlands	Corn flour	40–90	-	HPLC	[76]
Switzerland	Corn grits	0–790	0–160	HPLC	[77]
Turkey	Cornmeal	250–2660	550	HPLC	[78]
Ghana	Corn	11–1655	10–770	HPLC	[79]
Malawi	Corn	20–115	30	HPLC	[80]
Zambia	Corn inbred lines	20–1420	10–290	HPLC	[81]
Bahrain	Corn kernel	25	-	HPLC	[82]
Kenya	Corn kernel	110–120	-	HPLC	[83]
Venezuela	Yellow corn	40–15,050	-	HPLC	[84]
Korea	Corn for popping	23–1210	-	direct competitive (dcELISA) and HPLC	[85]
India	Corn seed samples	133 to 1617	-	HPLC	[86]
Iran	Corn	10–3980	<10–1180	HPLC	[87]
Thailand	Corn	63–18,800	50–1400	HPLC	[88]
Nepal	Corn kernels	50–4600	100–5500	HPLC	[89]
Indonesia	Corn kernels	51–2440	<376	HPLC and GCMS	[90]
Argentina	Durum wheat	10.50–987.20	15–258.50	HPLC-MS/MS	[91]
Brazil	Wheat	958–4906	-	HPLC-FL	[92]
Canada	Wheat	-	-	HPLC	[93]
Central Europe	Wheat/wheat bran	-	-	ELISA	[94]
China	Wheat flour	0.30–34.60	-	UPLC-MS-MS	[95]
France	Organic Oat, rye and wheat flakes with maple syrup	75.70–98.10	62.10–81.10	HPLC-MS/MS	[96]
Germany	Organic wheat flakes	20.20–59.80	25.40–41.80	HPLC-MS/MS	[96]
Iran	Stored wheat samples	15–155	12–86	HPLC	[97]
Italy	Cereals, whole meal flours	10–2870	10–420	LC-MS	[98]
Japan	Wheat	>10	-	LC-ESI-MSMS	[99]
Serbia	Wheat	750–5400	-	ELISA	[100]
South Africa	Wheat and wheat products	1000–30,000	-	TLC, HPLC, Ms/MS	[101]
South America	Wheat/wheat bran	-	-	ELISA-HPLC	[94]
South-East Asia	Wheat/wheat bran	-	-	ELISA-HPLC	[94]
Southern Europe	Wheat/wheat bran	-	-	ELISA-HPLC	[94]
Spain	Wheat Gofio	787.50–1001.40	645.20–952.10	HPLC-MS/MS	[96]
Syria	Durum wheat	5–6	12	HPLC-MS/MS	[102]
Tunisia	Wheat-based products	88.33–184	121–158	LC-MS/MS	[103]
United States	Wheat	5–2210	2-249	LC-MS	[104]
Zimbabwe	Wheat	2500–6000	-	HPLC	[105]

6. Effects on Agriculture and Food

Annually 25% of harvested crops are contaminated by mycotoxins, causing huge economic losses to agricultural and industrial commodities. These mycotoxins are stable in nature and do not eliminate during food processing, cooking, baking, roasting, and pasteurization. The meagre agricultural, as well as post-harvest practices like inappropriate drying techniques, handling procedure, packaging materials and methods, and storage and transport conditions, are responsible for the increased risk of fungal growth and fumonisin contamination [106]. Cao et al. [107] investigated the accumulation of fumonisins at different kernel developmental stages as well as during the drying of the kernel of hybrid varieties of white maize. They observed *Fusarium* (especially *F. verticillioides*) to be the most prevalent genus for growth and contamination as compared to *Aspergillus* and *Penicillium*. The lower humidity of kernels favoured damage by insects along with fungal growth and accumulation of fumonisins [107]. The occurrence of fumonisins have been reported in edible plants like onion, garlic, asparagus, and pea seed [108,109]; in other cereals, mainly in wheat [84,110] as well as in crops like sorghum, beans (white, adzuki, mung), barley, soybean, asparagus spears, and figs [111,112]. Besides this, fumonisins have been found to impact the performance of aquatic animals like the Nile tilapia fingerlings and juveniles [113]. Fumonisins affected the hepatic expression of growth hormone receptor (GHR) and insulin like growth factor 1 (IGF-1) in these species, which is an indication that other aquatic animals and plants could also be affected by fumonisins posing a serious threat to food safety and security.

Fumonisins are an important class of mycotoxins produced by *F. proliferatum* and *F. verticillioides* along with others such as *F. napiforme, F. oxysporum, F. dlamini, F. nygamai* and *F. anthophilum* that are widely distributed, having potential health hazards to humans and animals [9]. These toxins are widely distributed in crops like corn, rice, sorghum, barley, and coffee. The exact causes of ear rot and kernel rot diseases is not well known but may be due to changes in weather such as dry weather followed by warm wet weather during flowering. The damage caused by the insect at the time of maturity allows strains present in nature to enter the ear and kernels. Rain before harvest may intensify the contamination of fumonisins in corn. Sometimes there are substantial amounts of fumonisins present in the non-symptomatic kernels of corn [114]. Yoshizawa et al. [103] reported the occurrence of fumonisins and aflatoxins in eighteen samples of corn in Thailand and found FB1 and FB2 and isolated *F. moniliforme* and *F. proliferatum* from the corn grit samples. Studies carried out in the USA reported the presence of FB1 and moniliformin in 34% of corn samples and 53% of corn-based food products, respectively [115]. A study in Brazil was conducted (during 2007–2010) to detect fumonisins in corn-based food products and reported that FB1 and FB2 were present in 82% and 51% of the examined products, respectively [116]. Contaminations by FB1 and FB2 observed in poultry broiler and feed fatting calves in South Korea [117]. Abdallah et al. [118] found the co-occurrence of FB2 and ochratoxin A and B in the date palm. In Brazil, it was reported that the production of fumonisins by *F. verticillioides* is found in both symptomatic and asymptomatic grains [119].

Furthermore, a survey was conducted in Japan for aflatoxin, ochratoxin A, and fumonisins contamination using HPLC and LC-MS. Results revealed that peanut butter is contaminated by aflatoxin, while orchratoxin A infection in oatmeal, rye, buckwheat flour, green coffee beans, roasted coffee beans beers, wheat flour, and wine. However, fumonisins were observed in popcorn, frozen corn, corn flasks, and corn grits [120]. Noonim et al. [59] analyzed the aflatoxin and fumonisin contaminations in different samples of Thai dried coffee, and it was noted that no *Fusarium* spp. were observed; however, *A. niger* was present in the coffee beans and produced fumonisins along with aflatoxins. A variable range of acetyldeoxynivalenol, deoxynivalenol, neosolaniol, fumonisin B1, and ochratoxin A contaminations were observed in Spanish coffee, and this variation was due to different methods of coffee brewing [121].

7. Mechanism of Toxicity and Health Effects of Fumonisins

7.1. Mechanism of Toxicity

FB1 predominates in 70% of the total FBs naturally occurring in infected food and feed samples [122]. FB1 express both acute and chronic symptoms in infected animals. FB1, though being an initiator of cancer, is non-genotoxic [123]. The major organs affected are liver and kidney; however, the severity of infection depends upon the strain and species [124]. The intestine, on the other hand, is a possible target for fumonisin toxicity [125]. FBs contamination has raised higher concern because of their interference with sphingolipid metabolism that ultimately leads to serious health concerns. Fumonisins are also linked to esophagal cancer and defects of the neural tube in humans [126]. Further, FB1 is the major causative agent for porcine pulmonary edema (PPE) [39], the toxicity of the liver and nephron in rodents [127], as well as cancers of the liver and esophagus in humans [128].

Franceschi et al. [129] studied the relationship between maize consumption and the risk of cancer of the upper digestive tract in the Pordenone Province in the north-eastern part of Italy. The population of this province has a high incidence of these neoplasms and shows particularly elevated levels of alcohol and tobacco use, in addition to high maize consumption. They observed that there were highly significant associations with frequent intake of maize emerging for oral cancer, pharyngeal cancer, and esophageal cancer. Dragan et al. [130] showed that the FB1 caused renal carcinomas in male rats and liver cancer in female mice. FB1 also induces apoptosis in many kidney cell lines, primary cell cultures, and also in vivo in rat liver and kidney [130,131]. Sun et al. [132] reported high contamination of FB1 in the food of the Huaian and Fusui city of China and suggested that FB1 may have a contributing role in human esophageal- and hepatocarcinogenesis. Further, Alizadeh et al. [133] studied 66 samples of both corn and rice from the Golestan province of Iran and observed high levels of FB1 contamination in both corn (223.66 μg/g) and rice (21.59 μg/g). They found a significant relationship between FB1 contamination in rice and the risk of esophageal cancer. Besides this, FB1 was found to be toxic to other cell lines. For example, FB1 triggers dose-dependent apoptosis and necrosis in esophageal carcinoma (SNO) cell lines in humans. Similarly, FB1 inhibited the activity of ceramide (CER) synthase, which is responsible for the acylation of sphinganine (Sa) and the recycling of sphingosine (So). This leads to an increment in the intracellular cytotoxic Sa-compound. Therefore, the variation of Sa/So proportions in urine and blood samples may denote the exposure of FBs in several animals; however, this has not been accurately validated [134].

7.2. Health Effects of Fumonisin

Equine leucoencephalomalacia first reported in 1891 is now revealed to be caused by consuming fumonisin-contaminated maize [135]. Further, the consumption of maize culture material infected by *F. verticillioides* [136] is responsible for the occurrence of porcine pulmonary edema (PPE) [30]. Since then, the outbreaks of PPE in the USA have been identified because of fumonisin infection. Further intake of fumonisin-affected diets by pregnant women causes neural tube defects in the developing fetus [126,137]. Sadler et al. [138] reported that FB1 has the potential to inhibit embryonic sphingolipid synthesis, produce embryotoxicity, and block folate transport and has been associated with increased prevalence of cancer and neural tube defects. On the other hand, Missmer et al. [126] reported the prevalence of neural tube defects (NTDs) doubled between 1990–1991 in Mexican–American women because they consume large amounts of corn in the form of tortillas, due to which they may be exposed to high levels of fumonisin. Fumonisin exposure increases the risk of NTDs and a dose above the threshold level may cause fetal death. Similarly, the exposure of fumonisin and its effect on esophageal and liver cancer is rare [132,139]. While no direct evidence of fumonisin hazard is found, its prolonged exposure may lead to cancer and birth defects in humans [140]. Moreover, the co-contamination of foods by fumonisin and aflatoxin has imposed risks of occurrences of outbreaks in southwest Nigeria [140], and the rural areas of Malawi in sub-Saharan Africa [141].

Besides this, the contamination of breast milk by fumonisins has been reported in several studies [142–144]. Recent studies have revealed the relationship between exposure to FBs and growth impairment in children [145–147]. According to Shirima et al. [146], fumonisin exposure negatively impacted child growth among children in Tanzania, which was confirmed based on urinary biomarker levels of fumonisin (UFB1). On the other hand, aflatoxin exposure had no significant impact on child growth. Furthermore, breastfeeding and weaning practices were considered to be associated with growth impairment in children due to exposure to FB1 [147]. The fumonisin carry-over has been observed in cow's milk as well [69]. Therefore, the incidence of fumonisin in human breast milk and its consumption by infants cannot be ignored, as the milk is a crucial part of infants' nutrition [148].

8. Effects of Processing on Fumonisin

Fumonisins are known to be comparatively heat-stable and affected only when heated above 150–200 °C during food processing techniques like baking, frying, roasting, or extrusion cooking.

The degree of reduction in their chemical structure and toxicity depends on the cooking conditions and the composition of the food matrix [149]. However, this reduction could be due to the structural modifications of fumonisins while interacting with other components of food that leads to the conjugate's formation [150]. FB1 interacts with reducing sugars to form strong covalent bonds during heat treatments. For instance, FB1 reacts with D-glucose of corn grits during the extrusion cooking at 160–180 °C and forms a reaction product, N-(carboxymethyl) fumonisin B1 (NCM) [151]. However, the condensation reaction of FB1 and D-glucose forms N-(deoxy-Dfructos-1-yl) FB1 (NDF) [152].

Besides this, the wet milling causes the reduction of fumonisins to some extent in steep water. Further industrial milling processes reduce the fumonisin content significantly such that the fractions obtained (gluten, fiber, germ, and starch) are suitable for animal and human consumption [153]. However, during the dry milling process, there is a negligible reduction in fumonisin content as the fumonisins are embedded in the germ and pericarp in higher concentrations than in the endosperm and its derivatives [72,154,155]. Fumonisins are variably distributed in cereals and the fractions depending upon the type of cultivars, agricultural practices, and the method of milling processes [153,156]. The toxins might be degraded or modified during the processing of Tortillas at high temperatures and pH [157]. However, the industrial processing methods like roasting, frying, and extrusion cooking are effective in reducing the fumonisins to significantly low levels [158].

9. Effects of Environmental Temperature on Fumonisin Production

The two main factors impacting on the growth of fungus and the production of fumonisin are temperatures and water potential [159]. Therefore, the toxins are predominant in temperate and Mediterranean climatic regions [160–163]. The Mediterranean climate regions experience extreme temperature, rainfall patterns, as well as longer durations of drought. These conditions might lead to variation in the population of mycotoxigenic fungi and the fumonisin production by them which ultimately impacts the control strategies [164]. The infection of maize by *F. verticillioides* and accumulation of fumonisins is determined by the climatic conditions, insect damage, as well as the plant characteristics. The ear rot infection by *F. verticillioides* occurs during the flowering stage and is favored by warm and dry conditions; however, both warm and wet conditions following silking have been found to be favorable for disease development [165]. The weather conditions are critical for toxin accumulation during flowering as well as prior to harvesting [166,167]. It has been found that the less rainfall with maximum temperatures of 30–35°C during flowering induces disease development [168].

Cendoya et al. [169] evaluated the effect of different levels of temperature and water activity (a_w) on the fungal growth and fumonisin biosynthesis in wheat using three strains of *F. proliferatum*. Temperatures of 15, 25, and 30 °C and a_w of 0.99, 0.98, 0.96, 0.94, 0.92, and 0.88 were evaluated. They found maximum growth of fumonisins at the highest a_w of 0.99 at 15 °C for two strains while for the third strain, the maximum growth was observed at 25 °C at the same a_w level. Furthermore, environmental factors like light along with nutrients available impacted the growth of *F. proliferatum* and the production of fumonisin [48,170]. In addition, Li et al. [171] evaluated the impact of pH levels on the growth of *F. proliferatum* culture. It was found that the toxin production was significantly inhibited in culture maintained at pH 5 compared to the culture at pH 10. However, the acidic pH 3–4, was found to enhance FB1 production by the fungus *F. proliferatum* [172].

10. Detection Techniques

The FB1 presence was detected by the Association of Official Analytical Chemists (AOAC) official method in food and feed samples. The derivatization was done using precolumn with ortho-phthaldialdehyde (OPA) and the detection by chromatographic techniques like HPLC (high-performance liquid chromatography) coupled with a fluorescence detector (HPLC-FLD). However, the drawback of this method is the use of high sample size (around 50 g), more extraction solvent (methanol:water), and solid-phase extraction (SPE) cartridges [173]. Therefore, methods like QuEChERS (Quick, Easy, Cheap, Effective, Rugged, and Safe) proved to be ideal for the detection of

FB1 [174–176]. Some of the commonly used techniques for fumonisin extractions include: (i) solid-liquid extraction (SLE) [177–180], (ii) liquid-liquid extraction (LLE) [181,182], (iii) matrix solid-phase dispersion (MSPD) [87,183,184], and (iv) dispersive liquid-liquid microextraction (DLLME) [185]. Recently, it was observed that the extraction yields were higher in finer flours indicating the importance of sample particle size on the recovery of fumonisins [11].

The traditional analytical methods to detect and quantify fumonisin include HPLC or UPLC (ultra-performance liquid chromatography) coupled with detectors such as UV–Vis spectrophotometric [186], fluorescence [187,188], and mass spectrometry (MS) [176,189–191]; liquid chromatography-mass spectrometry (LC-MS), and thin-layer chromatography (TLC) [192–194]. As these methods are expensive, tedious, and time-consuming [195], other advanced methods like the detection of mycotoxins producing fungi, enzyme-linked immunosorbent assay (ELISA), surface plasmon resonance (SPR), lateral flow immunoassay (LFI), immunosensors, electronic nose, and hyperspectral imaging are found to be more efficient [194,196]. Fumonisins producing genes have been amplified by PCR to detect *Fusarium* species in freshly harvested maize kernels [197]. PCR-based methods are used for the detection of mycotoxins producing fungal genera *Fusarium, Aspergillus*, and, *Penicillium* [198,199].

Recently, Nagaraj et al. [196] used a multiplex PCR technique to detect fumonisin producing *F. verticillioides* strains. ELISA coupled with PCR, i.e., PCR-ELISA by Omor et al. [200] for the detection of *F. verticillioides* based on the FUM21 gene in corn. In addition to this, a highly sensitive indirect competitive enzyme-linked immunosorbent assay (icELISA) and gold nanoparticle-based gray imaging quantification immunoassay (GNPs-GI) has been developed to detect FB1 in agricultural products [201]. Another important and non-destructive way of identifying toxigenic fungi in maize is by the application of hyperspectral imaging processes [202,203]. Besides this, the color-encoded lateral flow immunoassay (LFIA) has emerged as a leading technique for simultaneous detection of aflatoxin B1 and type-B fumonisins in a single test line [204]. Nowadays, electrochemical immunosensors are employed for rapid and sensitive detection of FB1 [205]. Furthermore, a rapid and ultrasensitive molecularly imprinted photoelectrochemical (MIP-PEC) sensing technique has been recently developed to measure FB1 [206].

11. Masked Mycotoxins as a major concern in detection

The masked mycotoxins issue was initially seen during the mid-1980s due to several mysterious cases of mycotoxicosis occurrence; however, the symptoms of mycotoxins in affected animals did not connect with the low mycotoxins content detected in their feed. At the same time, the metabolic biotransformation of deoxynivalenol (DON) to the less toxic derivatives *in planta* was first reported to appear in corn inoculated with *F. graminerium* [207] and also in naturally infected winter wheat [208]. In vivo studies for masked mycotoxins were carried out in pig and reported that zearalenone-14-glucoside was decomposed during the digestion process and zearalenone (ZEN) and zearalenol (ZEL) were detected in urinary and fecal metabolites [209].

During infection in plants, the mycotoxins produced by fungi are modified by plant enzymes and often conjugated to more polar substances, like sugars. These form of toxins are often less toxic metabolites stored in the vacuole in the soluble form or bound to macromolecules and are not detectable during routine analysis processes; therefore, referred to as masked mycotoxins [210]. These mycotoxins may not be a homogeneous group of contaminants but somewhat a complex mixture of different plant metabolites of various classes of mycotoxins and they are overall termed as the 'maskedome' [211]. Detection of masked mycotoxins is difficult as they change the physiological properties of their molecules leading to modified chromatographic behavior [212]. Due to less detectability, these toxins are a serious concern for food safety and these toxins may be converted back to the parent toxin forms during the food digestion process [213]. De Boevre et al. [214] analyzed cereal-based food products and raw feed materials for the presence of mycotoxins including deoxynivalenol, 3-acetyldeoxynivalenol, 15-acetyldeoxynivalenol, zearalenone, α-zearalenol (α-ZEL), β-zearalenol, and their respective masked forms like α-zearalenol-1-3glucoside, zearalenone-4-glucoside, α-zearalenone-4-glucoside, β-zearalenone-4-glucoside, and zearalenone-4-sulfate in fiber-enriched bread, bran-enriched bread, cornflakes, popcorn, and oatmeal. Binder et al. [215] evaluated the absorption, distribution, metabolism, and excretion (ADME) of plant (ZEN-14-Glc, ZEN-16-Glc) and fungal (ZEN-14-S) ZEN metabolites in pigs and found that the total amounts of ZEN-14-GlcA, ZEN, and α-ZEL were excreted into urine after 0–48 hours of administration.

12. Degradation Kinetics

The degradation of FB1 was first revealed by Duvick et al. [216] to occur by microbes like *Exophiala spinifera*, *Rhinocladiella atrovirens*, and *Sphingomonas* or *Xanthomonas* having the capacity to metabolize FB1. These microbes were isolated from various tissues of maize. Further, the fumonisin metabolism by *E. spinifera* and the bacterium (deposited as ATCC55552 with the American Type Culture Collection) was studied by radiochemical and chromatographic (e.g., thin layer chromatography, TLC) methods. The initial two steps of biodegradation of FB1 were revealed to be due to de-esterification by a carboxylesterase releasing two tricarballylic acid (TCA) moieties leading to the formation of hydrolyzed FB1 (HFB1). The bacterial strain ATCC55552 further metabolized 14C-FB1 with the release of 14 molecules of CO_2. However, *E. spinifera* could not further metabolize the TCA moieties. Blackwell et al. [217] later studied the oxidative deamination process of HFB1 by *E. spinifera* through TLC and mass spectrometry. They found that the HFB1 gets converted to Nacetyl HFB1 and 2-oxo-12,16-dimethyl-3,5,10,14,15-icosanepentol hemiketal. A cluster of genes in the bacterium ATCC55552 responsible for the degradation of fumonisin is mentioned in a patent, WO 00/04158 by Duvick et al. [218].

FB1 can be degraded to the less toxic form of hydrolyzed FB1 (HFB1) by an enzymatic process which could be used to reduce intestinal inflammation in pigs [219]. Further, the gene that catalyzes the oxidative deamination process of HFB1 in *E. spinifera* was revealed; however, the responsible enzyme for the deamination reaction is still unknown [218]. Later, Benedetti et al. [220] screened and isolated a bacterium related to the Delftia/Comamonas group (known as NCB 1492) from the soil. It was able to hydrolyze and deaminate FB1, but still, the sequences of the responsible genes are unknown. A year before, *Sphingomonas* sp. MTA144 was shown to have fumonisin degrading activity [221]. Further, Heinl et al. [222] identified two genes (carboxylesterase and aminotransferase) having prominent fumonisin-degrading activity. In addition to this, essential oils from plants were found to inhibit as well as degrade FB1 for example anise, camphor, cinnamon, citral, clove, eucalyptus, *Litsea cubeba*, and spearmint [223,224].

13. Management and Control Strategies

13.1. Management and Control using Agricultural Practices

As the crop plants like maize are infected by fumonisins during their growth in fields [225], the implementation of good agricultural practices (GAP), good storage practices (GSP), and good manufacturing practices (GMP) can mitigate the fumonisin contamination [226]. Harvesting the crop at earlier stages could be one of the strategies to control fumonisin contamination [227]; however, this cannot be applied to crops that need to be harvested at full maturity. Instead, the early harvest can be done for forage maize to increase the digestibility of silage. These practices require careful study as the farmers prefer a delayed harvest because of advancement in technologies. For instance, the use of kernel processors during forage harvesting leads to the production of digestible silage from maize when harvested at later stages [228].

Recently, the Codex Alimentarius Commission has set maximum levels of fumonisin at 4000 μg/kg and 2000 μg/kg, respectively for raw maize and for maize flour and meal which have been implemented in South Africa. However, the lowering of fumonisin exposure in subsistence farmers need an integrated approach, and this cannot be solely achieved by regulatory measures [229]. Besides these approaches, the use of nanotechnology and genetic engineering should be encouraged in the field of agriculture to develop resistant varieties of crops to get rid of *Fusarium* infection and FB contamination. The creation of drought and insect-resistant crops can also play a significant role in the fumonisin control as these factors are responsible, in one or the other way, for the fungal infection [230]. In addition to this, educating the farmers about the importance of drying and sorting out of the contaminated kernels from the crops can manage and control the risk of infection to some extent [231]. The in vitro study of combinations of fungicides (fludioxonil + metalaxyl-M) showed that it was not sufficient in the growth inhibition of *F. verticillioides* and even the increase in the production of FB1 by their strains [232]. A similar study also showed that these fungicides inhibit the growth and extracellular material formation but enhance the sporulation and fumonisin production in liquid culture of *F. verticillioides* [233]. Masiello et al. [234] reported that prothioconazole and thiophanate-methyl were effective in reducing the *F. graminearum* (52% and 48%) and *F. proliferatum* contamination (44% and 27%) under the field trial.

Fumonisin production and *Fusarium* growth are the result of interactions with various biotic and abiotic factors. In the case of abiotic factor temperature, water stress was the most significant environmental factor which influenced the fumonisin production and *Fusarium* growth. Several other stress conditions such as osmotic stress, pH, and fungicides were reported for the production mycotoxins [235,236]. *F. verticillioides* isolates were found to exhibit better performance at higher temperatures and under water stress conditions in comparison to *F. proliferatum*, another fumonisin-producing species. Marin et al. [237] suggested that environmental conditions leading to water stress (drought) might result in an increased risk of fumonisin contamination of maize caused by *F. verticillioides*. Drought stress and excess irrigation favor *Fusarium* infection. Drought stress should be avoided during the period of wheat seed development and maturation [238]. Excess moisture during the flowering seasons and early grain-fill periods also supports the *Fusarium* infection and moisture also increases the DON contamination [239]. Fungicide treatments were found to be effective against wheat *Fusarium* infection and DON contaminations [240,241]. Azole fungicides were found to be effective in the reduction of DON and other emerging and modified mycotoxins [242]. Therefore, an integrated approach, involving good agricultural management practices, hazard analysis, and critical control point production, storage management along with selected biologically based treatments, and mild chemical and physical treatments could reduce the fumonisin contamination effectively [243].

13.2. Management and Control using Mycotoxin Binder

Mycotoxin binders or adsorbents are substances that bind to mycotoxins and prevent them from being absorbed through the gut and prevent their entrance into the blood circulation. The mycotoxin binders can be helpful and utilized when other preventive measures fail against molds and mycotoxins [244]. The main aim of mycotoxin binders is to prevent the absorption of the mycotoxins from the intestinal tract of animals by absorbing the toxin to their surface. These binders may be organic or inorganic in nature, such as clay and yeast derived products, respectively [245]. However, mycotoxin modifiers are used to alter the chemical structure of mycotoxins and reduce their toxicity. These are microbiological in origin containing whole bacterial and yeast culture and specifically extracted compound such as enzymes [246]. In the field during harvesting of the crop, the production of mycotoxins can be reduced by choosing varieties that are adapted to the growing area and have resistance to fungal diseases. Mycotoxin production can also be reduced in the field by proper irrigation and balanced fertilizer applications [247]. These binders bind to the mycotoxins strong enough to prevent toxic interactions with the consuming animals and their absorption across the digestive tract. Potential absorbent materials include activated carbon, aluminosilicates (bentonite, clay, montmorillonite, zeolite, pollyosilicates etc.), complex indigestible carbohydrates (Cellulose, polysaccharides in the cell wall of yeast and bacteria such as glucomannans, petidoglycans) and other synthetic polymers such as cholestryamine and polyvinylpyrrolidone and derivatives [247]. De Mil et al. [248] characterized 27 feed additives marketed as mycotoxin binders and screened them for their in vitro zearalenone (ZEN) adsorption. Recent studies showed that the addition of the commercial toxin binders to the aflatoxin B1 (AFB1) containing diets reduced the adverse effects of AFB1 and could be helpful as a solution to the aflatoxicosis problem in young broiler chicks [249].

14. Conclusion

The contamination of food and feed by fumonisin is a serious threat for disease outbreaks worldwide. The various techniques ranging from physical to biochemical as well as genetic engineering can be utilized in an efficient manner to mitigate fumonisin contamination of foods. However, a major issue of concern lies with the development of fungal and insect resistant crops to combat the fungal infection and fumonisin contamination. The naturally occurring soil microorganisms have been reported to have an immense capability of degrading and reducing the biosynthesis of fumonisins and its contamination in various agricultural crops. Moreover, the application of nanotechnology and genetic engineering should be given more emphasis to develop resistant varieties of crops and ensure the safety and quality of food for future generations.

Author Contributions: P.K. conceived and designed the manuscript; D.K.M., M.K., and P.K. wrote the manuscript; K.E.L. and S.D. helped in the editing of the manuscript; P.K. and S.G.K. critically reviewed the manuscript and did the required editing.

Funding: This work was supported by the Sunforce Inc. Republic of Korea.

Acknowledgments: All authors are highly grateful to the authority of the respective department and Institution for their support in doing this research. Author (P.K.) would like to thank the DST-SERB (file no ECR/2017/001143) and DBT-Twinning (No. BT/PR24741/NER/95/659/2017) for their financial support. This work was supported by the Sunforce Inc. Republic of Korea.

Conflicts of Interest: The authors declare no conflict of interest.

References

1. Rheeder, J.P.; Marasas, W.F.; Vismer, H.F. Production of fumonisin analogs by Fusarium species. *Appl. Environ. Microbiol.* **2002**, *68*, 2101–2105. [CrossRef] [PubMed]
2. Astoreca, A.; Magnoli, C.; Barberis, C.; Chiacchiera, S.; Combina, M.; Dalcero, A. Ochratoxin a production in relation to ecophysiological factors by Aspergillus section Nigri strains isolated from different substrates in Argentina. *Sci. Total Environ.* **2007**, *388*, 16–23. [CrossRef] [PubMed]
3. Astoreca, A.; Magnoli, C.; Ramirez, M.L.; Combina, M.; Dalcero, A. Water activity and temperature effects on growth of Aspergillus niger, A. awamori and A. carbonarius isolated from different substrates in Argentina. *Int. J. Food Microbiol.* **2007**, *119*, 314–318. [CrossRef] [PubMed]
4. Frisvad, J.C.; Smedsgaard, J.; Samson, R.A.; Larsen, T.O.; Thrane, U. Fumonisin B2 production by Aspergillus niger. *J. Agric. Food Chem.* **2007**, *55*, 9727–9732. [CrossRef] [PubMed]
5. Mogensen, J.M.; Frisvad, J.C.; Thrane, U.; Nielsen, K.F. Production of fumonisin B2 and B4 by Aspergillus niger on grapes and raisins. *J. Agric. Food Chem.* **2009**, *58*, 954–958. [CrossRef] [PubMed]
6. Kumar, P.; Mahato, D.K.; Kamle, M.; Mohanta, T.K.; Kang, S.G. Aflatoxins: A global concern for food safety, human health and their management. *Front. Microbiol.* **2017**, *7*, 2170. [CrossRef]
7. Dall'Asta, C.; Battilani, P. Fumonisins and their modified forms, a matter of concern in future scenario? *World Mycotoxin J.* **2016**, *9*, 727–739. [CrossRef]
8. Cendoya, E.; Chiotta, M.L.; Zachetti, V.; Chulze, S.N.; Ramirez, M.L. Fumonisins and fumonisin-producing *Fusarium* occurrence in wheat and wheat by products: A review. *J. Cereal Sci.* **2018**, *80*, 158–166. [CrossRef]
9. Braun, M.S.; Wink, M. Exposure, occurrence, and chemistry of fumonisins and their cryptic derivatives. *Compr. Rev. Food Sci. Food Saf.* **2018**, *17*, 769–791. [CrossRef]
10. Marasas, W.F. *Fumonisins in Food*; Springer: Berlin/Heidelberg, Germany, 1996.
11. Damiani, T.; Righetti, L.; Suman, M.; Galaverna, G.; Dall'Asta, C. Analytical issue related to fumonisins: A matter of sample comminution? *Food Control* **2019**, *95*, 1–5. [CrossRef]
12. Shephard, G. Chromatographic determination of the fumonisin mycotoxins. *J. Chromatogr. A* **1998**, *815*, 31–39. [CrossRef]

13. Corrêa, J.A.F.; Orso, P.B.; Bordin, K.; Hara, R.V.; Luciano, F.B. Toxicological effects of fumonisin B1 in combination with other *Fusarium* toxins. *Food Chem. Toxicol.* **2018**, *121*, 483–494. [CrossRef] [PubMed]
14. Garrido, C.; Pezzani, C.H.; Pacin, A. Mycotoxins occurrence in Argentina's maize (Zea mays L.), from 1999 to 2010. *Food Control.* **2012**, *25*, 660–665. [CrossRef]
15. Vargas, E.; Preis, R.; Castro, L.; Silva, C. Co-occurrence of aflatoxins B 1, B 2, G 1, G 2, zearalenone and fumonisin B 1 in Brazilian corn. *Food Addit. Contam.* **2001**, *18*, 981–986. [CrossRef] [PubMed]
16. Wang, Y.; Liu, S.; Zheng, H.; He, C.; Zhang, H. T-2 toxin, zearalenone and fumonisin B1 in feedstuffs from China. *Food Addit. Contam.* **2013**, *6*, 116–122. [CrossRef] [PubMed]
17. Gutleb, A.; Caloni, F.; Giraud, F.; Cortinovis, C.; Pizzo, F.; Hoffmann, L.; Bohn, T.; Pasquali, M. Detection of multiple mycotoxin occurrences in soy animal feed by traditional mycological identification combined with molecular species identification. *Toxicol. Rep.* **2015**, *2*, 275–279. [CrossRef] [PubMed]
18. Almeida, I.; Martins, H.M.; Santos, S.; Costa, J.M.; Bernardo, F. Co-occurrence of mycotoxins in swine feed produced in Portugal. *Mycotoxin Res.* **2011**, *27*, 177–181. [CrossRef] [PubMed]
19. Cano-Sancho, G.; Ramos, A.J.; Marín, S.; Sanchis, V. Presence and co-occurrence of aflatoxins, deoxynivalenol, fumonisins and zearalenone in gluten-free and ethnic foods. *Food Control* **2012**, *26*, 282–286. [CrossRef]
20. Kamala, A.; Ortiz, J.; Kimanya, M.; Haesaert, G.; Donoso, S.; Tiisekwa, B.; De Meulenaer, B. Multiple mycotoxin co-occurrence in maize grown in three agro-ecological zones of Tanzania. *Food Control.* **2015**, *54*, 208–215. [CrossRef]
21. Tansakul, N.; Jala, P.; Laopiem, S.; Tangmunkhong, P.; Limsuwan, S. Co-occurrence of five *Fusarium* toxins in corn-Dried Distiller's Grains with Solubles in Thailand and comparison of ELISA and LC-MS/MS for fumonisin analysis. *Mycotoxin Res.* **2013**, *29*, 255–260. [CrossRef]
22. Chu, F.S.; Li, G.Y. Simultaneous occurrence of fumonisin B1 and other mycotoxins in moldy corn collected from the People's Republic of China in regions with high incidences of esophageal cancer. *Appl. Environ. Microbiol.* **1994**, *60*, 847–852. [PubMed]
23. Gelderblom, W.; Jaskiewicz, K.; Marasas, W.; Thiel, P.; Horak, R.; Vleggaar, R.; Kriek, N. Fumonisins–novel mycotoxins with cancer-promoting activity produced by *Fusarium moniliforme*. *Appl. Environ. Microbiol.* **1988**, *54*, 1806–1811. [PubMed]
24. Carlson, D.B.; Williams, D.E.; Spitsbergen, J.M.; Ross, P.F.; Bacon, C.W.; Meredith, F.I.; Riley, R.T. Fumonisin B1 promotes aflatoxin B1 and N-methyl-N'-nitro-nitrosoguanidine-initiated liver tumors in rainbow trout. *Toxicol. Appl. Pharmacol.* **2001**, *172*, 29–36. [CrossRef] [PubMed]
25. Qian, G.; Tang, L.; Lin, S.; Xue, K.S.; Mitchell, N.J.; Su, J.; Gelderblom, W.C.; Riley, R.T.; Phillips, T.D.; Wang, J.-S. Sequential dietary exposure to aflatoxin B1 and fumonisin B1 in F344 rats increases liver preneoplastic changes indicative of a synergistic interaction. *Food Chem. Toxicol.* **2016**, *95*, 188–195. [CrossRef] [PubMed]
26. Xue, K.S.; Qian, G.; Lin, S.; Su, J.; Tang, L.; Gelderblom, W.C.; Riley, R.T.; Phillips, T.D.; Wang, J.-S. Modulation of pre-neoplastic biomarkers induced by sequential aflatoxin B1 and fumonisin B1 exposure in F344 rats treated with UPSN clay. *Food Chem. Toxicol.* **2018**, *114*, 316–324. [CrossRef] [PubMed]
27. International Agency for Research on Cancer (IARC), World Health Organisation (WHO). Fumonisin B1. In *IARC Monographs on the Evaluation of Carcinogenic Risks to Humans, Some Traditional Herbal Medicines, Some Mycotoxins, Naphthalene and Styrene*; IARC Press: Lyon, France, 2002; Volume 82, pp. 301–366.
28. Joint FAO WHO Expert Committee on Food Additives, World Health Organization. Safety evaluation of certain food additives and contaminants: Prepared by the Seventy fourth meeting of the Joint FAO/WHO Expert Committee on Food Additives (JECFA). Available online: https://apps.who.int/iris/bitstream/handle/10665/171781/9789240693982_eng.pdf;jsessionid=79EFFBD803B75293027EDA351F998A18?sequence=3 (accessed on 7 June 2019).
29. Burgess, L. General ecology of the fusaria. In *Fusarium: Diseases, Biology, and Taxonomy*; Nelson, P.E., Toussoun, T.A., Cook, R.J., Eds.; Pennsylvania State University Press: University Park, PA, USA, 1981; pp. 225–235.
30. Marasas, W. Discovery and occurrence of the fumonisins: A historical perspective. *Environ. Health Perspect.* **2001**, *109*, 239–243. [PubMed]
31. Gullino, M.L.; Minuto, A.; Gilardi, G.; Garibaldi, A. Efficacy of azoxystrobin and other strobilurins against *Fusarium* wilts of carnation, cyclamen and Paris daisy. *Crop. Prot.* **2002**, *21*, 57–61. [CrossRef]
32. Booth, C. The genus Fusarium. *Fusarium*; CAB, 1971. Available online: http://www.mycobank.org/BioloMICS.aspx?TableKey=14682616000000061&Rec=744&Fields=All (accessed on 7 June 2019).

33. Vujanovic, V.; St-Arnaud, M.; Barabé, D.; Thibeault, G. Viability testing of orchid seed and the promotion of colouration and germination. *Ann. Bot.* **2000**, *86*, 79–86. [CrossRef]
34. Alabouvette, C.; Lemanceau, P.; Steinberg, C. Recent advances in the biological control of *Fusarium* wilts. *Pestic. Sci.* **1993**, *37*, 365–373. [CrossRef]
35. Louvet, J.; Rouxel, F.; Alabouvette, C. Recherches sur la résistance des sols aux maladies. I. Mise en évidence de la nature microbiologique de la résistance d'un sol au développement de la fusariose vasculaire du melon. *Ann. Phytopathol.* **1976**, *8*, 425–436.
36. Coleman, J.J. The *Fusarium solani* species complex: Ubiquitous pathogens of agricultural importance. *Mol. Plant Pathol.* **2016**, *17*, 146–158. [CrossRef] [PubMed]
37. Chulze, S. Strategies to reduce mycotoxin levels in maize during storage: A review. *Food Addit. Contam.* **2010**, *27*, 651–657. [CrossRef]
38. Ross, P.F.; Rice, L.G.; Osweiler, G.D.; Nelson, P.E.; Richard, J.L.; Wilson, T.M. A review and update of animal toxicoses associated with fumonisin-contaminated feeds and production of fumonisins by *Fusarium* isolates. *Mycopathologia* **1992**, *117*, 109–114. [CrossRef] [PubMed]
39. Harrison, L.R.; Colvin, B.M.; Greene, J.T.; Newman, L.E.; Cole Jr, J.R. Pulmonary edema and hydrothorax in swine produced by fumonisin B1, a toxic metabolite of *Fusarium moniliforme*. *J. Vet. Diagn. Investig.* **1990**, *2*, 217–221. [CrossRef] [PubMed]
40. Voss, K.A.; Plattner, R.D.; Riley, R.T.; Meredith, F.I.; Norred, W.P. In vivo effects of fumonisin B 1-producing and fumonisin B 1-nonproducing *Fusarium moniliforme* isolates are similar: Fumonisins B 2 and B 3 cause hepato-and nephrotoxicity in rats. *Mycopathologia* **1998**, *141*, 45–58. [CrossRef] [PubMed]
41. Jones, C.; Ciacci-Zanella, J.R.; Zhang, Y.; Henderson, G.; Dickman, M. Analysis of fumonisin B1-induced apoptosis. *Environ. Health Perspect.* **2001**, *109* (Suppl. 2), 315–320. [CrossRef]
42. Burgess, K.M.; Renaud, J.B.; McDowell, T.; Sumarah, M.W. Mechanistic insight into the biosynthesis and detoxification of fumonisin mycotoxins. *ACS Chem. Biol.* **2016**, *11*, 2618–2625. [CrossRef]
43. Chandrasekhar, S.; Sreelakshmi, L. Formal synthesis of fumonisin B1, a potent sphingolipid biosynthesis inhibitor. *Tetrahedron Lett.* **2012**, *53*, 3233–3236. [CrossRef]
44. Wang, E.; Norred, W.; Bacon, C.; Riley, R.; Merrill, A.H. Inhibition of sphingolipid biosynthesis by fumonisins. Implications for diseases associated with *Fusarium moniliforme*. *J. Biol. Chem.* **1991**, *266*, 14486–14490.
45. Gurjar, M.K.; Rajendran, V.; Rao, B.V. Chiron approach towards a potent toxin fumonisin B1 backbone: Synthesis of its hexaacetate derivative. *Tetrahedron Lett.* **1998**, *39*, 3803–3806. [CrossRef]
46. Oikawa, H.; Yamawaki, D.; Kagawa, T.; Ichihara, A. Total synthesis of AAL-toxin TA1. *Tetrahedron Lett.* **1999**, *40*, 6621–6625. [CrossRef]
47. Pereira, C.L.; Chen, Y.-H.; McDonald, F.E. Total synthesis of the sphingolipid biosynthesis inhibitor fumonisin B1. *J. Am. Chem. Soc.* **2009**, *131*, 6066–6067. [CrossRef] [PubMed]
48. Fanelli, F.; Schmidt-Heydt, M.; Haidukowski, M.; Geisen, R.; Logrieco, A.; Mulè, G. Influence of light on growth, fumonisin biosynthesis and FUM1 gene expression by *Fusarium proliferatum*. *Int. J. Food Microbiol.* **2012**, *153*, 148–153. [CrossRef] [PubMed]
49. Stępień, Ł.; Waśkiewicz, A.; Wilman, K. Host extract modulates metabolism and fumonisin biosynthesis by the plant-pathogenic fungus *Fusarium proliferatum*. *Int. J. Food Microbiol.* **2015**, *193*, 74–81. [CrossRef]
50. Alexander, N.J.; Proctor, R.H.; McCormick, S.P. Genes, gene clusters, and biosynthesis of trichothecenes and fumonisins in *Fusarium*. *Toxin Rev.* **2009**, *28*, 198–215. [CrossRef]
51. Proctor, R.H.; Brown, D.W.; Plattner, R.D.; Desjardins, A.E. Co-expression of 15 contiguous genes delineates a fumonisin biosynthetic gene cluster in *Gibberella moniliformis*. *Fungal Genet. Biol.* **2003**, *38*, 237–249. [CrossRef]
52. Desjardins, A.; Proctor, R. Molecular biology of *Fusarium* mycotoxins. *Int. J. Food Microbiol.* **2007**, *119*, 47–50. [CrossRef]
53. Bojja, R.S.; Cerny, R.L.; Proctor, R.H.; Du, L. Determining the biosynthetic sequence in the early steps of the fumonisin pathway by use of three gene-disruption mutants of *Fusarium verticillioides*. *J. Agric. Food Chem.* **2004**, *52*, 2855–2860. [CrossRef]
54. López-Errasquín, E.; Vázquez, C.; Jiménez, M.; González-Jaén, M.T. Real-time RT-PCR assay to quantify the expression of FUM1 and FUM19 genes from the fumonisin-producing *Fusarium verticillioides*. *J. Microbiol. Methods* **2007**, *68*, 312–317. [CrossRef]
55. Seo, J.-A.; Proctor, R.H.; Plattner, R.D. Characterization of four clustered and coregulated genes associated with fumonisin biosynthesis in *Fusarium verticillioides*. *Fungal Genet. Biol.* **2001**, *34*, 155–165. [CrossRef]

56. Baker, S.E. Aspergillus niger genomics: Past, present and into the future. *Med. Mycol.* **2006**, *44*, S17–S21. [CrossRef] [PubMed]
57. Pel, H.J.; De Winde, J.H.; Archer, D.B.; Dyer, P.S.; Hofmann, G.; Schaap, P.J.; Turner, G.; De Vries, R.P.; Albang, R.; Albermann, K. Genome sequencing and analysis of the versatile cell factory *Aspergillus niger* CBS 513.88. *Nat. Biotechnol.* **2007**, *25*, 221–231. [CrossRef]
58. Proctor, R.H.; Plattner, R.D.; Desjardins, A.E.; Busman, M.; Butchko, R.A. Fumonisin production in the maize pathogen *Fusarium verticillioides*: Genetic basis of naturally occurring chemical variation. *J. Agric. Food Chem.* **2006**, *54*, 2424–2430. [CrossRef] [PubMed]
59. Noonim, P.; Mahakarnchanakul, W.; Nielsen, K.F.; Frisvad, J.C.; Samson, R.A. Fumonisin B2 production by *Aspergillus niger* in Thai coffee beans. *Food Addit. Contam.* **2009**, *26*, 94–100. [CrossRef]
60. Mansson, M.; Klejnstrup, M.L.; Phipps, R.K.; Nielsen, K.F.; Frisvad, J.C.; Gotfredsen, C.H.; Larsen, T.O. Isolation and NMR characterization of fumonisin B2 and a new fumonisin B6 from *Aspergillus niger*. *J. Agric. Food Chem.* **2009**, *58*, 949–953. [CrossRef] [PubMed]
61. Susca, A.; Proctor, R.H.; Butchko, R.A.; Haidukowski, M.; Stea, G.; Logrieco, A.; Moretti, A. Variation in the fumonisin biosynthetic gene cluster in fumonisin-producing and nonproducing black aspergilli. *Fungal Genet. Biol.* **2014**, *73*, 39–52. [CrossRef]
62. Kim, H.; Woloshuk, C.P. Functional characterization of fst1 in *Fusarium verticillioides* during colonization of maize kernels. *Mol. Plant Microbe Interact.* **2011**, *24*, 18–24. [CrossRef]
63. Ridenour, J.B.; Bluhm, B.H. The novel fungal-specific gene FUG1 has a role in pathogenicity and fumonisin biosynthesis in *Fusarium verticillioides*. *Mol. Plant Pathol.* **2017**, *18*, 513–528. [CrossRef]
64. Niehaus, E.-M.; Münsterkötter, M.; Proctor, R.H.; Brown, D.W.; Sharon, A.; Idan, Y.; Oren-Young, L.; Sieber, C.M.; Novák, O.; Pěnčík, A. Comparative "omics" of the *Fusarium fujikuroi* species complex highlights differences in genetic potential and metabolite synthesis. *Genome Biol. Evol.* **2016**, *8*, 3574–3599. [CrossRef]
65. Seefelder, W.; Gossmann, M.; Humpf, H.-U. Analysis of fumonisin B1 in *Fusarium proliferatum*-infected asparagus spears and garlic bulbs from Germany by liquid chromatography– electrospray ionization mass spectrometry. *J. Agric. Food Chem.* **2002**, *50*, 2778–2781. [CrossRef]
66. Park, J.; Kim, E.; Shon, D.; Kim, Y. Natural co-occurrence of aflatoxin B1, fumonisin B1 and ochratoxin A in barley and corn foods from Korea. *Food Addit. Contam.* **2002**, *19*, 1073–1080. [CrossRef] [PubMed]
67. Kawashima, L.M.; Vieira, A.P.; Soares, L.M.V. Fumonisin B1 and ochratoxin A in beers made in Brazil. *Food Sci. Technol.* **2007**, *27*, 317–323. [CrossRef]
68. Heperkan, D.; Güler, F.K.; Oktay, H. Mycoflora and natural occurrence of aflatoxin, cyclopiazonic acid, fumonisin and ochratoxin A in dried figs. *Food Addit. Contam. Part A* **2012**, *29*, 277–286. [CrossRef] [PubMed]
69. Gazzotti, T.; Lugoboni, B.; Zironi, E.; Barbarossa, A.; Serraino, A.; Pagliuca, G. Determination of fumonisin B1 in bovine milk by LC–MS/MS. *Food Control* **2009**, *20*, 1171–1174. [CrossRef]
70. Stępień, Ł.; Koczyk, G.; Waśkiewicz, A. Genetic and phenotypic variation of *Fusarium proliferatum* isolates from different host species. *J. Appl. Genet.* **2011**, *52*, 487–496. [CrossRef] [PubMed]
71. Scudamore, K.; Scriven, F.; Patel, S. *Fusarium* mycotoxins in the food chain: Maize-based snack foods. *World Mycotoxin J.* **2009**, *2*, 441–450. [CrossRef]
72. Castells, M.; Marín, S.; Sanchis, V.; Ramos, A.J. Distribution of fumonisins and aflatoxins in corn fractions during industrial cornflake processing. *Int. J. Food Microbiol.* **2008**, *123*, 81–87. [CrossRef] [PubMed]
73. Lino, C.; Silva, L.; Pena, A.; Fernández, M.; Mañes, J. Occurrence of fumonisins B1 and B2 in broa, typical Portuguese maize bread. *Int. J. Food Microbiol.* **2007**, *118*, 79–82. [CrossRef] [PubMed]
74. Omuttang, G.Z.; Yaziciogilu, D. Determination of fumonisins B1 and B2 in herbal tea and medicinal plants in Turkey by high-performance liquid chromatography. *J. Food Prot.* **2004**, *67*, 1782–1786.
75. Preis, R.; Vargas, E. A method for determining fumonisin B1 in corn using immunoaffinity column clean-up and thin layer chromatography/densitometry. *Food Addit. Contam.* **2000**, *17*, 463–468. [CrossRef] [PubMed]
76. De Nijs, M.; Sizoo, E.; Vermunt, A.; Notermans, S.; Van Egmond, H. The occurrence of fumonisin B1 in maize-containing foods in the Netherlands. *Food Addit. Contam.* **1998**, *15*, 385–388. [CrossRef] [PubMed]
77. Pittet, A.; Parisod, V.; Schellenberg, M. Occurrence of fumonisins B1 and B2 in corn-based products from the Swiss market. *J. Agric. Food Chem.* **1992**, *40*, 1352–1354. [CrossRef]
78. Omurtag, G.Z. Determination of fumonisin B1 and B2 in corn and corn-based products in Turkey by high-performance liquid chromatography. *J. Food Prot.* **2001**, *64*, 1072–1075. [CrossRef] [PubMed]

79. Kpodo, K.; Thrane, U.; Hald, B. Fusaria and fumonisins in maize from Ghana and their co-occurrence with aflatoxins. *Int. J. Food Microbiol.* **2000**, *61*, 147–157. [CrossRef]
80. Doko, M.B.; Canet, C.; Brown, N.; Sydenham, E.W.; Mpuchane, S.; Siame, B.A. Natural co-occurrence of fumonisins and zearalenone in cereals and cereal-based foods from Eastern and Southern Africa. *J. Agric. Food Chem.* **1996**, *44*, 3240–3243. [CrossRef]
81. Doko, M.B.; Rapior, S.; Visconti, A.; Schjoth, J.E. Incidence and levels of fumonisin contamination in maize genotypes grown in Europe and Africa. *J. Agric. Food. Chem.* **1995**, *43*, 429–434. [CrossRef]
82. De Nijs, M.; Sizoo, E.; Rombouts, F.; Notermans, S.; Van Egmond, H. Fumonisin B1 in maize for food production imported in The Netherlands. *Food Addit. Contam.* **1998**, *15*, 389–392. [CrossRef]
83. Kedera, C.; Plattner, R.; Desjardins, A. Incidence of *Fusarium* spp. and levels of fumonisin B1 in maize in western Kenya. *Appl. Environ. Microbiol.* **1999**, *65*, 41–44.
84. Medina-Martínez, M.S.; Martínez, A.J. Mold occurrence and aflatoxin B1 and fumonisin B1 determination in corn samples in Venezuela. *J. Agric. Food. Chem.* **2000**, *48*, 2833–2836. [CrossRef]
85. Kim, E.-K.; Shon, D.-H.; Chung, S.-H.; Kim, Y.-B. Survey for fumonisin B1 in Korean corn-based food products. *Food Addit. Contam.* **2002**, *19*, 459–464. [CrossRef]
86. Nayaka, S.C.; Shankar, A.U.; Niranjana, S.; Wulff, E.G.; Mortensen, C.; Prakash, H. Detection and quantification of fumonisins from *Fusarium verticillioides* in maize grown in southern India. *World J. Microbiol. Biotechnol.* **2010**, *26*, 71. [CrossRef]
87. Shephard, G.S.; Marasas, W.F.; Leggott, N.L.; Yazdanpanah, H.; Rahimian, H.; Safavi, N. Natural occurrence of fumonisins in corn from Iran. *J. Agric. Food. Chem.* **2000**, *48*, 1860–1864. [CrossRef]
88. Yoshizawa, T.; Yamashita, A.; Chokethaworn, N. Occurrence of fumonisins and aflatoxins in corn from Thailand. *Food Addit. Contam.* **1996**, *13*, 163–168. [CrossRef]
89. Ueno, Y.; Aoyama, S.; Sugiura, Y.; Wang, D.; Lee, U.; Hirooka, E.; Hara, S.; Karki, T.; Chen, G.; Yu, S. A limited survey of fumonisins in corn and corn-based products in Asian countries. *Mycotoxin Res.* **1993**, *9*, 27–34. [CrossRef]
90. Ali, N.; Sardjono; Yamashita, A.; Yoshizawa, T. Natural co-occurrence of aflatoxins and *Fusavium* mycotoxins (fumonisins, deoxynivalenol, nivalenol and zearalenone) in corn from Indonesia. *Food Addit. Contam.* **1998**, *15*, 377–384. [CrossRef]
91. Palacios, S.A.; Ramirez, M.L.; Cabrera Zalazar, M.; Farnochi, M.C.; Zappacosta, D.; Chiacchiera, S.M.; Reynoso, M.M.; Chulze, S.N.; Torres, A.M. Occurrence of *Fusarium* spp. and fumonisin in durum wheat grains. *J. Agric. Food Chem.* **2011**, *59*, 12264–12269. [CrossRef]
92. Mendes, G.D.R.L.; Reis, T.A.D.; Corrêa, B.; Badiale-Furlong, E. Mycobiota and occurrence of Fumonisin B1 in wheat harvested in Southern Brazil. *Ciênc. Rural.* **2015**, *45*, 1050–1057. [CrossRef]
93. Roscoe, V.; Lombaert, G.; Huzel, V.; Neumann, G.; Melietio, J.; Kitchen, D.; Kotello, S.; Krakalovich, T.; Trelka, R.; Scott, P. Mycotoxins in breakfast cereals from the Canadian retail market: A 3-year survey. *Food Addit. Contam.* **2008**, *25*, 347–355. [CrossRef]
94. Rodrigues, I.; Naehrer, K. A three-year survey on the worldwide occurrence of mycotoxins in feedstuffs and feed. *Toxins* **2012**, *4*, 663–675. [CrossRef]
95. Li, F.; Jiang, D.; Zheng, F.; Chen, J.; Li, W. Fumonisins B1, B2 and B3 in corn products, wheat flour and corn oil marketed in Shandong province of China. *Food Addit. Contam. Part B.* **2015**, *8*, 169–174. [CrossRef]
96. Rubert, J.; Soriano, J.M.; Mañes, J.; Soler, C. Occurrence of fumonisins in organic and conventional cereal-based products commercialized in France, Germany and Spain. *Food Chem. Toxicol.* **2013**, *56*, 387–391. [CrossRef]
97. Chehri, K.; Jahromi, S.T.; Reddy, K.; Abbasi, S.; Salleh, B. Occurrence of *Fusarium* spp. and fumonisins in stored wheat grains marketed in Iran. *Toxins* **2010**, *2*, 2816–2823. [CrossRef]
98. Cirillo, T.; Ritieni, A.; Galvano, F.; Amodio Cocchieri, R. Natural co-occurrence of deoxynivalenol and fumonisins B1 and B2 in Italian marketed foodstuffs. *Food Addit. Contam.* **2003**, *20*, 566–571. [CrossRef]
99. Kushiro, M.; Zheng, Y.; Nagata, R.; Nakagawa, H.; Nagashima, H. Limited surveillance of fumonisins in brown rice and wheat harvested in Japan. *J. Food Prot.* **2009**, *72*, 1327–1331. [CrossRef]
100. Stanković, S.; Lević, J.; Ivanović, D.; Krnjaja, V.; Stanković, G.; Tančić, S. Fumonisin B1 and its co-occurrence with other fusariotoxins in naturally-contaminated wheat grain. *Food Control* **2012**, *23*, 384–388. [CrossRef]
101. Mashinini, K.; Dutton, M.F. The incidence of fungi and mycotoxins in South Africa wheat and wheat-based products. *J. Environ. Sci. Health B.* **2006**, *41*, 285–296. [CrossRef]

102. Alkadri, D.; Rubert, J.; Prodi, A.; Pisi, A.; Mañes, J.; Soler, C. Natural co-occurrence of mycotoxins in wheat grains from Italy and Syria. *Food Chem.* **2014**, *157*, 111–118. [CrossRef]
103. Serrano, A.; Font, G.; Ruiz, M.; Ferrer, E. Co-occurrence and risk assessment of mycotoxins in food and diet from Mediterranean area. *Food Chem.* **2012**, *135*, 423–429. [CrossRef]
104. Busman, M.; Desjardins, A.; Proctor, R. Analysis of fumonisin contamination and the presence of *Fusarium* in wheat with kernel black point disease in the United States. *Food Addit. Contam. Part A* **2012**, *29*, 1092–1100. [CrossRef]
105. Gamanya, R.; Sibanda, L. Survey of *Fusarium moniliforme* (*F. verticillioides*) and production of fumonisin B1 in cereal grains and oilseeds in Zimbabwe. *Int. J. Food Microbiol.* **2001**, *71*, 145–149. [CrossRef]
106. Marin, S.; Ramos, A.; Cano-Sancho, G.; Sanchis, V. Mycotoxins: Occurrence, toxicology, and exposure assessment. *Food Chem. Toxicol.* **2013**, *60*, 218–237. [CrossRef] [PubMed]
107. Cao, A.; Santiago, R.; Ramos, A.J.; Marín, S.; Reid, L.M.; Butrón, A. Environmental factors related to fungal infection and fumonisin accumulation during the development and drying of white maize kernels. *Int. J. Food Microbiol.* **2013**, *164*, 15–22. [CrossRef] [PubMed]
108. Irzykowska, L.; Bocianowski, J.; Waśkiewicz, A.; Weber, Z.; Karolewski, Z.; Goliński, P.; Kostecki, M.; Irzykowski, W. Genetic variation of Fusarium oxysporum isolates forming fumonisin B 1 and moniliformin. *J. Appl. Genet.* **2012**, *53*, 237–247. [CrossRef] [PubMed]
109. Waśkiewicz, A.; Stępień, Ł.; Wilman, K.; Kachlicki, P. Diversity of pea-associated F. proliferatum and F. verticillioides populations revealed by FUM1 sequence analysis and fumonisin biosynthesis. *Toxins* **2013**, *5*, 488–503. [CrossRef] [PubMed]
110. Cendoya, E.; Monge, M.P.; Palacios, S.A.; Chiacchiera, S.M.; Torres, A.M.; Farnochi, M.C.; Ramirez, M.L. Fumonisin occurrence in naturally contaminated wheat grain harvested in Argentina. *Food Control.* **2014**, *37*, 56–61. [CrossRef]
111. Wong, J.; Jeffries, P. Diversity of pathogenic *Fusarium* populations associated with asparagus roots in decline soils in Spain and the UK. *Plant Physiol.* **2006**, *55*, 331–342. [CrossRef]
112. Karbancıoglu-Güler, F.; Heperkan, D. Natural occurrence of fumonisin B1 in dried figs as an unexpected hazard. *Food Chem. Toxicol.* **2009**, *47*, 289–292. [CrossRef] [PubMed]
113. da Silva, S.C.C.; Lala, B.; Carniato, C.; Schamberd, C.R.; Nascimento, C.S.; Braccini, G.L.; Porto, C.; Roldi, G.; Tanamati, F.; Gasparino, E. Fumonisin affects performance and modulates the gene expression of IGF-1 and GHR in Nile tilapia fingerlings and juveniles. *Aquaculture* **2019**, *507*, 233–237. [CrossRef]
114. Richard, J.L. Some major mycotoxins and their mycotoxicoses—An overview. *Int. J. Food Microbiol.* **2007**, *119*, 3–10. [CrossRef] [PubMed]
115. Gutema, T.; Munimbazi, C.; Bullerman, L.B. Occurrence of fumonisins and moniliformin in corn and corn-based food products of US origin. *J. Food Prot.* **2000**, *63*, 1732–1737. [CrossRef]
116. Martins, F.A.; Ferreira, F.M.D.; Ferreira, F.D.; Bando, É.; Nerilo, S.B.; Hirooka, E.Y.; Machinski Jr, M. Daily intake estimates of fumonisins in corn-based food products in the population of Parana, Brazil. *Food Control.* **2012**, *26*, 614–618. [CrossRef]
117. Seo, D.-G.; Phat, C.; Kim, D.-H.; Lee, C. Occurrence of *Fusarium* mycotoxin fumonisin B 1 and B 2 in animal feeds in Korea. *Mycotoxin Res.* **2013**, *29*, 159–167. [CrossRef] [PubMed]
118. Abdallah, M.F.; Krska, R.; Sulyok, M. Occurrence of Ochratoxins, Fumonisin B2, Aflatoxins (B1 and B2), and Other Secondary Fungal Metabolites in Dried Date Palm Fruits from Egypt: A Mini-Survey. *J. Food Sci.* **2018**, *83*, 559–564. [CrossRef] [PubMed]
119. Rosa Junior, O.F.; Dalcin, M.S.; Nascimento, V.L.; Haesbaert, F.M.; Ferreira, T.P.S.; Fidelis, R.R.; Sarmento, R.A.; Aguiar, R.W.S.; Oliveira, E.E.; Santos, G.R. Fumonisin Production by *Fusarium verticillioides* in Maize Genotypes Cultivated in Different Environments. *Toxins* **2019**, *11*, 215. [CrossRef] [PubMed]
120. Sugita-Konishi, Y.; Nakajima, M.; Tabata, S.; Ishikuro, E.; Tanaka, T.; Norizuki, H.; Itoh, Y.; Aoyama, K.; Fujita, K.; Kai, S. Occurrence of aflatoxins, ochratoxin A, and fumonisins in retail foods in Japan. *J. Food Prot.* **2006**, *69*, 1365–1370. [CrossRef] [PubMed]
121. García-Moraleja, A.; Font, G.; Mañes, J.; Ferrer, E. Analysis of mycotoxins in coffee and risk assessment in Spanish adolescents and adults. *Food Chem. Toxicol.* **2015**, *86*, 225–233. [CrossRef] [PubMed]
122. Larsen, J.C. Opinion of the Scientific Panel on Contaminants in Food Chain on a request from the Commission related to ergot as undesirable substance in animal feed: Question No EFSA-Q-2003-38. *EFSA J.* **2005**. [CrossRef]

123. Norred, W.; Plattner, R.; Vesonder, R.; Bacon, C.; Voss, K. Effects of selected secondary metabolites of *Fusarium moniliforme* on unscheduled synthesis of DNA by rat primary hepatocytes. *Food Chem. Toxicol.* **1992**, *30*, 233–237. [CrossRef]
124. Voss, K.; Smith, G.; Haschek, W. Fumonisins: Toxicokinetics, mechanism of action and toxicity. *Anim. Feed Sci.Technol.* **2007**, *137*, 299–325. [CrossRef]
125. Bouhet, S.; Oswald, I.P. The intestine as a possible target for fumonisin toxicity. *Mol. Nutr. Food Res.* **2007**, *51*, 925–931. [CrossRef]
126. Missmer, S.A.; Suarez, L.; Felkner, M.; Wang, E.; Merrill Jr, A.H.; Rothman, K.J.; Hendricks, K.A. Exposure to fumonisins and the occurrence of neural tube defects along the Texas–Mexico border. *Environ. Health Perspect.* **2005**, *114*, 237–241. [CrossRef] [PubMed]
127. Gelderblom, W.C.; Kriek, N.; Marasas, W.; Thiel, P. Toxicity and carcinogenicity of the *Fusanum monilzforine* metabolite, fumonisin B1, in rats. *Carcinogenesis* **1991**, *12*, 1247–1251. [CrossRef] [PubMed]
128. Marasas, D.; WFO, J. *Fusarium moniliforme* contamination of maize in oesophageal cancer areas in Transkei. *S. Afr. Med. J.* **1988**, *74*, 110–114. [PubMed]
129. Franceschi, S.; Bidoli, E.; Barón, A.E.; La Vecchia, C. Maize and risk of cancers of the oral cavity, pharynx, and esophagus in northeastern Italy. *J. Natl. Cancer Inst.* **1990**, *82*, 1407–1411. [CrossRef] [PubMed]
130. Dragan, Y.P.; Bidlack, W.R.; Cohen, S.M.; Goldsworthy, T.L.; Hard, G.C.; Howard, P.C.; Riley, R.T.; Voss, K.A. Implications of apoptosis for toxicity, carcinogenicity, and risk assessment: Fumonisin B1 as an example. *Toxicol. Sci.* **2001**, *61*, 6–17. [CrossRef] [PubMed]
131. Rumora, L.; Kovačić, S.; Rozgaj, R.; Čepelak, I.; Pepeljnjak, S.; Grubišić, T.Ž. Cytotoxic and genotoxic effects of fumonisin B 1 on rabbit kidney RK13 cell line. *Arch. Toxicol.* **2002**, *76*, 55–61. [CrossRef] [PubMed]
132. Sun, G.; Wang, S.; Hu, X.; Su, J.; Huang, T.; Yu, J.; Tang, L.; Gao, W.; Wang, J.-S. Fumonisin B1 contamination of home-grown corn in high-risk areas for esophageal and liver cancer in China. *Food Addit. Contam.* **2007**, *24*, 181–185. [CrossRef] [PubMed]
133. Alizadeh, A.M.; Roshandel, G.; Roudbarmohammadi, S.; Roudbary, M.; Sohanaki, H.; Ghiasian, S.A.; Taherkhani, A.; Semnani, S.; Aghasi, M. Fumonisin B1 contamination of cereals and risk of esophageal cancer in a high risk area in northeastern Iran. *Asian Pac. J. Cancer Prev.* **2012**, *13*, 2625–2628. [CrossRef] [PubMed]
134. Solfrizzo, M.; Chulze, S.; Mallmann, C.; Visconti, A.; De Girolamo, A.; Rojo, F.; Torres, A. Comparison of urinary sphingolipids in human populations with high and low maize consumption as a possible biomarker of fumonisin dietary exposure. *Food Addit. Contam.* **2004**, *21*, 1090–1095. [CrossRef] [PubMed]
135. Haliburton, J.C.; Buck, W.B. *Equine leucoencephalomalacia: An historical review. In Diagnosis of Mycotoxicoses*; Springer: Berlin/Heidelberg, Germany, 1986; pp. 75–79.
136. Kriek, N.; Kellerman, T.S.; Marasas, W.F.O. A comparative study of the toxicity of Fusarium verticillioides (=F. moniliforme) to horses, primates, pigs, sheep and rats. *Onderstepoort J. Vet. Res.* **1981**, *48*, 129–131.
137. Marasas, W.F.; Riley, R.T.; Hendricks, K.A.; Stevens, V.L.; Sadler, T.W.; Gelineau-van Waes, J.; Missmer, S.A.; Cabrera, J.; Torres, O.; Gelderblom, W.C. Fumonisins disrupt sphingolipid metabolism, folate transport, and neural tube development in embryo culture and in vivo: A potential risk factor for human neural tube defects among populations consuming fumonisin-contaminated maize. *J. Nutr.* **2004**, *134*, 711–716. [CrossRef] [PubMed]
138. Sadler, T.; Merrill, A.H.; Stevens, V.L.; Sullards, M.C.; Wang, E.; Wang, P. Prevention of fumonisin B1-induced neural tube defects by folic acid. *Teratology* **2002**, *66*, 169–176. [CrossRef] [PubMed]
139. Sun, G.; Wang, S.; Hu, X.; Su, J.; Zhang, Y.; Xie, Y.; Zhang, H.; Tang, L.; Wang, J.-S. Co-contamination of aflatoxin B1 and fumonisin B1 in food and human dietary exposure in three areas of China. *Food Addit. Contam.* **2011**, *28*, 461–470. [CrossRef] [PubMed]
140. Liverpool-Tasie, L.; Turna, N.S.; Ademola, O.; Obadina, A.; Wu, F. The occurrence and co-occurrence of aflatoxin and fumonisin along the maize value chain in southwest Nigeria. *Food Chem. Toxicol.* **2019**, *129*, 458–465. [CrossRef] [PubMed]
141. Mwalwayo, D.S.; Thole, B. Prevalence of aflatoxin and fumonisins (B1+ B2) in maize consumed in rural Malawi. *Toxicol. Rep.* **2016**, *3*, 173–179. [CrossRef]
142. Polychronaki, N.; West, R.M.; Turner, P.C.; Amra, H.; Abdel-Wahhab, M.; Mykkänen, H.; El-Nezami, H. A longitudinal assessment of aflatoxin M1 excretion in breast milk of selected Egyptian mothers. *Food Chem. Toxicol.* **2007**, *45*, 1210–1215. [CrossRef]

143. Mahdavi, R.; Nikniaz, L.; Arefhosseini, S.; Jabbari, M.V. Determination of Aflatoxin M 1 in Breast Milk Samples in Tabriz–Iran. *Matern. Child Health J.* **2010**, *14*, 141–145. [CrossRef]
144. Magoha, H.; Kimanya, M.; De Meulenaer, B.; Roberfroid, D.; Lachat, C.; Kolsteren, P. Association between aflatoxin M1 exposure through breast milk and growth impairment in infants from Northern Tanzania. *Matern. World Mycotoxin J.* **2014**, *7*, 277–284. [CrossRef]
145. Kimanya, M.E.; De Meulenaer, B.; Roberfroid, D.; Lachat, C.; Kolsteren, P. Fumonisin exposure through maize in complementary foods is inversely associated with linear growth of infants in Tanzania. *Mol. Nutr. Food Res.* **2010**, *54*, 1659–1667. [CrossRef]
146. Shirima, C.P.; Kimanya, M.E.; Routledge, M.N.; Srey, C.; Kinabo, J.L.; Humpf, H.-U.; Wild, C.P.; Tu, Y.-K.; Gong, Y.Y. A prospective study of growth and biomarkers of exposure to aflatoxin and fumonisin during early childhood in Tanzania. *Environ. Health Perspect.* **2014**, *123*, 173–178. [CrossRef]
147. Chen, C.; Mitchell, N.J.; Gratz, J.; Houpt, E.R.; Gong, Y.; Egner, P.A.; Groopman, J.D.; Riley, R.T.; Showker, J.L.; Svensen, E. Exposure to aflatoxin and fumonisin in children at risk for growth impairment in rural Tanzania. *Environ. Int.* **2018**, *115*, 29–37. [CrossRef] [PubMed]
148. Michaelsen, K.F. *Feeding and Nutrition of Infants and Young Children: Guidelines for the WHO European Region, with Emphasis on the Former Soviet Countries*; WHO Regional Office Europe: Copenhagen, Denmark, 2000.
149. Humpf, H.U.; Voss, K.A. Effects of thermal food processing on the chemical structure and toxicity of fumonisin mycotoxins. *Mol. Nutr. Food Res.* **2004**, *48*, 255–269. [CrossRef] [PubMed]
150. Falavigna, C.; Cirlini, M.; Galaverna, G.; Dall'Asta, C. Masked fumonisins in processed food: Co-occurrence of hidden and bound forms and their stability under digestive conditions. *World Mycotoxin J.* **2012**, *5*, 325–334. [CrossRef]
151. Seefelder, W.; Hartl, M.; Humpf, H.-U. Determination of N-(carboxymethyl) fumonisin B1 in corn products by liquid chromatography/electrospray ionization–mass spectrometry. *J. Agric. Food Chem.* **2001**, *49*, 2146–2151. [CrossRef] [PubMed]
152. Poling, S.M.; Plattner, R.D.; Weisleder, D. N-(1-Deoxy-D-fructos-1-yl) fumonisin B1, the initial reaction product of fumonisin B1 and D-glucose. *J. Agric. Food. Chem.* **2002**, *50*, 1318–1324. [CrossRef] [PubMed]
153. Saunders, D.S.; Meredith, F.I.; Voss, K.A. Control of fumonisin: Effects of processing. *Environ. Health Perspect.* **2001**, *109*, 333–336. [PubMed]
154. Scudamore, K.; Patel, S. *Fusarium* mycotoxins in milling streams from the commercial milling of maize imported to the UK, and relevance to current legislation. *Food Addit. Contam.* **2009**, *26*, 744–753. [CrossRef] [PubMed]
155. Burger, H.; Shephard, G.; Louw, W.; Rheeder, J.; Gelderblom, W. The mycotoxin distribution in maize milling fractions under experimental conditions. *Int. J. Food Microbiol.* **2013**, *165*, 57–64. [CrossRef]
156. Scudamore, K. Fate of *Fusarium* mycotoxins in the cereal industry: Recent UK studies. *World Mycotoxin J.* **2008**, *1*, 315–323. [CrossRef]
157. Schaarschmidt, S.; Fauhl-Hassek, C. Mycotoxins during the Processes of Nixtamalization and Tortilla Production. *Toxins* **2019**, *11*, 227. [CrossRef]
158. Bullerman, L.B.; Ryu, D.; Jackson, L.S. Stability of fumonisins in food processing. In *Mycotoxins and Food Safety*; Springer: Berlin/Heidelberg, Germany, 2002; pp. 195–204.
159. Magan, N. Fungi in extreme environments. *Mycota* **2007**, *4*, 85–103.
160. Jurado, M.; Vázquez, C.; Callejas, C.; González-Jaén, M. Occurrence and variability of mycotoxigenic *Fusarium* species associated to wheat and maize in the South West of Spain. *Mycotoxin Res.* **2006**, *22*, 87–91. [CrossRef] [PubMed]
161. Aliakbari, F.; Mirabolfathy, M.; Emami, M.; Mazhar, S.F.; Karami-Osboo, R. Natural occurrence of *Fusarium* species in maize kernels at Gholestan province in northern Iran. *Asian J. Plant Sci.* **2007**, *8*, 1276–1281.
162. Cavaglieri, L.; Keller, K.; Pereyra, C.; Pereyra, M.G.; Alonso, V.; Rojo, F.; Dalcero, A.; Rosa, C. Fungi and natural incidence of selected mycotoxins in barley rootlets. *J. Stored Prod. Res.* **2009**, *45*, 147–150. [CrossRef]
163. Gil-Serna, J.; Mateo, E.; González-Jaén, M.; Jiménez, M.; Vázquez, C.; Patiño, B. Contamination of barley seeds with *Fusarium* species and their toxins in Spain: An integrated approach. *Food Addit. Contam. Part A* **2013**, *30*, 372–380. [CrossRef] [PubMed]
164. Magan, N.; Medina, A.; Aldred, D. Possible climate-change effects on mycotoxin contamination of food crops pre-and postharvest. *Plant Pathol.* **2011**, *60*, 150–163. [CrossRef]

165. Munkvold, G.P. Epidemiology of *Fusarium* diseases and their mycotoxins in maize ears. *Eur. J. Plant Pathol.* **2003**, *109*, 705–713. [CrossRef]
166. Maiorano, A.; Reyneri, A.; Magni, A.; Ramponi, C. A decision tool for evaluating the agronomic risk of exposure to fumonisins of different maize crop management systems in Italy. *Agric. Syst.* **2009**, *102*, 17–23. [CrossRef]
167. Cao, A.; Santiago, R.; Ramos, A.J.; Souto, X.C.; Aguín, O.; Malvar, R.A.; Butrón, A. Critical environmental and genotypic factors for *Fusarium verticillioides* infection, fungal growth and fumonisin contamination in maize grown in northwestern Spain. *Int. J. Food Microbiol.* **2014**, *177*, 63–71. [CrossRef]
168. Czembor, E.; Waśkiewicz, A.; Piechota, U.; Puchta, M.; Czembor, J.H.; Stepien, L. Differences in ear rot resistance and *Fusarium verticillioides*-produced fumonisin contamination between Polish currently and historically used maize inbred lines. *Front. Microbiol.* **2019**, *10*, 449. [CrossRef]
169. Cendoya, E.; del Pilar Monge, M.; Chiacchiera, S.M.; Farnochi, M.C.; Ramirez, M.L. Influence of water activity and temperature on growth and fumonisin production by *Fusarium proliferatum* strains on irradiated wheat grains. *Int. J. Food Microbiol.* **2018**, *266*, 158–166. [CrossRef] [PubMed]
170. Kohut, G.; Ádám, A.L.; Fazekas, B.; Hornok, L. N-starvation stress induced FUM gene expression and fumonisin production is mediated via the HOG-type MAPK pathway in *Fusarium proliferatum*. *Int. J. Food Microbiol.* **2009**, *130*, 65–69. [CrossRef] [PubMed]
171. Li, T.; Gong, L.; Wang, Y.; Chen, F.; Gupta, V.K.; Jian, Q.; Duan, X.; Jiang, Y. Proteomics analysis of *Fusarium proliferatum* under various initial pH during fumonisin production. *J. Proteom.* **2017**, *164*, 59–72. [CrossRef] [PubMed]
172. Keller, S.; Sullivan, T.; Chirtel, S. Factors affecting the growth of *Fusarium proliferatum* and the production of fumonisin B 1: Oxygen and pH. *J. Ind. Microbiol. Biotechnol.* **1997**, *19*, 305–309. [CrossRef] [PubMed]
173. Horwitz, W.; Latimer, J.G. (Eds.) *Official Methods of Analysis of AOAC International*; AOAC International: Gaithersburg, MD, USA, 2005.
174. Arroyo-Manzanares, N.; Huertas-Pérez, J.F.; Gámiz-Gracia, L.; García-Campaña, A.M. Simple and efficient methodology to determine mycotoxins in cereal syrups. *Food Chem.* **2015**, *177*, 274–279. [CrossRef]
175. Bolechová, M.; Benešová, K.; Běláková, S.; Čáslavský, J.; Pospíchalová, M.; Mikulíková, R. Determination of seventeen mycotoxins in barley and malt in the Czech Republic. *Food Control.* **2015**, *47*, 108–113. [CrossRef]
176. Nielsen, K.F.; Ngemela, A.F.; Jensen, L.B.; De Medeiros, L.S.; Rasmussen, P.H. UHPLC-MS/MS determination of ochratoxin A and fumonisins in coffee using QuEChERS extraction combined with mixed-mode SPE purification. *J. Agric. Food Chem.* **2015**, *63*, 1029–1034. [CrossRef] [PubMed]
177. Wang, Y.; Xiao, C.; Guo, J.; Yuan, Y.; Wang, J.; Liu, L.; Yue, T. Development and Application of a Method for the Analysis of 9 Mycotoxins in Maize by HPLC-MS/MS. *J. Food Sci.* **2013**, *78*, M1752–M1756. [CrossRef] [PubMed]
178. Ediage, E.N.; Van Poucke, C.; De Saeger, S. A multi-analyte LC–MS/MS method for the analysis of 23 mycotoxins in different sorghum varieties: The forgotten sample matrix. *Food Chem.* **2015**, *177*, 397–404. [CrossRef] [PubMed]
179. Jung, S.-Y.; Choe, B.-C.; Choi, E.-J.; Jeong, H.-J.; Hwang, Y.-S.; Shin, G.-Y.; Kim, J.-H. Survey of mycotoxins in commonly consumed Korean grain products using an LC-MS/MS multimycotoxin method in combination with immunoaffinity clean-up. *Food Sci. Biotechnol.* **2015**, *24*, 1193–1199. [CrossRef]
180. Bryła, M.; Roszko, M.; Szymczyk, K.; Jędrzejczak, R.; Obiedziński, M.W. Fumonisins and their masked forms in maize products. *Food Control* **2016**, *59*, 619–627. [CrossRef]
181. Beltrán, E.; Ibáñez, M.; Portolés, T.; Ripollés, C.; Sancho, J.V.; Yusà, V.; Marín, S.; Hernández, F. Development of sensitive and rapid analytical methodology for food analysis of 18 mycotoxins included in a total diet study. *Anal. Chim. Acta* **2013**, *783*, 39–48. [CrossRef] [PubMed]
182. García-Moraleja, A.; Font, G.; Mañes, J.; Ferrer, E. Development of a new method for the simultaneous determination of 21 mycotoxins in coffee beverages by liquid chromatography tandem mass spectrometry. *Food Res. Int.* **2015**, *72*, 247–255. [CrossRef]
183. Rubert, J.; Dzuman, Z.; Vaclavikova, M.; Zachariasova, M.; Soler, C.; Hajslova, J. Analysis of mycotoxins in barley using ultra high liquid chromatography high resolution mass spectrometry: Comparison of efficiency and efficacy of different extraction procedures. *Talanta* **2012**, *99*, 712–719. [CrossRef] [PubMed]

184. Blesa, J.; Moltó, J.-C.; El Akhdari, S.; Mañes, J.; Zinedine, A. Simultaneous determination of *Fusarium* mycotoxins in wheat grain from Morocco by liquid chromatography coupled to triple quadrupole mass spectrometry. *Food Control.* **2014**, *46*, 1–5. [CrossRef]
185. Arroyo-Manzanares, N.; Huertas-Pérez, J.F.; Gámiz-Gracia, L.; García-Campaña, A.M. A new approach in sample treatment combined with UHPLC-MS/MS for the determination of multiclass mycotoxins in edible nuts and seeds. *Talanta* **2013**, *115*, 61–67. [CrossRef]
186. Ye, H.; Lai, X.; Liu, C. Determination of Fumonisin B 1 and B 2 in Corn Using Matrix-Phase Dispersion Coupled to High Performance Liquid Chromatography. *Asian J. Chem.* **2013**, *25*, 6807–6810. [CrossRef]
187. Petrarca, M.H.; Rodrigues, M.I.; Rossi, E.A.; de Sylos, C.M. Optimisation of a sample preparation method for the determination of fumonisin B1 in rice. *Food Chem.* **2014**, *158*, 270–277. [CrossRef]
188. Petrarca, M.H.; Rossi, E.A.; de Sylos, C.M. In-house method validation, estimating measurement uncertainty and the occurrence of fumonisin B1 in samples of Brazilian commercial rice. *Food Control* **2016**, *59*, 439–446. [CrossRef]
189. Zhang, K.; Wong, J.W.; Hayward, D.G.; Vaclavikova, M.; Liao, C.-D.; Trucksess, M.W. Determination of mycotoxins in milk-based products and infant formula using stable isotope dilution assay and liquid chromatography tandem mass spectrometry. *J. Agric. Food Chem.* **2013**, *61*, 6265–6273. [CrossRef]
190. Azaiez, I.; Giusti, F.; Sagratini, G.; Mañes, J.; Fernández-Franzón, M. Multi-mycotoxins analysis in dried fruit by LC/MS/MS and a modified QuEChERS procedure. *Food Anal. Methods* **2014**, *7*, 935–945. [CrossRef]
191. Liao, C.-D.; Wong, J.W.; Zhang, K.; Yang, P.; Wittenberg, J.B.; Trucksess, M.W.; Hayward, D.G.; Lee, N.S.; Chang, J.S. Multi-mycotoxin analysis of finished grain and nut products using ultrahigh-performance liquid chromatography and positive electrospray ionization–quadrupole orbital ion trap high-resolution mass spectrometry. *J. Agric. Food Chem.* **2015**, *63*, 8314–8332. [CrossRef] [PubMed]
192. Soares, C.; Rodrigues, P.; Freitas-Silva, O.; Abrunhosa, L.; Venâncio, A. HPLC method for simultaneous detection of aflatoxins and cyclopiazonic acid. *World Mycotoxin J.* **2010**, *3*, 225–231. [CrossRef]
193. Liu, X.; Xu, Y.; He, Q.-H.; He, Z.-Y.; Xiong, Z.-P. Application of mimotope peptides of fumonisin B1 in Peptide ELISA. *J. Agric. Food Chem.* **2013**, *61*, 4765–4770. [CrossRef] [PubMed]
194. Ran, R.; Wang, C.; Han, Z.; Wu, A.; Zhang, D.; Shi, J. Determination of deoxynivalenol (DON) and its derivatives: Current status of analytical methods. *Food Control.* **2013**, *34*, 138–148. [CrossRef]
195. Lee, N.A.; Wang, S.; Allan, R.D.; Kennedy, I.R. A rapid aflatoxin B1 ELISA: Development and validation with reduced matrix effects for peanuts, corn, pistachio, and soybeans. *J. Agric. Food Chem.* **2004**, *52*, 2746–2755. [CrossRef] [PubMed]
196. Nagaraj, D.; Adkar-Purushothama, C.R.; Yanjarappa, S.M. Multiplex PCR for the early detection of fumonisin producing *Fusarium verticillioides*. *Food Biosci.* **2016**, *13*, 84–88. [CrossRef]
197. Sreenivasa, M.; Dass, R.S.; Raj, A.C.; Janardhana, G. Molecular detection of fumonisin producing *Fusarium* species of freshly harvested maize kernels using polymerase chain reaction (PCR). *Taiwania* **2006**, *51*, 251–257.
198. Bintvihok, A.; Treebonmuang, S.; Srisakwattana, K.; Nuanchun, W.; Patthanachai, K.; Usawang, S. A rapid and sensitive detection of aflatoxin-producing fungus using an optimized polymerase chain reaction (PCR). *Toxicol. Res.* **2016**, *32*, 81–87. [CrossRef]
199. Niessen, L. PCR-based diagnosis and quantification of mycotoxin-producing fungi. In *Advances in Food and Nutrition Research*; Elsevier: Amsterdam, The Netherlands, 2008; Volume 54, pp. 81–138.
200. Omori, A.M.; Ono, E.Y.S.; Bordini, J.G.; Hirozawa, M.T.; Fungaro, M.H.P.; Ono, M.A. Detection of *Fusarium verticillioides* by PCR-ELISA based on FUM21 gene. *Food Microbiol.* **2018**, *73*, 160–167. [CrossRef]
201. Tang, X.; Li, P.; Zhang, Z.; Zhang, Q.; Guo, J.; Zhang, W. An ultrasensitive gray-imaging-based quantitative immunochromatographic detection method for fumonisin B1 in agricultural products. *Food Control.* **2017**, *80*, 333–340. [CrossRef]
202. Del Fiore, A.; Reverberi, M.; Ricelli, A.; Pinzari, F.; Serranti, S.; Fabbri, A.; Bonifazi, G.; Fanelli, C. Early detection of toxigenic fungi on maize by hyperspectral imaging analysis. *Int. J. Food Microbiol.* **2010**, *144*, 64–71. [CrossRef] [PubMed]
203. Kimuli, D.; Wang, W.; Lawrence, K.C.; Yoon, S.-C.; Ni, X.; Heitschmidt, G.W. Utilisation of visible/near-infrared hyperspectral images to classify aflatoxin B1 contaminated maize kernels. *Biosyst. Eng.* **2018**, *166*, 150–160. [CrossRef]

204. Di Nardo, F.; Alladio, E.; Baggiani, C.; Cavalera, S.; Giovannoli, C.; Spano, G.; Anfossi, L. Colour-encoded lateral flow immunoassay for the simultaneous detection of aflatoxin B1 and type-B fumonisins in a single Test line. *Talanta* **2019**, *192*, 288–294. [CrossRef] [PubMed]
205. Lu, L.; Seenivasan, R.; Wang, Y.-C.; Yu, J.-H.; Gunasekaran, S. An electrochemical immunosensor for rapid and sensitive detection of mycotoxins fumonisin B1 and deoxynivalenol. *Electrochim. Acta* **2016**, *213*, 89–97. [CrossRef]
206. Mao, L.; Ji, K.; Yao, L.; Xue, X.; Wen, W.; Zhang, X.; Wang, S. Molecularly imprinted photoelectrochemical sensor for fumonisin B1 based on GO-CdS heterojunction. *Biosens. Bioelectron.* **2019**, *127*, 57–63. [CrossRef] [PubMed]
207. Miller, J.D.; Young, J.C.; Trenholm, H.L. *Fusarium* toxins in field corn. I. Time course of fungal growth and production of deoxynivalenol and other mycotoxins. *Can. J. Bot.* **1983**, *61*, 3080–3087. [CrossRef]
208. Scott, P.M.; Nelson, K.; Kanhere, S.R.; Karpinski, K.F.; Hayward, S.; Neish, G.A.; Teich, A.H. Decline in deoxynivalenol (vomitoxin) concentrations in 1983 Ontario winter wheat before harvest. *Appl. Environ. Microbiol.* **1984**, *48*, 884–886.
209. Gareis, M.; Bauer, J.; Thiem, J.; Plank, G.; Grabley, S.; Gedek, B. Cleavage of zearalenone-glycoside, a "masked" mycotoxin, during digestion in swine. *J. Vet. Med. B* **1990**, *37*, 236–240. [CrossRef]
210. Berthiller, F.; Maragos, C.M.; Dall'Asta, C. Introduction to masked mycotoxins. In *Masked Mycotoxins in Food: Formation, Occurrence and Toxicological Relevance*; Royal Society of Chemistry, RSC Publishing: Cambridge, UK, 2015; pp. 1–13. [CrossRef]
211. Dellafiora, L.; Dall'Asta, C. Masked mycotoxins: An emerging issue that makes renegotiable what is ordinary. *Food Chem.* **2016**, *213*, 534–535. [CrossRef]
212. Tran, S.; Smith, T. Determination of optimal conditions for hydrolysis of conjugated deoxynivalenol in corn and wheat with trifluoromethanesulfonic acid. *Anim. Feed Sci. Technol.* **2011**, *163*, 84–92. [CrossRef]
213. McCormick, S.P.; Kato, T.; Maragos, C.M.; Busman, M.; Lattanzio, V.M.; Galaverna, G.; Dall-Asta, C.; Crich, D.; Price, N.P.; Kurtzman, C.P. Anomericity of T-2 toxin-glucoside: Masked mycotoxin in cereal crops. *J. Agric. Food Chem.* **2015**, *63*, 731–738. [CrossRef] [PubMed]
214. De Boevre, M.; Di Mavungu, J.D.; Landschoot, S.; Audenaert, K.; Eeckhout, M.; Maene, P.; Haesaert, G.; De Saeger, S. Natural occurrence of mycotoxins and their masked forms in food and feed products. *World Mycotoxin J.* **2012**, *5*, 207–219. [CrossRef]
215. Binder, S.; Schwartz-Zimmermann, H.; Varga, E.; Bichl, G.; Michlmayr, H.; Adam, G.; Berthiller, F. Metabolism of zearalenone and its major modified forms in pigs. *Toxins* **2017**, *9*, 56. [CrossRef] [PubMed]
216. Duvick, J.; Rood, T.; Maddox, J.; Gilliam, J. *Molecular Genetics of Host-Specific Toxins in Plant Disease*; Springer: Berlin/Heidelberg, Germany, 1998; pp. 369–381.
217. Blackwell, B.A.; Gilliam, J.T.; Savard, M.E.; David Miller, J.; Duvick, J.P. Oxidative deamination of hydrolyzed fumonisin B1 (AP1) by cultures of *Exophiala spinifera*. *Nat. Toxins* **1999**, *7*, 31–38. [CrossRef]
218. Duvick, J.; Maddox, J.; Gilliam, J. Compositions and methods for fumonisin detoxification. U.S. Patent US6482621B1, 19 November 2002.
219. Gu, M.J.; Han, S.E.; Hwang, K.; Mayer, E.; Reisinger, N.; Schatzmayr, D.; Park, B.-C.; Han, S.H.; Yun, C.-H. Hydrolyzed fumonisin B1 induces less inflammatory responses than fumonisin B1 in the co-culture model of porcine intestinal epithelial and immune cells. *Toxicol. Lett.* **2019**, *305*, 110–116. [CrossRef] [PubMed]
220. Benedetti, R.; Nazzi, F.; Locci, R.; Firrao, G. Degradation of fumonisin B1 by a bacterial strain isolated from soil. *Biodegradation* **2006**, *17*, 31–38. [CrossRef]
221. Täubel, M. Isolierung und Charakterisierung von Mikroorganismen zur biologischen Inaktivierung von Fumonisinen. Doctoral thesis, University of Natural Resources and Applied Life Sciences, Vienna, Austria, 2005.
222. Heinl, S.; Hartinger, D.; Thamhesl, M.; Vekiru, E.; Krska, R.; Schatzmayr, G.; Moll, W.-D.; Grabherr, R. Degradation of fumonisin B1 by the consecutive action of two bacterial enzymes. *J. Biotechnol.* **2010**, *145*, 120–129. [CrossRef]
223. Velluti, A.; Sanchis, V.; Ramos, A.; Egido, J.; Marın, S. Inhibitory effect of cinnamon, clove, lemongrass, oregano and palmarose essential oils on growth and fumonisin B1 production by *Fusarium proliferatum* in maize grain. *Int. J. Food Microbiol.* **2003**, *89*, 145–154. [CrossRef]

224. Patil, J.R.; Jayaprakasha, G.; Murthy, K.C.; Tichy, S.E.; Chetti, M.B.; Patil, B.S. Apoptosis-mediated proliferation inhibition of human colon cancer cells by volatile principles of *Citrus aurantifolia*. *Food Chem.* **2009**, *114*, 1351–1358. [CrossRef]
225. Driehuis, F.; Te Giffel, M.; Van Egmond, H.; Fremy, J.; Blüthgen, A. Feed-associated mycotoxins in the dairy chain: Occurrence and control. *Fil-Idf Bull. Fed. Int. Lait. Int. Dairy Fed. Brussels – Belgium* **2010**, *444*, 2.
226. Okabe, I.; Hiraoka, H.; Miki, K. Influence of harvest time on fumonisin contamination of forage maize for whole-crop silage. *Mycoscience* **2015**, *56*, 470–475. [CrossRef]
227. Bush, B.; Carson, M.; Cubeta, M.; Hagler, W.; Payne, G. Infection and fumonisin production by *Fusarium verticillioides* in developing maize kernels. *Phytopathology* **2004**, *94*, 88–93. [CrossRef] [PubMed]
228. Johnson, L.; Harrison, J.; Hunt, C.; Shinners, K.; Doggett, C.; Sapienza, D. Nutritive value of corn silage as affected by maturity and mechanical processing: A contemporary review. *J. Dairy Sci.* **1999**, *82*, 2813–2825. [CrossRef]
229. Shephard, G.S.; Burger, H.-M.; Rheeder, J.P.; Alberts, J.F.; Gelderblom, W.C. The effectiveness of regulatory maximum levels for fumonisin mycotoxins in commercial and subsistence maize crops in South Africa. *Food Control* **2019**, *97*, 77–80. [CrossRef]
230. Miller, J.D. Factors that affect the occurrence of fumonisin. *Environ. Health Perspect.* **2001**, *109*, 321–324. [PubMed]
231. van der Westhuizen, L.; Shephard, G.S.; Burger, H.M.; Rheeder, J.P.; Gelderblom, W.C.; Wild, C.P.; Gong, Y.Y. Fumonisin B1 as a urinary biomarker of exposure in a maize intervention study among South African subsistence farmers. *Cancer Epidemiol. Biomark. Prev.* **2011**, *20*, 483–489. [CrossRef] [PubMed]
232. Falcão, V.C.A.; Ono, M.A.; de Ávila Miguel, T.; Vizoni, E.; Hirooka, E.Y.; Ono, E.Y.S. *Fusarium verticillioides*: Evaluation of fumonisin production and effect of fungicides on in vitro inhibition of mycelial growth. *Mycopathologia* **2011**, *171*, 77–84. [CrossRef]
233. Miguel, T.Á.; Bordini, J.G.; Saito, G.H.; Andrade, C.G.J.; Ono, M.A.; Hirooka, E.Y.; Vizoni, É.; Ono, E. Effect of fungicide on *Fusarium verticillioides* mycelial morphology and fumonisin B1 production. *Braz. J. Microbiol.* **2015**, *46*, 293–299. [CrossRef] [PubMed]
234. Masiello, M.; Somma, S.; Ghionna, V.; Logrieco, A.F.; Moretti, A. In Vitro and in Field Response of Different Fungicides against *Aspergillus flavus* and *Fusarium* Species Causing Ear Rot Disease of Maize. *Toxins* **2019**, *11*, 11. [CrossRef]
235. Schmidt-Heydt, M.; Geisen, R. Gene expression as an indication for ochratoxin A biosynthesis in Penicillium nordicum. *Mycotoxin Res.* **2007**, *23*, 13–21. [CrossRef] [PubMed]
236. Schmidt-Heydt, M.; Magan, N.; Geisen, R. Stress induction of mycotoxin biosynthesis genes by abiotic factors. *FEMS Microbiol. Lett.* **2008**, *284*, 142–149. [CrossRef] [PubMed]
237. Marín, P.; Magan, N.; Vázquez, C.; González-Jaén, M.T. Differential effect of environmental conditions on the growth and regulation of the fumonisin biosynthetic gene FUM1 in the maize pathogens and fumonisin producers Fusarium verticillioides and Fusarium proliferatum. *FEMS Microbiol. Ecol.* **2010**, *73*, 303–311. [CrossRef] [PubMed]
238. Bernhoft, A.; Torp, M.; Clasen, P.-E.; Løes, A.-K.; Kristoffersen, A. Influence of agronomic and climatic factors on *Fusarium* infestation and mycotoxin contamination of cereals in Norway. *Food Addit. Contam. Part A* **2012**, *29*, 1129–1140. [CrossRef] [PubMed]
239. Lemmens, M.; Buerstmayr, H.; Krska, R.; Schuhmacher, R.; Grausgruber, H.; Ruckenbauer, P. The effect of inoculation treatment and long-term application of moisture on *Fusarium* head blight symptoms and deoxynivalenol contamination in wheat grains. *Eur. J. Plant Pathol.* **2004**, *110*, 299–308. [CrossRef]
240. Haidukowski, M.; Pascale, M.; Perrone, G.; Pancaldi, D.; Campagna, C.; Visconti, A. Effect of fungicides on the development of *Fusarium* head blight, yield and deoxynivalenol accumulation in wheat inoculated under field conditions with *Fusarium graminearum* and *Fusarium culmorum*. *J. Sci. Food Agric.* **2005**, *85*, 191–198. [CrossRef]
241. Yoshida, M.; Nakajima, T.; Tomimura, K.; Suzuki, F.; Arai, M.; Miyasaka, A. Effect of the timing of fungicide application on *Fusarium* head blight and mycotoxin contamination in wheat. *Plant Dis.* **2012**, *96*, 845–851. [CrossRef]
242. Scarpino, V.; Reyneri, A.; Sulyok, M.; Krska, R.; Blandino, M. Effect of fungicide application to control Fusarium head blight and 20 *Fusarium* and *Alternaria* mycotoxins in winter wheat (*Triticum aestivum* L.). *World Mycotoxin J.* **2015**, *8*, 499–510. [CrossRef]

243. Alberts, J.F.; Van Zyl, W.H.; Gelderblom, W.C. Biologically based methods for control of fumonisin-producing *Fusarium* species and reduction of the fumonisins. *Front. Microbiol.* **2016**, *7*, 548. [CrossRef]
244. Jacela, J.Y.; DeRouchey, J.M.; Tokach, M.D.; Goodband, R.D.; Nelssen, J.L.; Renter, D.G.; Dritz, S.S. Feed additives for swine: Fact sheets–flavors and mold inhibitors, mycotoxin binders, and antioxidants. *Kansas Agric. Exp. Station Res. Rep.* **2010**, *10*, 27–32. [CrossRef]
245. Kolosova, A.; Stroka, J. Substances for reduction of the contamination of feed by mycotoxins: A review. *World Mycotoxin J.* **2011**, *4*, 225–256. [CrossRef]
246. Kabak, B.; Dobson, A.D. Biological strategies to counteract the effects of mycotoxins. *J. Food Prot.* **2009**, *72*, 2006–2016. [CrossRef] [PubMed]
247. Whitlow, L.W. Evaluation of mycotoxin binders. In Proceedings of the 4th Mid-Atlantic Nutrition Conference, Timonium, Maryland, 2006; pp. 132–143.
248. De Mil, T.; Devreese, M.; De Baere, S.; Van Ranst, E.; Eeckhout, M.; De Backer, P.; Croubels, S. Characterization of 27 mycotoxin binders and the relation with in vitro zearalenone adsorption at a single concentration. *Toxins* **2015**, *7*, 21–33. [CrossRef] [PubMed]
249. Nazarizadeh, H.; Pourreza, J. Evaluation of three mycotoxin binders to prevent the adverse effects of aflatoxin B1 in growing broilers. *J. Appl. Anim. Res.* **2019**, *47*, 135–139. [CrossRef]

toxins

MDPI

Review

Co-Occurrence and Combinatory Effects of *Alternaria* Mycotoxins and Other Xenobiotics of Food Origin: Current Scenario and Future Perspectives

Francesco Crudo [1], Elisabeth Varga [2], Georg Aichinger [2], Gianni Galaverna [1], Doris Marko [1,2], Chiara Dall'Asta [1] and Luca Dellafiora [1,*]

1 Department of Food and Drug, University of Parma, Parco Area delle Scienze 27/A, 43124 Parma, Italy; francesco.crudo1@studenti.unipr.it (F.C.); gianni.galaverna@unipr.it (G.G.); doris.marko@univie.ac.at (D.M.); chiara.dallasta@unipr.it (C.D.)

2 Department of Food Chemistry and Toxicology, Faculty of Chemistry, University of Vienna, Währinger Str. 38, 1090 Vienna, Austria; elisabeth.varga@univie.ac.at (E.V.); georg.aichinger@univie.ac.at (G.A.)

* Correspondence: luca.dellafiora@unipr.it; Tel.: +39-0521-906-196

Received: 6 September 2019; Accepted: 31 October 2019; Published: 3 November 2019

Abstract: Mycotoxins are low-molecular weight compounds produced by diverse genera of molds that may contaminate food and feed threatening the health of humans and animals. Recent findings underline the importance of studying the combined occurrence of multiple mycotoxins and the relevance of assessing the toxicity their simultaneous exposure may cause in living organisms. In this context, for the first time, this work has critically reviewed the most relevant data concerning the occurrence and toxicity of mycotoxins produced by *Alternaria* spp., which are among the most important emerging risks to be assessed in food safety, alone or in combination with other mycotoxins and bioactive food constituents. According to the literature covered, multiple *Alternaria* mycotoxins may often occur simultaneously in contaminated food, along with several other mycotoxins and food bioactives inherently present in the studied matrices. Although the toxicity of combinations naturally found in food has been rarely assessed experimentally, the data collected so far, clearly point out that chemical mixtures may differ in their toxicity compared to the effect of toxins tested individually. The data presented here may provide a solid foothold to better support the risk assessment of *Alternaria* mycotoxins highlighting the actual role of chemical mixtures on influencing their toxicity.

Keywords: *Alternaria* mycotoxins; combinatory effects; food safety; combined toxicity; co-occurrence; bioactive compounds

Key Contribution: This work provides for the first time an extensive and critical analysis of the most relevant literature concerning the occurrence and toxicity of *Alternaria* mycotoxins, studied either individually or in combination with other mycotoxins or bioactive compounds of food origin. Overall, this review pinpoints the need to investigate the simultaneous occurrence of diverse mycotoxins in food and to assess their combined toxicity to better support the risk assessment of *Alternaria* mycotoxins.

1. Introduction

Mycotoxins are low-molecular-weight toxic compounds synthetized by different types of molds belonging mainly to the genera *Aspergillus*, *Penicillium*, *Fusarium* and *Alternaria* [1]. They may enter the food chain worldwide as a consequence of the ability of mycotoxin-producing molds to infect a wide number of crops and food commodities [2]. It has been reported that up to 25 % of world crops may be contaminated with mycotoxins and over 4.5–5.0 billion people are thought to be chronically exposed to these food contaminants [3]. However, a much higher prevalence of detected mycotoxins can be found depending either on the considered mycotoxin or crop (up to 80% in certain circumstances), as recently reported [4]. Although the highest levels of food contamination are more frequently found in low-income countries, mycotoxins actually represent a growing threat also on account of climate changes [5]. The contamination of food and feed by mycotoxins results in significant economic losses worldwide, not only in terms of food and feed spoilage, but also in terms of a burden on human health, animal productivity and international trade [6]. In particular, mycotoxins may pose a toxicological concern for humans and animals since they may exert a wide number of effects including acute toxic, mutagenic, carcinogenic, teratogenic, estrogenic and immunotoxic actions [7]. Among the various categories of mycotoxins, those produced by the genus *Alternaria* are gaining increasing interest due to their frequent occurrence in food, the recent insights on their genotoxic potential and mechanisms of action, and their consequent possible effects on human health [2,7]. The *Alternaria* toxins belong to the group of the so called "emerging" mycotoxins. They are compounds of possible concern due to their abundance, occurrence or toxicity, but the limited available data do not allow a comprehensive risk assessment with an acceptable degree of certainty.

Alternaria species are ubiquitous plant pathogens and saprophytes that may contaminate a wide variety of crops and raw materials due to their environmental adaptability, particularly to their tolerance to low temperature and water stress conditions. They produce a cocktail of secondary metabolites and more than 70 *Alternaria* toxins have been characterized so far [2]. Based on their chemical structures, *Alternaria* toxins may be divided into five groups (Figure 1): (i) dibenzo-α-pyrones, including alternariol (AOH), alternariol monomethyl ether (AME), and altenuene (ALT); (ii) perylene quinones, including the altertoxins I, II, III (ATX-I, ATX-II and ATX-III, respectively), stemphyltoxin I and III (STTX-I and STTX-III, respectively), and alterperylenol/alteichin (ALP); (iii) tetramic acid derivatives, including tenuazonic acid (TeA) and iso-tenuazonic acid (iso-TeA); (iv) *A. alternata* f. sp. *lycopersici* toxins, which includes several phytotoxins such as AAL-TA and ALL-TB sub-groups (v) miscellaneous structures, as tentoxin (TEN), which has a cyclic tetrapeptidic structure [2,8]. However, many other mycotoxins might be produced by *Alternaria* spp. such as dihydrotentoxin, isotentoxin, altenuisol (ALTSOH), altenusin, infectopyrone, altersetin, macrosporin A, altersolanol A, monocerin, altenuic acids I, II, and III [9].

Due to the broad spectrum of adverse effects observed in vitro (e.g., genotoxic, mutagenic, clastogenic, androgenic, and estrogenic effects) and in vivo (e.g., fetotoxic and teratogenic effects), some of the *Alternaria* mycotoxins most frequently found in food may pose a severe threat to human health, especially for the most exposed categories such as infants, toddler and vegetarians [10]. Nevertheless, for most *Alternaria* mycotoxins, neither the toxicity nor the occurrence in food is adequately described. The current limitation of data hinders the proper assessment of risks to human health and, consequently, it prevents the establishment of specific regulations [11]. Therefore, the need of additional representative data to support the proper risk assessment of *Alternaria* toxins, especially for AOH, AME, TeA, TEN and ALT, was claimed by the expert Committee "Agricultural Contaminants" of the EU commission in 2012 [12]. In 2016, a call to collect data for the human exposure assessment to *Alternaria* toxins (AOH, AME, TeA and TEN) was published by the European Food Safety Authority (EFSA) [13].

In this respect, the chemical risk assessment of food-related compounds is currently based on the integration of knowledge about the single exposure to a given substance and its potential to individually cause harmful effects [14]. However, food is typically contaminated simultaneously by more than one mycotoxin. It is noteworthy that the simultaneous occurrence of compounds (either toxicants or bioactive food constituents) may lead to combinatory interactions (namely, additive, synergistic or antagonistic effects) that may significantly change the final toxicological outcome depending on the overall composition of chemical mixtures (see Section 3.2). In addition, mycotoxins may be present in food along with a high number of bioactive compounds, showing a huge variety of chemical structures and mechanisms of action, which may further modify their toxic impact. On this basis, risk assessment studies should take into account this complexity rather than relying on individual evidences, to better evaluate the overall risk associated with the consumption of mycotoxins-contaminated food.

Therefore, in the framework of supporting a better risk assessment of *Alternaria* mycotoxins, this work aims at consolidating the current knowledge on occurrence and combined actions of *Alternaria* mycotoxins. The relevance of investigating the effects and occurrence of chemical mixtures to support the thorough assessment of the actual risk this class of mycotoxins may pose to humans is pointed out. In more detail, this work presents the current state-of-the art in terms of co-occurrence and combinatory effects of: (i) different *Alternaria* toxins; (ii) *Alternaria* toxins in combination with other mycotoxins; (iii) *Alternaria* toxins in combination with bioactive compounds of food origin.

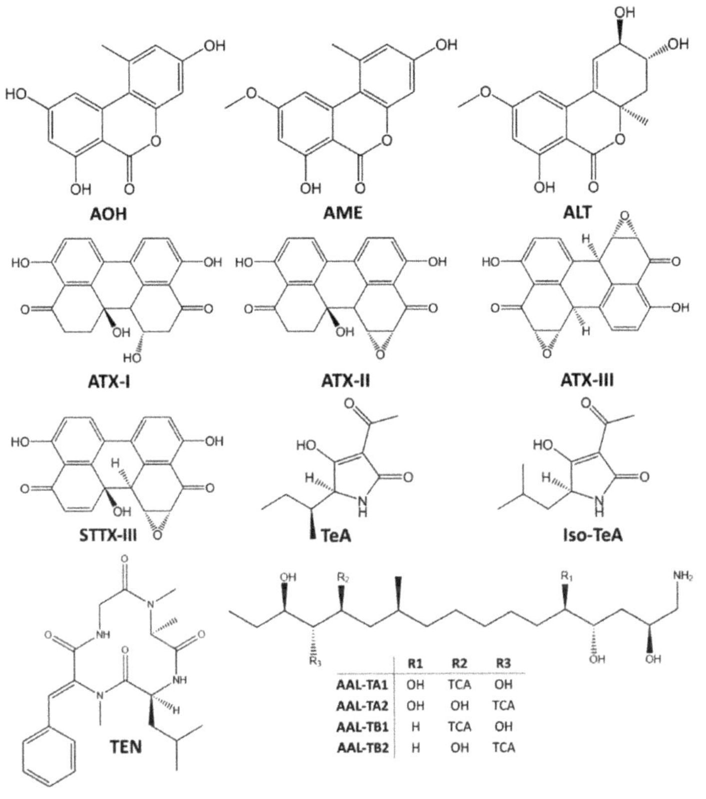

Figure 1. Chemical structures of the main *Alternaria* mycotoxins. AOH – alternariol; AME – alternariol monomethyl ether; ALT – altenuene; ATX-I, ATX-II, ATX-III – altertoxin I, II and III; STTX-III – stemphyltoxin III; TeA – tenuazonic acid; Iso-TeA – iso-tenuazonic acid; TEN – tentoxin; AAL-TA1-2 *Alternaria alternata* f. sp. *lycopersici* toxins sub-group A 1 and 2; AAL-TB1-2 *Alternaria alternata* f. sp. *lycopersici* toxins sub-group B 1 and 2; TCA - tricarballylic acid.

2. Natural Occurrence and Co-Occurrence of *Alternaria* Mycotoxins in Food

The occurrence of *Alternaria* mycotoxins in food and feed has been reviewed over the years [8,15–18]. However, in most cases, the occurrence and the relative concentrations of single or a small group of toxins has been reported, whilst the simultaneous co-occurrence of a high number of mycotoxins likely co-occurring together was not systematically assessed.

This section presents a collection of the co-occurrence of multiple *Alternaria* toxins in food commodities. In addition, data on the co-occurrence of *Alternaria* mycotoxins along with other mycotoxins and food constituents are reviewed. The key references covered in this review addressing the natural co-occurrence of different *Alternaria* mycotoxins are summarized in Table 1, while a schematic overview of the literature concerning the study of the co-occurrence of *Alternaria* and other mycotoxins is provided in Table 2. Detailed information concerning the number of samples analyzed, mycotoxin concentrations, as well as the methods and instruments used are reported in the Supplementary Materials (Table S1).

2.1. Co-Occurrence of Different Alternaria Toxins in Food

With regard to the co-contamination of food by different *Alternaria* toxins, AOH, AME, ALT, TeA, TEN, and ATX-I are the most frequently investigated compounds, while broader sets of compounds, including for instance ATX-II, IsoALT, AAL-TA1, AAL-TA2, ALP, macrosporin, ALTSOH, and Val-TeA, are rarely reported.

As shown in Table 1, the presence of *Alternaria* mycotoxins has been well-documented both in fresh and processed food, including fruits and vegetables, nuts, seeds, cereals, and fermented beverages. Among the food commodities investigated so far, apples, tomato, and their derivative products have been more frequently explored than other types of fruits and vegetables. Notably, most of them were found simultaneously contaminated by both AOH and AME, and, in some cases, also by up to five different mycotoxins. One of the first investigations were performed by Stinson and co-workers [19] who reported the contamination of apples and tomatoes with several *Alternaria* toxins already back in 1981. The observed contamination determined by HPLC-UV was in the low mg/kg range for AOH and AME, and in the μg/kg range for ALT and TeA in the case of apple samples. In tomatoes, TeA showed the highest contamination levels with up to 139 mg/kg. Furthermore, the presence or absence of ATX-I was assessed by thin layer chromatography. In the last ten years, multi-analyte measurements using liquid chromatography coupled to mass spectrometry became more and more important. The contamination with seven different *Alternaria* mycotoxins (AOH, AME, ALT, TeA, TEN, ATX-I, and ALP) and two phase-II metabolites (AOH-3-sulfate and AME-3-sulfate) was reported in tomato sauce, sunflower seed oil and wheat flour samples by Puntscher et al. [20]. In this study, the simultaneous contamination in the μg/kg range was reported in sample(s) from Austria, Croatia and Italy.

Infant foods were also found to be contaminated by multiple *Alternaria* mycotoxins. As an example, Gotthard and co-workers reported that tomato sauce and apple-pear-cherry puree were simultaneously contaminated by AOH, AME, TeA, and TEN [21]. In addition, those mycotoxins were also found in cereal-based infant formulas and they were reported along with ATX-I in wheat- and spelt-based food. These results are particularly relevant considering that the young population (infants and toddlers) show a higher exposure to *Alternaria* toxins in comparison to the other population categories due to their high food consumption in relation to body weight [10]. The most important dietary contributors to these mycotoxins were fruits and fruit products, vegetable oil, cereal-based foods and fruiting vegetables (tomatoes) wherein multiple mycotoxins were often found simultaneously, as shown in Table 1.

This scenario is further complicated by the possible presence of so called "masked mycotoxins". This term refers to modified forms of mycotoxins as a result of their metabolic transformations in plants. Masked mycotoxins have been reported to abundantly co-occur in contaminated food and raw materials along with their respective parent counterparts [22]. The most common masked mycotoxins covalently link sulfate or glucoside groups as a result of plant phase-II metabolism [23]. After ingestion, these phase II plant metabolites can be hydrolyzed during the digestion releasing the respective toxic parental compounds [1]. The transformation of masked mycotoxins to metabolites with higher toxicity than the parent compounds was also described in vitro [24,25], further highlighting the toxicological potential of the masked forms of mycotoxins (referred to as "maskedome"). Nevertheless, masked mycotoxins are not routinely screened, and this may result in an underestimation of the actual amounts of mycotoxins in foods. In this respect, Puntscher et al. [26] reported the presence of some modified forms of AOH and AME (i.e., AOH-3-glucoside, AOH-9-glucoside, AOH-3-sulfate and AME-3-sulfate) in tomato sauce samples from Italy. In particular, one sample was found contaminated not only with AOH, AME, TeA and TEN, but also with AOH-3-glucoside, AOH-3-sulfate and AME-3-sulfate. Similarly, Walravens and co-workers found tomato products (juices, sauces and concentrates) contaminated with AOH-3-sulfate and AME-3-sulfate, with a prevalence ranging from 11% to 26% and from 32% to 78%, respectively [27]. The authors reported the highest prevalence of AOH and AME in tomato sauces (86% and 78%, respectively), while ALT was most frequently detected in tomato concentrates (56%). In addition, a prevalence of TEN-contaminated products, ranging from 21% to 64% (in sauces and juices, respectively), was also reported and, interestingly, all the tested samples showed a high contamination with TeA. More recently, another study highlighted the contamination of both fresh and dried tomato samples by different *Alternaria* toxins, among which TeA was found the most frequent and abundant compound [28].

The frequent co-occurrence of multiple *Alternaria* mycotoxins was also described in many other foods, including peppers. As an example, Gambacorta and co-workers [29] analyzed samples of fresh, dried, grounded, and fried sweet pepper, wherein AOH, AME, TeA, and TEN were found together (limit of quantifications in the low μg/kg range). In particular, TeA was detected in all samples, while AOH was detected in 86%, 43%, 100% and 14% of fresh, dried, grounded and fried products, respectively. Fresh pepper samples were mostly contaminated by AME (57% of fresh pepper samples), while fried peppers were the least AME-contaminated samples (14% of fried peppers samples). ALT was detected only in 43% and 13% of fresh and grounded samples, respectively.

Beside fruits and vegetables, cereals and derived products play an important role in the exposure to *Alternaria* toxins, representing the main source of exposure for infants and toddlers [10]. According to EFSA [2], the highest mean concentrations of AOH, AME, TeA and TEN in grains were observed as follows: AOH (spelt, oats, rice); AME (oats, rice); TeA (wheat, barley, rye, spelt, oats and rice); TEN (rye). Nevertheless, in addition to the above-mentioned mycotoxins, some authors reported also the presence of other compounds in grains, although the actual co-occurrence was not clearly specified. Specifically, ragi, sorghum and spelt were found contaminated by ALT [30,31], while ATX-I was detected in spelt and wheat [20,21]. Among the least investigated mycotoxins, macrosporin, which is produced primarily by the *Stemphylium* genus but it can be produce by *Alternaria* spp. too [32], was found in corn and wheat silage [33], while ALP was detected in wheat flour samples [20]. The presence of macrosporin was also detected in dried fruits and nuts, such as almonds, dried grape berries, hazelnuts, peanuts, and pistachios [34], often in combination with other *Alternaria* mycotoxins. In a study performed by Mikušová et al. [35], dried grape berries from three Slovak winemaking regions were simultaneously contaminated by up to eight *Alternaria* mycotoxins, i.e., AOH, AME, ALT, TeA, TEN, ATX-I, ATX-II, and macrosporin, whose highest concentrations were 1308 μg/kg, 776 μg/kg, 4120 μg/kg, 159.6 μg/kg, 43.1 μg/kg, 31175 μg/kg, 624 μg/kg, and 762 μg/kg, respectively. Notably, TEN was detected in all the analyzed samples.

Alternaria toxins can be found also in beverages such as fruit juices, beers and wines [36–41], as well as in food supplements used for various purposes [42]. Milk thistle-based supplements for liver diseases were simultaneously contaminated by AOH, AME, TEN, and TeA with maximum concentrations of 4560 μg/kg, 3200 μg/kg, 1280 μg/kg, and 2140 μg/kg, respectively. The same mycotoxins were detected, even though at a lower concentration, in supplements used to treat menopause symptoms (containing red clover, flax seeds and soy) or for general health support (containing among others green barley, nettle, goji berries and yucca). The maximum concentration of TeA was found in supplements for general health support (6780 μg/kg), while milk thistle-based supplements showed the highest average concentrations of all mycotoxins. Notably, the beneficial effects of health-promoting compounds of food supplements might be impaired to various extents by the presence of mycotoxins. In addition, taking into account that food supplements are thought to supply specific deficiencies, the presence of mycotoxins might have a higher impact on specific categories of consumers. These aspects require urgent investigations to timely support the enforcement of specific regulations.

Table 1. Co-occurrence of *Alternaria* toxins in food.

Food/Foodstuff	*Alternaria* Mycotoxins							Reference
	AOH	AME	ALT	TeA	TEN	ATX-I	Other	
Fruits, Vegetables and Derivatives								
Apple	X	X	X	X		X		[19]
Apple juice	X	X						[36,43]
Apple juice (concentrated)	X	X						[44]
Apple-pear-cherry (puree infant formula)	X	X		X	X	–	ALP (–)	[21]
Berry juice	X	X			–			[37]
Cherry-banana (puree infant formula)	X	X		X	–	–	ALP (–)	[21]
Cranberry juice	X	X						[39]
Cranberry nectar	X	X						[43]
Citrus juice	–	X [a]		X [a]	–			[38]
Grape juice	X	X						[39]
Ketchup	X [a]	–	X [a]					[45]
Ketchup	X	X		X	X			[38]
Mixed juice (fruits and vegetables)	X	X [a]	X [a]	X		–	Iso-ALT (–), AAL TA1 (–), AAL TA2(–)	[46]
Orange juice	X	X						[36]
Pepper	X	X		X				[47]
Prune nectar	X	X						[43]
Soya beans	X	X						[48]
Strawberry	X [a]	X [a]						[49]
Sweet pepper	X	X	X	X				[29]
Tangerine (flavedo)	X	X						[50]
Tomato	X	X	X	X		–		[19]
Tomato	X [a]	X [a]		X [a]		–	ATX-II (–)	[51]
Tomato	X	X	X					[45]
Tomato (dried)	X [a]	X [a]	X [a]		X [a]			[52]
Tomato (puree and ketchup)	X	X	–	X	X [a]	–	Iso-ALT (–), AAL TA1 (–), AAL TA2(–)	[46]
Tomato (sun-dried)	X	X	X					[45]
Tomato juice	–	X		X	X			[38]
Tomato sauce	X	X	X [a]	X	X [a]	X	ALP (X), AOH-3-S (X [a]), AME-3-S (X)	[20]
Tomato sauce (puree infant formula)	X	X		X	X	–	ALP (–)	[21]
Tomato soup (puree infant formula)	–	X		X	–	–	ALP (–)	[21]
Vegetable juice	X	X						[36]

Table 1. *Cont.*

Food/Foodstuff	*Alternaria* Mycotoxins							Reference
	AOH	AME	ALT	TeA	TEN	ATX-I	Other	
Cereals and Derivatives								
Bakery products (wheat- and rye- based)	X	X	–	X	X	–	Iso-ALT (–), AAL TA1 (–), AAL TA2(–)	[46]
Bread	X [a]	X		X	X			[53]
Cereal grains	X [a]	X [a]	–		X [a]			[41]
Corn silage	X [a]	X [a]			X [a]		MACRO (X [a])	[33]
Dried noodles	X [a]	X		X	X			[53]
Maize-based snacks	X	X						[54]
Millet (infant formula)	X	X		X	X	–	ALP (–)	[21]
Oat (infant formula)	–	X		X	X	–	ALP (–)	[21]
Ragi	–	X	X	X		–		[30]
Rice (infant formula)	X	X		X	X	–	ALP (–)	[21]
Sorghum	–	X	X	X		–		[30]
Spelt (infant formula)	X	X		X	X	X	ALP (–)	[21]
Wheat	X [a]	X [a]	X [a]	X [a]				[31]
Wheat	X [a]	X [a]		X [a]				[55]
Wheat (infant formula)	X	X		X	X	X	ALP (–)	[21]
Wheat flour	X [a]	X		X	X			[53]
Wheat flour	X [a]	X	–	X	X [a]	X	ALP (X), AOH-3-S (-), AME-3-S (-)	[20]
Wheat silage	X [a]	X [a]			X [a]		MACRO (X [a])	[33]
Weathered wheat	X	X		X				[56]

Table 1. *Cont.*

Food/Foodstuff	*Alternaria* Mycotoxins							Reference
	AOH	AME	ALT	TeA	TEN	ATX-I	Other	
Dried Fruits and Nuts								
Almonds	X [a]	X [a]			X [a]			[57]
Almonds	X [a]	X [a]			X [a]	–	MACRO (X [a])	[34]
Chestnuts	X [a]	X [a]			X [a]			[57]
Dried figs	X [a]	X [a]			–			[57]
Dried grape berries	X	X	X	X	X	X	ATX-II (X), MACRO (X)	[35]
Dried jujubes	X [a]	X [a]			X [a]			[57]
Dried persimmons	X [a]	X [a]			–			[57]
Dried raisins	X [a]	X [a]			–			[57]
Dried raisins	X	X	–	X	–			[58]
Dried wolfberries	X [a]	X [a]	–	X	X			[58]
Hazelnuts	X [a]	X [a]			X [a]			[57]
Hazelnuts	X	X			X	X [a]	MACRO (X)	[34]
Peanuts	X [a]	X [a]			X [a]	–	MACRO (X [a])	[34]
Pine nuts	X [a]	X [a]			X [a]			[57]
Pistachios	–	–			–	–	MACRO (X [a])	[34]
Walnuts	X [a]	X [a]			X [a]			[57]
Other Food and Foodstuff								
Beer	X [a]	–	X [a]	–	X [a]			[40]
Food supplement (antioxidants)	X [a]	X [a]		X [a]	X [a]			[42]
Food supplement (milk thistle)	X	X		X	X			[42]
Food supplement (phytoestrogens)	X	X		X [a]	X			[42]
Red wines	X	X						[39]
Sesame seeds	X	X		X				[59]
Sunflower seed oil	X	X	–	X	X	X [a]	ALP (X [a]), AOH-3-S (-), AME-3-S (-)	[20]
Sunflower seeds	–	–	–	X [a]	X [a]			[41]
Sunflower seeds	X	X		X				[60]
Sunflower seeds	X	X	X [a]	X	X	X [a]	Iso-ALT (X [a]), AAL TA1 (–), AAL TA2(–)	[46]
Sunflower seeds	X [a]	X [a]		X	X		ALTSOH (X [a]), Val-TeA (X [a])	[61]
Vegetable oils (rapeseed and sunflower seeds)	X	X	–	X [a]	X	–	Iso-ALT (–), AAL TA1 (–), AAL TA2(–)	[46]
White wines	X	X						[39]
Wines	X [a]	–	–	X [a]	–			[41]

X: certain co-occurrence; X [a]: uncertain co-occurrence; –: checked but not detected.

2.2. Co-Occurrence of Alternaria Toxins with Other Mycotoxins

As discussed above, many food categories may be contaminated by more than one *Alternaria* mycotoxin. However, food commodities can be simultaneously contaminated by a high number of different mycotoxins produced by molds other than *Alternaria*. In particular, mycotoxins produced by *Aspergillus*, *Fusarium*, and *Penicillium* genera frequently co-occur with *Alternaria* mycotoxins (Table 2). Among them, the most investigated and frequently detected were those produced by the genera *Fusarium* and *Aspergillus* [e.g., aflatoxins, enniatins (ENNs) and beauvericin], while the least frequently examined or detected were ochratoxins (ochratoxin A, OTA; ochratoxin B, OTB).

A study conducted by Gambacorta et al. [29] investigated the co-occurrence of 17 different mycotoxins in fresh, fried, dried or grounded sweet pepper products. Notably, all of them were contaminated by more than one mycotoxin simultaneously. In more detail, 6 out of 39 samples contained 2, 3 or 4 different mycotoxins, while the remaining samples were positive for a number of mycotoxins ranging from 5 to 16. The fried peppers showed the lowest average level of contamination (with an average mycotoxin contamination of 231 μg/kg), while the fresh pepper samples were the most contaminated (27,280 μg/kg). TeA was the most frequently detected mycotoxin (100% of samples) with an average concentration of 4817.9 μg/kg. With regard to the other *Alternaria* toxins, 93%, 56%, 33%, and 9% of pepper samples were found to be contaminated by TEN, AOH, AME and ALT, respectively. These compounds (except for ALT) were found to co-occur along with 7 other *Fusarium* mycotoxins (nivalenol, HT-2 toxin, T-2 toxin, fumonisin B_1, fumonisin B_2, deoxynivalenol (DON) and zearalenone (ZEN)), 4 other *Aspergillus* mycotoxins (the aflatoxins B_1, B_2, G_1, and G_2), and OTA in the most contaminated sample. It is worth mentioning the average low level of contamination of fried samples. In this respect, the frying process might have a role in lowering the content of *Alternaria* mycotoxins, though it was not directly assessed by the authors. It would be in agreement with other studies pointing to a significant reduction of mycotoxin content upon fry cooking [62]. In addition, high-temperature treatments already proved to be effective in mitigating the content of certain *Alternaria* mycotoxins [63], supporting the possible role of fry cooking in reducing the content of *Alternaria* mycotoxins. The effects of three extrusion processing parameters (moisture content, feeding rate and screw speed) on the degradation of TeA, AOH and AME in whole wheat flour have been investigated. With the optimal parameters, a reduction of 65.6, 87.9 and 94.5% was achieved for TeA, AOH and AME, respectively [63]. As a general remark, the thermal stability of *Alternaria* mycotoxins needs to be further investigated, along with the possible formation of toxic by-products, to identify effective food processing for reducing their content in food.

The co-occurrence of AOH with the *Fusarium* mycotoxins ZEN and DON and, with the ergot alkaloid ergometrine was described in beer [64]. In particular, ergometrine, a toxin produced by *Claviceps* spp. used in pharmaceutical applications [65], was detected at low concentrations in 93% of the beer samples (0.07–0.47 μg/L, median 0.15 μg/ L). AOH (0.23–1.6 μg/L, median 0.45 μg/L) and ZEN (0.35–2.0 μg/L, median 0.88 μg/L) were detected in all the beer samples, while DON was found in 75% of samples (2.2–20 μg/L, median 3.7 μg/L). In the light of the low concentrations reported above, the authors concluded that beer should not be considered among the most important source of dietary intake of AOH, ZEN and DON.

In another study, 253 samples of dried fruits and nuts were analyzed for the presence of 16 mycotoxins (aflatoxins, ochratoxins, *Alternaria* toxins and trichothecenes) [57]. The authors reported that 124 samples were contaminated with at least one mycotoxin, while more than half (66 out of 124 samples) were contaminated by at least two mycotoxins. AME was the most frequently detected mycotoxin (44/124), followed by AOH (found in 31 out of 124 samples) and enniatin B_1 (found in 30 out of 124 samples). The most contaminated sample contained eight different mycotoxins (i.e., aflatoxins B_1 and B_2, enniatins B and B_1, beauvericin (BEA), TEN, AOH, and AME). Among the number of combinations found, the most common were binary (such as BEA + AME) and tertiary (such as BEA + AME + AOH) combinations. Ochratoxin B was found occurring along with the *Alternaria* toxins AOH, AME and TEN only in two samples.

The co-occurrence of ochratoxin A with AOH and aflatoxin B_2 was described with a low frequency in berry juice (only 1 out of 32 samples was found positive) [37]. Additionally, although 47% of berry juices were negative for all the investigated mycotoxins, at least one mycotoxin was present in 53% of the samples, with percentage distributions of 9%, 9%, 22%, and 13% for 1, 2, 3 and 4 co-occurring mycotoxins, respectively. Moreover, TEN and aflatoxin B_1 were not detected in any of the analyzed samples, while aflatoxin B_2 + aflatoxin G_2 + AME + AOH and aflatoxin G_2 + AME + AOH were the most frequently found combinations. Importantly, in 87% of the contaminated samples at least one *Alternaria* mycotoxin was detected: AOH was most frequently found (73%; concentrations from 2.5 to 85 ng/mL) followed by AME (67%; concentrations from 267 to 308 ng/mL). Similarly, the co-occurrence of *Alternaria* toxins with other mycotoxins was also reported in dried fruit samples from China (apricots, raisins, dates, and wolfberries) [58]. In particular, 64.6% of the samples were contaminated by at least one mycotoxin, while 31.4% of the samples were contaminated with two to four compounds. TeA was the most abundant (from 6.9 to 5665.3 μg/kg) and frequently detected compound, followed by TEN (20.5% of samples) and mycophenolic acid (MPA; 19.5% of samples). MPA is produced by various *Penicillium* species and it is used as an immunosuppressant drug to prevent organ rejection after transplantation. In terms of safety, its occurrence in food may raise concern on account of its potential to predispose susceptible individuals to infectious diseases [58]. The combinations TeA + TEN and TeA + MPA were found with a prevalence of 13.2% and 11.4%, respectively [58]. In addition, TeA was simultaneously detected along with OTA in 7% of samples, with an apparently inverse relationship: the higher the concentration of TeA, the lower the concentration of OTA. This might be due to competition phenomena between mycotoxin-producing fungi or due to degrading processes, as reported by Müller et al. [66]. They described an inverse correlation between the increase of AOH, AME and TeA production and the decrease of *Fusarium* toxins (DON and ZEN) possibly due to the degradation of the latter by *Alternaria* strains. In this context, in vitro studies on the synthesis of mycotoxins during the co-incubation of *Alternaria* strains with other fungi may be useful to investigate the existence of a possible mutual influence, which seems likely to exist on the basis of low level of co-occurring mycotoxins reported so far in the literature.

As already reported in Section 2.1, food supplements might be highly contaminated by *Alternaria* toxins. However, *Alternaria* toxins can be found in food supplements also along with other mycotoxins. As an example, Veprikova and co-workers found 66 out of 69 samples contaminated by more than one mycotoxin. Specifically, 58% of milk thistle-based supplements contained more than 12 different mycotoxins simultaneously, while one of the most contaminated samples contained 14 different mycotoxins, i.e., AOH, AME, TEN, 3-acetyl-DON, beauvericin, fusarenon-X, ZEN, HT-2 toxin, T-2 toxin and enniatins B, B_1, A and A_1 [42]. The most common combinations described were ENNs + HT-2/T-2 + AOH + AME + TEN and ENNs + AOH + AME + TEN + MPA. As a general remark, the state-of the-art of food supplements contamination warns about a potentially dangerous scenario. Indeed, although to date no maximum limits of *Alternaria* mycotoxins have been defined for food, the relatively high concentrations of mycotoxins occasionally detected in food supplements might suggest the need to perform dedicated risk assessment studies. Therefore, further occurrence and exposure studies have to be done urgently paving the ground to timely enact specific regulations for food supplements.

Table 2. Co-occurrence of *Alternaria* toxins with other mycotoxins.

Food/Foodstuff	Co-Occurring Mycotoxins				Reference
	2 Mycotoxins	3 Mycotoxins	4 Mycotoxins	>4 Mycotoxins	
Berry juices	AFB2, AME AFB2, AOH AOH, AME	AFB2, AFG2, AOH AFB2, AOH, OTA AFB2, AFG2, AME AFB2, AFG2, AOH AFG2, AME, AOH AFB2, AME, AOH	AFB2, AFG2, AME, AOH AFG1, AFG2, AME, AOH AFB2, AFG1, AFG2, AME		[37]
Sweet pepper (*Capsicum annuum*)	AFB1, TeA	ZEN, TEN, TeA	FB2, TEN, TeA, ZEN	*n* 16 (NIV, AOH, TeA, HT-2, FB2, OTA, T-2, FB1, TEN, AME, AFB1, DON, AFG1, AFB2, AFG2 and ZEN)	[29]
Durum wheat	n.a.	n.a.	n.a.	*n* 7 (EN B, EN B1, EN A1, AME, DON, HT2 and T2)	[67]
Dried fruits (raisins, dried apricots, dates and wolfberries)	TeA, MPA TeA, TEN	n.a.	n.a.	n.a.	[58]
Maize-based snacks	n.a.	n.a.	n.a.	*n* 6 (FB1, FB2, FB3, BEAU, AME, EMOD)	[54]
Nuts and dried fruits	AFB2, TEN AFG1, AME ZEN, AOH BEA, AME T-2, AME ENB1, TEN	AFB2, TEN, AME AFB2, AOH, AME ENA1, ENB1, AME BEA, AOH, AME T-2, BEA, AME AFB2, ENB, AOH	ZEN, TEN, AOH, AME ENA1, ENB, TEN, AME AFB2, TEN, AOH, AME AFB1, BEA, AOH, AME AFG1, AFG2, ENB1, TEN AFG1, ENB1, AOH, AME	*n* 8 (AFB1, AFB2, ENB, ENB1, OTB, TEN, AOH, AME)	[57]
Beer	AOH, ZEN	n.a.	Ergometrine, AOH, ZEN, DON	n.a.	[64]
Food supplements (milk thistle - based)	n.a.	n.a.	AOH, AME, TEN, MPA Other	*n* 14 (AOH, AME, TEN, 3-ADON, FUS-X, ENN-B, ENN-B1, ENN-A, ENN-A1, BEA, DON, HT-2, T-2, ZEN) etc.	[42]

n.a.: information not available.

3. Individual Toxicity of Main *Alternaria* Toxins and Combined Toxicity with Other Mycotoxins and Bioactive Compounds of Food Origin

Alternaria species may produce a huge variety of different mycotoxins showing a great variability in terms of chemical structures [68]. AOH, AME, TeA, ALT, and altertoxins (I, II, III) are considered the most relevant for food toxicology, taking into account their occurrence and/or toxicity. Nevertheless, in vivo toxicological data currently available are not adequate for a proper risk assessment and, therefore, they are not sufficient to define toxicological standard values for the establishment of maximum limits in food and feed. At present, the only LD_{50} values are available, even if they refer to a limited number of compounds (Table 3).

Table 3. LD_{50} values of *Alternaria* mycotoxins currently available.

Mycotoxin	Animal Species	Route of Exposure	LD_{50} (mg/kg b.w.)	Reference
AOH	Mouse (DBA/2)	intraperitoneal	>400 [1]	[69]
AME	Mouse (DBA/2)	intraperitoneal	>400 [1]	
TeA	Mouse	intravenous	115 (female)	[70]
			162 (male)	
		oral	81 (female)	
			186 (male)	
	Mouse (ICR)	intravenous	125 (male)	[71]
		intraperitoneal	150 (male)	
		subcutaneous	145 (male)	
		oral	225 (male)	
	Rat	intravenous	157 (female)	[70]
			146 (male)	
		oral	168 (female)	
			180 (male)	
	Chicken embryo	injection	548 [2]	[72]
	White leghorn chicken	oral	37.5 [3]	[73]

[1] LD_{50} values of AOH and AME were not reached at the maximum dose tested, corresponding to 400 mg/kg, [2] Unit of measurement: µg/egg, [3] Information about sex not available.

As a general remark, except for these few mycotoxins, very few data are available for the other members of the *Alternaria* mycotoxin family, which still remain largely uncharacterized in terms of toxicity and mechanisms of action.

As already discussed, the simultaneous occurrence of more than one *Alternaria* mycotoxin, also in combination with other mycotoxins produced by different fungi, is common in food. In this respect, it is important to remark that the risk assessment of mycotoxins currently relies on single substance effects [2,74], neglecting any possible mutual combined actions due to simultaneous exposure. These mycotoxin-mycotoxin interactions might modify the individual toxicity of compounds, likely resulting in a final toxic outcome different from the single compound tested alone. In addition, it must be considered that many extra-nutritional constituents (such as bioactive food constituents) are widely present in food, and their biological activity may also interfere with mycotoxin activity. The combined actions can be referred to as: (i) additive effects, when the final toxicity is the sum of the individual toxic effects of compounds; (ii) synergistic effects, when the resulting total toxicity is greater than the sum of individual effects or iii) antagonistic effects, when the opposite is the case and the combinatory effect is less than additive [75]. Several mathematical models and methods are commonly used to evaluate the nature of the combined effects of toxic compounds. Among them, the most common are the independent joint action model and the combination index-isobologram method. The first one allows to calculate an expected additive value from the effects of the single compounds [76] that can in turn be compared to a measured combinatory effect. The combination index-isobologram method allows to take into account the shape of dose-response curves when determining the type of interaction (synergism, additive effect and antagonism) [75,77]. This is considered the state-of-the-art model; however it can be challenging to meet the requirements to apply it.

As shown below, the evidence collected so far clearly states that synergistic effects of mycotoxins in mixtures with other compounds (either mycotoxins or other food components) may have important consequences on the single-compound activity. This might have an impact on the assessment of risk related to the presence of *Alternaria* mycotoxins in food, which should consider the mixtures, rather than focusing on single-compound evidences. The individual toxicity of the main *Alternaria* mycotoxins and the effects of their combination with other mycotoxins or food constituents are reported in the following sections.

3.1. *Individual Toxicity of Alternaria Mycotoxins*

3.1.1. Genotoxic Effects

Among the best characterized *Alternaria* toxins, those with genotoxic properties are considered of most concern for human health by regulatory authorities. This particularly applies to AOH and AME, for which the EFSA concluded that "the estimated mean chronic dietary exposures at the upper bound and 95th percentile dietary exposures exceeded the TTC value" in their latest exposure assessment [10], and thus called for more data regarding exposure and toxicity of those metabolites [13].

In human cells, both AOH and AME have been reported to induce DNA strand breaks in the comet assay at concentrations ≥1 μM [78], to act clastogenic at ≥2.5 μM [79] and to possess mutagenic potential at ≥10 μM, as measured by HPRT and TK gene mutation assays [80]. An in vivo study on mice did not find AOH to cause systemic DNA damages in liver tissue and bone marrow [81]. However, the authors argue that any toxicity of the substance would probably be limited to the gastrointestinal tract due to poor bioavailability, but did not include corresponding organs in their survey.

Concerning the mechanisms of action, both AOH and AME were found to act as a topoisomerase (TOP) poison at micromolar concentrations, affecting the activity of both TOP I and TOP II, with a certain preference for the α isoform of TOP II [78]. Those enzymes are needed to untangle the DNA for replication or transcription, a process which involves the induction of a transient DNA strand break that is re-ligated at the end of the catalytic cycle. Poisoning of these enzymes by small molecules results in a toxin-dependent stabilization of the covalent DNA–topoisomerase complex (i.e., the so-called "cleavable complex"). Stabilization of the cleavable complex by TOP "poisons" hinders release of TOP in the catalytic cycle and re-ligation of the DNA, thus resulting in a persistence of the initially induced strand break. Thus, TOP poisons are commonly described to act genotoxic [82].

An additional mechanism contributing to the toxicity of *Alternaria* toxins is the induction of intracellular reactive oxygen species (ROS), which indicate oxidative stress. ROS production induced by AOH and AME might play an important role in the inhibitory effects on cell proliferation observed in different cellular models [83,84].

Of note, ALT and iso-ALT were not found to affect topoisomerase activity [78], probably due to their less planar structure not allowing for DNA intercalation in comparison to AOH/AME [85].

However, it was observed that extracts from cultured *Alternaria* strains by far exceeded the genotoxicity of their dibenzo-α-pyrone contents [86]. This has led to the discovery of the epoxide-carrying perylene quinone ATX-II as a major contributing factor to the genotoxicity of naturally occurring mixtures of *Alternaria* toxins [87,88]. Later on, not only ATX II, but also the structurally related STTX-III was found to be more mutagenic then AOH. Regarding their mode of action, these mycotoxins were also found to act as inhibitors of TOPs at high concentrations. However, their main genotoxic mode of action is thought to be the formation of DNA adducts, a hypothesis which still awaits experimental confirmation [87–89].

Of note, there is speculation that yet not characterized secondary metabolites might also possess genotoxic properties, as an *Alternaria* extract very low on dibenzo-α-pyrones, which was additionally stripped off ATX-II and STTX-III, still maintained substantial DNA-damaging properties [90].

3.1.2. Endocrine-Modulating and Other Toxic Effects

AOH and AME, as well as other related metabolites, were reported to elicit estrogenic effects in cellular systems. In particular, AOH was described to be able to activate both ER-α and β but with a greater affinity (approximately ten-fold higher) for ER-β [79,91], although the binding strength is 10,000-fold weaker than the endogenous hormone estradiol. AME was found to be slightly more potent than AOH at 10 μM, and the methylation at the 9-OH group was thought to improve the molecular fitting within the estrogen receptor pocket [92]. AOH was additionally found to induce androgenic effects in the yeast androgen bioassay [93]. Recently, computational studies reported that mutations of the androgen receptors might affect the capability of AOH to bind and possibly stimulate the activation of receptors [94]. Moreover, increases in progesterone and estradiol levels, as well as in progesterone receptor expression, were reported in human adrenocarcinoma H295R cells treated with AOH, supporting its actual role as endocrine disruptor [95]. However, in naturally occurring mixtures of *Alternaria* toxins, endocrine-disrupting effects of AOH and related metabolites might be "quenched" by cytotoxic and anti-estrogenic properties of co-occurring compounds, as recently demonstrated in Ishikawa cells [90].

In addition to the above listed toxic effects, AOH and AME were found to modulate innate immunity in both human bronchial epithelial BEAS-2B cells and mouse macrophages RAW264.7, through the suppression of the lipopolysaccharide-induced innate immune responses [96]. This activity was also confirmed in THP-1 derived macrophages by Kollarova et al. [97]: AOH, in fact, suppressed lipopolysaccharide (LPS)-induced NF-κB pathway activation, induced transcription of the anti-inflammatory cytokine IL-10, and reduced the transcription of the pro-inflammatory cytokines IL-8, IL-6 and TNF-α.

TeA deserves a particular mention as, unlike the other *Alternaria* mycotoxins, it exerts toxic effects mainly by inhibiting the release of proteins from the ribosome. Although a low toxicity of this mycotoxin has been reported in vitro [86,98], in vivo studies carried out on several animal models highlighted more severe effects such as emesis, tachycardia and haemorrhages [18].

3.2. Combinatory Effects of Alternaria Mycotoxins

There are only a few studies investigating the combinatory effects of *Alternaria* mycotoxins, though food may be quite often simultaneously contaminated by more than one single compound as shown, for instance, for AOH and AME (Section 2.1). Notably, these two mycotoxins are not of particular concern in terms of cytotoxic effects, also on account of the high concentrations required to cause harmful effects when tested individually. However, the simultaneous exposure to AOH and AME may have significant effects on the overall toxicity in respect to their individual testing. In more detail, their combined effects (1:1 concentration ratio) were invested by Bensassi et al. on the human intestinal cell line HCT-116 [99]. No significant difference in cell viability was detected at 25 μM up to 24 h of exposure when mycotoxins were tested either individually or in combination. Conversely, both mycotoxins reduced cell viability about 30% after 24 h of exposure when tested individually, while they reduced viability about 50% when tested in combination. In this study, the nature of interactive effects was described to be additive, while Fernández-Blanco and co-workers reported synergistic effects in Caco-2 cells after 24 h of exposure to AOH and AME in a 1:1 binary combination and in a concentration range from 3.125 to 30 μM [83]. Moreover, the AOH-AME binary combination reduced cell proliferation to a greater extent than AOH alone at all tested concentrations, while it had greater effects than AME alone at 15 and 30 μM. The binary mixture also caused a greater dose-dependent reduction of cell proliferation after 48 h of incubation (in the concentration range 7.5–30 μM) than AOH or AME tested alone. In this case, the nature of the interactive effects was described as synergistic or additive at small or higher fraction affected, respectively.

The effects exerted by the simultaneous exposure to AOH and the genotoxic *Alternaria* mycotoxin ATX-II were investigated by Vejdovszky et al. [100] on two intestinal (HT-29, HCEC-1CT) and one hepatic (HepG2) cell line. Seven different concentrations, ranging from 500 nM to 10 μM for ATX-II and from 5 μM to 100 μM for AOH were tested for binary combinations (constant ratio of 1:10, ATX-II:AOH). As a result, the HT-29 cell line was found to be the least sensitive to cytotoxic effects mediated by the two tested mycotoxins and significant differences in cell viability were found starting from the combination 5 μM:50 μM (ATX-II:AOH). Among the different concentrations tested, the highest decrease in cell viability observed was of nearly 40%. Notably, the cell treatment at low mycotoxin concentrations led to an increase in mitochondrial activity in the co-treated samples. HepG2 cells were found the most sensitive to the cytotoxic effects exerted by AOH, while HCEC-1CT cells proved to be the most sensitive to the effects of ATX-II. Combining these two mycotoxins, an increased sensitivity to cytotoxic effects was also found in the HepG2 cell line, leading to a reduction in cell viability starting from the combination 1 μM:10 μM (ATX-II:AOH). Although most of the tested 1:10 combinations showed additive effects, antagonistic effects were reported in HCEC-1CT and HepG2 cell lines, while only one of the combinations analyzed showed synergistic effects on HepG2 cell line (750 nM ATX-II:750 nM AOH, 1:1 ratio). Modifications of microRNAs expression profile after incubation of HepG2 cells with the mixture 10 μM AOH:1 μM ATX-II may partially explains such effects. The combined exposure caused a significant increase of miR-224 expression after 12 h of exposure, which was no longer over-expressed after 24 h, while miR-192 and miR-29a were respectively down-regulated and up-regulated after 24 h. In addition, miR-29a was up-regulated also in samples treated with AOH alone, suggesting a possible role in the up-regulation of this miRNA by the binary mixture. Interestingly, these three microRNAs are involved in the regulation of apoptotic processes and the observed modifications led the authors to conclude that such miRNAs may be in part involved in the antagonistic effects observed for some of the combinations tested.

As previously described, *Alternaria* mycotoxins are often found in food commodities along with *Fusarium* mycotoxins. In a recent study [101], the cytotoxic effects and the type of interactions of AOH combined with *Fusarium* mycotoxins enniatin B and DON were evaluated after 24, 48, and 72 h of exposure in Caco-2 cells. For binary and tertiary combinations, five different concentrations, ranging from 0.3125 to 5 μM for enniatin B and DON, and from 1.875 to 30 μM for AOH, were tested. The binary combinations enniatin B + AOH (1:6 ratio) led to higher cytotoxic effects compared to AOH tested alone at all the timepoints and concentrations tested. However, no difference between enniatin B tested alone and in mixture was observed, suggesting that the cytotoxic effects were mainly mediated by enniatin B. With regard to the binary combinations DON + AOH (1:6 ratio), the resulting cytotoxicity after 24 h of exposure was lower than that exerted by DON tested alone. On the contrary, an opposite trend was observed after 48 and 72 h of exposure. As expected, the tertiary mixtures enniatin B + DON + AOH (ratio 1:1:6) led to a greater decrease, albeit of slight intensity, of cell viability compared to the binary combinations. Although the pattern was not uniform along the fraction affected, the application of the isobologram analysis described the interactions in the binary mixtures as additive and synergistic, depending on the concentrations and timepoints tested. Interestingly, the ternary combinations showed antagonistic effects, which were described as due to competition mechanisms at the same receptor site. In this respect, it is worth mentioning the marked diversity of these mycotoxins in terms of chemical structures. Taking into account that the competition to the same protein site usually requires strict conservation of key structural motifs [102], the inherent structural heterogeneity among enniatin B, DON and AOH is not fully compatible with their capability to physically compete with the same site. Therefore, both the molecular mechanisms and the network of biological targets involved in such antagonistic behavior need to be precisely described to better understand the effects of the enniatin B/DON/AOH ternary combination.

The effects of binary and ternary combinations of AOH with the DON's acetylated derivatives 3-ADON and 15-ADON were also investigated on HepG2 cells up to 72 h of incubation [103]. Constant ratios of 16:1 (AOH: 3-acetyl-ADON and AOH:15-acetyl-DON) and 16:1:1 (AOH:3-acetyl-DON:15-acetyl-DON) were chosen to test these mixtures, with concentrations ranging from 3.2μM to 24μM for AOH, and from 0.2 μM to 1.5 μM for DON's derivatives. Cytotoxicity ranking was found to be the same for all tested time points (AOH+3-acetyl-DON + 15-acetyl-DON > AOH + 3-acetyl-DON > AOH + 15-acetyl-DON) and a concentration-dependent decrease in HepG2 cell viability was found in all tested mixtures. The effects caused by binary and ternary mixtures were described to be mainly synergistic, but some exceptions were found for AOH + 3-acetyl-DON at 72 h (where additive effects were observed at higher fraction affected), and for AOH + 15-acetyl-DON (where additive or antagonistic effects were observed depending on the concentration and timepoint tested).

Binary effects of TeA with the *Fusarium* mycotoxins enniatin B, ZEN, DON, nivalenol and aurofusarin (AURO) were also evaluated on Caco-2 cells with two different concentration sets, named "low concentrations" (none or slight cytotoxic effect) and "high concentrations" (pronounced cytotoxic effect) [104]. TeA combinations at "low concentrations" of mycotoxins did not show significant differences between the measured and expected effects (calculated on the basis of the Independent Joint Action model). This indicates that the combinations of TeA at "low concentrations of mycotoxins" only determined additive effects. On the contrary, binary combinations at "high concentrations" led to lower cytotoxic effects then the calculated additive effects. Additional investigations allowed getting more details about the type of interactions between TeA and *Fusarium* mycotoxins. No difference in cytotoxicity was found in samples co-treated with enniatin B and ZEN keeping the concentration of *Fusarium* mycotoxins constant (from 5 to 50 μM depending on the mycotoxin) and varying that of TeA (from 1 μM to 250 μM). Indeed, the cytotoxicity of binary mixtures with TeA was found to be equivalent to the toxicity of toxins tested individually. Notably, the toxic effect induced by 10μM DON was reduced in a concentration-independent manner by the combination with TeA at concentrations between 10 μM and 200 μM. A similar trend was found for the combination with 10 μM nivalenol, although differences were not statistically significant. Keeping in mind that TeA and the *Fusarium* mycotoxins DON and nivalenol are known to inhibit protein synthesis in vitro [104], the lower cytotoxic effects of binary mixtures might be due to a molecular interplay at the level of protein synthesis inhibition. Nevertheless, considering that nivalenol and DON inhibit protein synthesis by different mechanisms (i.e., by inhibiting the initiation or elongation-termination steps, respectively) [105], the observed effects cannot be straightforwardly explained in terms of mechanisms of action pointing out the need of investigating further the molecular basis of such interaction. In this respect, the inhibition of protein synthesis by TeA may modify the expression of specific factors, including metabolizing enzymes, and consequences on the pattern of metabolites produced by cells are thought likely. This is of particular relevance as some trichothecenes metabolites might be involved in mediating ribotoxic effects of parent mycotoxins, as supported recently by in silico studies [106]. On this basis, TeA might have indirect effects on trichothecenes toxicity acting on their metabolism and changing the relative abundance of ribotoxic metabolites produced.

Recently, an interesting study was performed by Solhaug et al. that investigated the ability of AOH, DON and ZEN in binary and tertiary mixtures to affect immune response checking the differentiation of monocytes to macrophages [107]. The differentiation process leads to several changes, including modifications of the expression of some cell surface markers such as CD14, CD11b and CD71. AOH, DON and ZEN were able to modify the expression of these markers in THP-1 monocytes, but with some differences: while AOH affected the expression of the all set of markers, DON did not modify the expression of CD71 and ZEN altered only the expression of CD-14. Since CD-14 was the only marker modified by all the three mycotoxins, its expression was used to evaluate the type of interactions in binary and ternary mycotoxins mixtures by applying the "Concentration Addition" (CA) and the "Independent Joint Action" (IA) models. Since authors did not find significant differences between the experimental data and the predicted models, the type of interaction was described to be additive. Remarkably, at the lowest concentrations of the AOH + ZEN combination, the confidence interval of the predicted CA model did not overlap with the experimental values, suggesting a possible synergistic effect. The same results were obtained for the binary combinations through the application of the isobologram analysis. To verify if the observed inhibitory effects of AOH, DON, and ZEN on the up-regulation of CD14 led to a real reduction in macrophage activation, the pro-inflammatory cytokine TNFα and its gene expression were quantified after incubation with single mycotoxins. Contrary to what was observed for AOH and ZEN, DON induced an increased secretion of TNFα following the increase of TNFα gene expression, in spite of its inhibitory action on the up-regulation of CD14. The expression of NF-kB, a protein complex involved in TNFα expression, might provide a plausible explanation to these differences. Indeed, ZEN was reported to reduce the expression of NF-kB [108], and, recently, also AOH showed the ability to suppress the lipopolysaccharide-induced NF-kB pathway activation, resulting in the reduction of TNFα [97]. In contrast, DON was found to induce both NF-kB activation and TNF-α expression, but the signaling pathway was different from those activated by ZEN and AOH [109].

3.3. *Combined Effects with Bioactive Food Constituents*

Beside the combined action of the different members of *Alternaria* mycotoxins group, also in combination with mycotoxins produced by fungi other than *Alternaria*, it is important to take into consideration even the complex interactions that these mycotoxins may have with the other bioactive compounds of food origin.

In this contest, Vejdovszky et al. recently investigated the combinatory estrogenic effects of the isoflavone genistein (GEN) in combination with ZEN and AOH [110]. To elucidate the combinatory effects, the human endometrial adenocarcinoma Ishikawa cell line was chosen as a model system and the phosphatase alkaline (ALP) activity assay was used to measure estrogen receptor activation. The xenoestrogens under investigation were tested at different concentrations (ranging from pM to μM) after 48 h of incubation. All of them increased the ALP activation when tested individually, with the following order of potency in terms of EC50: E2 (17β-estradiol; used as positive control) > ZEN > GEN > AOH. Moreover, these xenoestrogens did not only differ in terms of potency, but also in terms of efficacy as none of them (at any concentration) was able to determine the same effects induced by 1 nM E2. A possible explanation for this finding is that AOH, ZEN and GEN might act as partial agonists. The lower capability to satisfy the pharmacophoric requirements of estrogen receptors pockets in comparison to E2 [111,112] might provide a structural rational to explain such evidence. With regards to binary mixtures of GEN with ZEN or AOH, some of them resulted in significantly higher effects than the respective compounds tested individually, clearly pointing out the existence of synergistic effects. However, combinations of GEN-AOH activated ALP to a lower extent than ZEN-AOH mixtures. It must be highlighted that in many studies ZEN was found to be more estrogenic than AOH, and this could partly justify the lowering of estrogenic effect observed in combinations [110]. In addition, while the authors noted the preference of AOH and GEN to ERβ, ZEN was previously described with a higher affinity for ERα [113]. The simultaneous activation of both α and β estrogen receptor isoforms in the ZEN-GEN and ZEN-AOH binary mixtures may explain the stronger synergistic effects observed. Although some GEN-AOH combinations showed synergistic effects, other combinations at very low doses led to antagonistic effects. Indeed, anti-estrogenic effects were found testing the combination 0.001 μM GEN-0.1 μM AOH and observing a reduction of ALP activation (10.9%) compared to the control (vehicle). A subsequent more-in-depth analysis of the combinatory effects, performed through the combination index and the isobologram method, allowed to determine the type of interactions occurring in the different combinations. Both methods showed that the combinatory effects of GEN and ZEN in the constant ratio of 1000:1 were mainly synergistic and, only at very low or very high effect levels, additive or antagonistic effects were observed. In the constant ratios of 100:1 and 10:1, the substances led to a strong antagonism at low effect levels, and to a strong synergism at higher effects.

Comparable outcomes were reported for the 1:10 GEN:AOH ratio (which showed antagonistic or synergistic effects at low or high effect levels, respectively), while the 1:5 combination ratio determined mainly antagonistic effects. Additionally, the 1:1 GEN:AOH ratio resulted in the onset of synergistic effects up to about 65% of the maximum ALP activation observed (E2 1nM). Above, additive or antagonistic effects were observed depending on the concentrations tested. Thus, the nature of the interactions seemed to depend on both the ratio of substances and the specific concentrations tested.

It was also established that AOH is able to cause oxidative stress and to exert genotoxic effects in different cellular models, mainly by acting as a topoisomerase poison [78]. Aichinger et al. investigated the effects of AOH in combination with the two polyphenols GEN and delphinidin (DEL) [114]. These two compounds are known for their antioxidant effects at specific concentrations, although pro-oxidant effects at certain concentrations were also demonstrated [115,116]. Both GEN and DEL were found to interact, albeit with different mechanisms, with topoisomerases: while GEN usually acts as a topoisomerase poison, turning the enzyme into a DNA-damaging agent, DEL acts as a catalytic inhibitor of topoisomerase hindering the formation of the TOP-DNA intermediate. Therefore, considering both the antioxidant effects and the interaction with the topoisomerases, a modification of the effects induced by AOH may be expected when the mycotoxin is combined with these two polyphenols. Preliminary investigations on the combinatory cytotoxic effects were conducted in HT-29 colon carcinoma cells with concentrations ranging from 1 to 100 μM (1:1 ratio): cytotoxicity was observed starting from 25 μM for AOH and GEN, and from 50 μM for DEL. Both AOH/GEN and AOH/DEL combinations led to cytotoxic effects starting from 25 μM (1:1 ratio) and the type of interactions was described as synergistic, with a tendency to lose synergism when increasing cytotoxic effects. DNA strand breaks and oxidative DNA damages of the combinations of AOH (50 μM) with DEL (10–100 μM) or GEN (25–250 μM) were evaluated by performing an alkaline comet assay with or without treatment with formamidopyrimidin-DNA-glycosylase (FPG). When combined, DEL and AOH showed marked antagonistic effects at 50 μM in the FPG-untreated samples, while lower oxidative DNA damages were observed at 25 and 100 μM. Similar results were found for the combination AOH/GEN at 25 and 100 μM, which showed a lower oxidative damage than AOH tested individually. The authors also evaluated the influence of the co-incubations on the stabilization of the topoisomerases/DNA intermediate (the so-called "cleavable complexes"), which is typically due to the action of topoisomerase poisons (such as AOH). The AOH/GEN combination did not increase the formation of cleavable complexes, rather an antagonistic effect was found at the highest GEN concentration tested (100 μM). Antagonistic effects were also found in AOH/DEL combinations starting from 25 μM. These results were partially attributed to the dual anti-oxidant or pro-oxidant properties of the polyphenols. In this respect, simultaneous short-time incubations with AOH and DEL led to a reduction of AOH-induced ROS generation at concentrations of DEL starting from 1μM. On the contrary, GEN induced oxidative stress per se and did not suppress the pro-oxidative effects induced by AOH. Moreover, 24-h pre-incubations with polyphenols followed by incubation with AOH, did not result in any change in pro-oxidant effects of AOH. This evidence led to exclude any possible modulations of anti-oxidant defense systems as a mechanism underlying the observed antagonistic effects. Therefore, direct anti- or pro-oxidant activities are reasonably as the base of the effects observed during the co-incubations with DEL and GEN. On this basis, DEL could help in preventing the genotoxic effects of AOH, but, considering the low systemic bioavailability of DEL, these protective effects may be limited to the gastrointestinal tract only [117,118].

The same authors also investigated the effects of DEL in combination with ATX-II, one of the most genotoxic *Alternaria* toxins [119]. As reported for the combination with AOH, DEL reduced both DNA strand breaks and oxidative damage in HT-29 cells after short-time co-incubation with ATX-II. The type of interaction was found to be antagonistic according to the applied "independent joint action" model. The production of ROS induced by 10 μM ATX-II was also reduced by DEL in concentrations from 1 μM to 100 μM, but these reductions cannot fully explain the huge reduction of genotoxic effects observed following the co-incubation with DEL. Indeed, no increase of ROS production was observed at the concentration of ATX-II used in the comet assay (1 μM). In cell-free conditions, a reduction of the concentration of ATX-II was found upon co-incubation with DEL. The authors suggested that DEL, after being degraded to phloroglucinol aldehyde (PGA) and gallic acid (GA), might react with ATX-II neutralizing its epoxy group, which is the reactive chemical moiety presumably responsible for genotoxicity. Considering the hypothesis that PGA can react with ATX-II, it is important to underline that the reduction of adverse effects of this mycotoxin may actually occur in subjects that follow diets with a high content of anthocyanins as they are prone to release PGA during digestion.

In the context of the evaluation of combinatory effects between *Alternaria* toxins and bioactive compounds of food origin, polyphenols represent a class of compounds of great interest since they are widely distributed in those food categories which are prone to contamination with *Alternaria* mycotoxins. Quercetin (QUE) is one of the most abundant flavonoids in human diets. QUE has been previously associated to several potential health benefits mainly related to its antioxidant properties, although pro-oxidant effects at certain concentrations have also been described [120]. The potential ability of QUE to reduce the cytotoxicity of AOH and AME was investigated by Fernàndez-Blanco et al. [83]. Although cytoprotective effects were attributed to QUE [121], simultaneous exposure of Caco-2 cells to AOH and QUE (at concentrations ranging from 3.125 to 100 μM) did not result in any cytoprotective effect. In particular, no significant differences were found between the QUE-AOH combination and AOH tested alone after 48 h of exposure. However, the combination significantly affected cell viability at 24 h of treatment in comparison to AOH tested alone. Similarly, no difference between the binary combinations QUE + AME and AME tested alone were detected and, additionally, no cytoprotective effect was found in the tertiary combination AOH + AME + QUE at any of the tested concentrations. Therefore, QUE was not effective in reducing the effects of AOH and AME.

Possible cytoprotective properties of food components against the effects of AOH were also evaluated by Vila-Donat et al. in Caco-2 cells [122]. Keeping in mind that AOH may contaminate legumes (including soybeans and lentils), the authors investigated the effects of AOH in combination with soy saponin I (Ss-I), which was previously found to possess antioxidant activity, or with a lentils extract. In particular, the authors used two different approaches to evaluate the effects of Ss-I and lentil extract: (i) the first one consisted in pre-treating cells with Ss-I (6.25 μM) or with the extract, and then refreshing the growth medium and testing different dilutions of AOH (ranging from 3.125 to 50 μM); (ii) the second approach aimed at evaluating the combinatory effects and the type of interaction co-incubating AOH with Ss-I or lentil extract. By using the first approach, no differences were found between samples pre-treated with Ss-I and samples treated only with AOH. As an exception, the highest AOH concentration tested (50 μM) caused an increase in cell viability in the pre-treated samples. In contrast, co-treatments with AOH + Ss-I (1:1 ratio) above 6.25 μM resulted in an increase in cell viability compared to AOH tested alone. These results suggested that Ss-I likely acted via a direct interaction rather than modulating intracellular defense systems. With regard to cytoprotective effects of the lentils extract, only one single combination was tested and about 30% increase in cell viability was found in comparison to AOH tested alone.

4. The Key Role of Bioactive Compounds

Food is a complex matrix composed by macro- and micro-nutrients, containing also a huge number of non-nutrient compounds that may exert several biological activities. These compounds can interfere at different levels with mycotoxin activities. For instance, they can: (i) activate or inhibit enzymes involved in the metabolism of xenobiotics; (ii) act as anti-oxidant or pro-oxidant compounds; (iii) act as receptor agonists or antagonists targeting, in some cases, the same biological targets of mycotoxins; (iv) modify the expression of genes encoding proteins involved in the regulation of important physiological functions. On this basis, bioactive compounds of food origin may determine the onset of additive, synergistic or antagonistic effects when combined with *Alternaria* mycotoxins. Keeping in mind that the application of mitigating strategies along the food chain are supposed to progressively reduce the dietary exposure to toxicants, the assessment of combinatory effects of mycotoxins with other food constituents will be the most accurate and realistic, but also highly challenging tasks to achieve in the next decades. The challenge will be even harsher taking into account that many food constituents potentially interplaying with mycotoxins are generally recognized as health promoting (i.e., polyphenols) and the consumption of foods rich in such compounds is typically recommended in healthy diet habits. In this framework, this section focuses on the modulation of *Alternaria* mycotoxins toxicity by bioactive compounds.

One of the best characterized toxicological endpoints of *Alternaria* mycotoxins likely affected by food constituents is the estrogenic activity. As a matter of fact, estrogenic and anti-estrogenic effects of bioactive compounds might markedly modify the overall estrogenicity of the *Alternaria* mycotoxins AOH and AME. In terms of risk characterization, this might change the toxicological relevance of such mycotoxins case by case, though they show a weak estrogenicity per se, depending on the composition of chemical mixtures in given foods. In this respect, foods prone to *Alternaria* contamination with a high content of potentially interfering constituents (e.g., polyphenolic phytoestrogens) are legumes (especially soy) and some alcoholic beverages (especially wine and beer). In particular, soybeans and derived products are among the richest dietary sources of phytoestrogens, and many of the isoflavones of soy (including genistein, daidzein, glycitein, and coumestrol) induce estrogen-receptor dependent estrogenic stimuli [123]. As a matter of fact, combinations of GEN-AOH at specific concentrations have been demonstrated to determine synergistic or antagonistic effects in Ishikawa cell line [110]. Similarly to soybeans, hops used to produce beer is characterized by the presence of some prenylflavonoids (e.g., naringenin, 8-prenylnaringenin, 6-prenylnaringenin, 6,8-diprenylnaringenin, and 8-geranylnaringenin) that are potent phytoestrogens with a dual effect being able to bind both estrogen receptor isoforms and to inhibit specific enzymes involved in the estrogenic cellular responses [124,125]. In this context, Aichinger et al. [126] demonstrated the ability of the phytoestrogens from hops xanthohumol and 8-prenylnaringenin to antagonize the estrogenic effects of the *Fusarium* mycotoxins ZEN and α-ZEL. Therefore, possible interactions can be expected also in combination with the estrogenic *Alternaria* toxins AOH and AME. Other important food constituents able to modulate estrogen receptor activity are resveratrol and β-sitosterol, whose primary dietary sources are peanuts, grapes, and wine. Resveratrol, in particular, may exhibit a super-agonist activity inducing a stimulation higher than the endogenous ligand 17β-estradiol in estrogenic gene report assay, even if anti-estrogenic effects were found in the MCF-7 cell line [127]. Although evidences have been not yet collected, these compounds are likely to affect the estrogenicity of *Alternaria* mycotoxins.

Another focal point of the cross-talk between mycotoxins and food components that requires further investigations is the modulation of the aryl hydrocarbon receptor (AhR) [128]. The cascade of events following the activation of AhR is of particular interest in toxicological investigations as it modulates the expression of genes involved in detoxification and transport of various xenobiotics, including the expression of cytochrome P450 family members. Interestingly, AOH and AME were able to bind and activate AhR, causing the increase of CYP1A1 expression and promoting their own metabolism [129]. This process was not affecting the mycotoxin-dependent production of ROS in murine hepatoma cells (Hepa1c1c7). In addition, the authors showed that mycotoxins reduced the number of cells via an AhR-independent process, although the apoptotic phenotype was found only in cells with functional AhR and ARNT [129]. With regard to the ability of AOH to suppress the lipopolysaccharide-induced inflammation previously mentioned, Grover & Lawrence did not find any correlation between AOH-mediated AhR activation and the suppression of the inflammation found in BEAS-2B cells [96]. Thus, despite the increased metabolism of AOH and AME, AhR activation does not seem to raise much concern for ROS production, cytotoxic and immunosuppressive effects, further studies are needed to determine the toxicity of hydroxylated metabolites (e.g., estrogenic properties). In particular, Dellafiora and co-workers showed that hydroxylated forms of AOH and AME cannot interact with estrogen receptors in vitro, pointing to the relevance of phase-I metabolism to modify the toxicodynamic of these mycotoxins. However, methylation of respective catecholic metabolites might reactivate the estrogenic potential [92].

Besides AOH and AME, many food constituents have been described to activate or inhibit AhR. Thus, they are likely to interfere with the ability of AOH and AME to bind AhR and/or with the metabolic processes following the activation of AhR. Foods consumed worldwide such as potatoes, cruciferous, bread, hamburgers, and citrus juices were investigated for the presence of natural AhR-agonists (NAhRAs) [128]. Among these, indole-3-carbinol, and many polyphenols and furocoumarins were found to be responsible for the activities shown by cruciferous vegetables (Brussels sprouts, broccoli, cabbage) and citrus juices, respectively. On the contrary, the activation of AhR induced by the baked or fried foods tested is thought due to secondary chemicals originating from the high-temperature processing, such as polycyclic aromatic hydrocarbons (PAHs), heterocyclic amines or Maillard products [128]. In addition, many dietary flavonoids showed a significant context–dependent AhR agonist or antagonist activities, depending on the concentration and cell types tested [130]. As an example, galangin, GEN, daidzein, and diosmin were found to be AhR agonist only in Hepa-1 cells, while cantharidin acted as an agonist only in human HepG2 and MCF-7 cells. On the contrary, AhR antagonist activities were shown both in MCF-7 and HepG2 cells by luteolin, while the antagonistic activity of kaempferol, quercetin and myricetin was strictly dependent on the cell context [130]. Many other flavones, flavonols, flavanones, isoflavones, and catechins also showed a high affinity to the AhR at dietary exposure levels [131]: apigenin, luteolin, quercetin, kaempferol, and myricetin were found to inhibit the activation of AhR induced by the most potent AhR activator identified so far (2,3,7,8-tetrachlorodibenzo-*p*-dioxin at 5 nM in MCF-7 cells) [131]. Taken together, these findings suggest that the AhR-dependent effects of food constituents strongly depend on both the chemical environment (which may significantly change among the different type of food) and on the cell type tested. Therefore, both the metabolism of *Alternaria* mycotoxins in vivo and their ability to modulate AhR could change depending on the food-specific chemical mixture.

An additional noteworthy activity of AOH and AME common with a number of food components is the capability to poison topoisomerases. In particular, many food bioactives naturally occurring in fruits, vegetables and legumes have been shown to affect the activity of both topoisomerase I and II. Taking into consideration that some *Alternaria* mycotoxins exert important genotoxic effects via either the inhibition or poisoning of these enzyme (see Section 3 for further details), the co-occurrence of other compounds targeting topoisomerases may reasonably change the overall topoisomerase-dependent genotoxic effects of *Alternaria* mycotoxins. Several studies demonstrated the ability of some polyphenols to poison topoisomerase I and/or topoisomerase II, albeit their specific mechanism of action has been poorly investigated. Kaempferol and quercetin were reported to be, at specific concentrations, non-covalently binders of topoisomerase IIα, while myricetin showed the ability to covalently bind to topoisomerase IIα and cleaving DNA in a redox-dependent way [132]. Additionally, the flavonoids quercetin, myricetin, fisetin, and apigenin were highlighted by other authors as poisons of topoisomerase I [133], whilst genistein, daidzein, biochanin A, chrysin, have shown poisoning effects also against topisomerases II [134]. Interestingly, genistein and especially delphinidin (that acts as catalytic topoisomerase inhibitor) were found to protect cells from AOH-induced genotoxicity [114]. Grapes and red wines are characterized by a large amount of resveratrol, belonging to polyphenols' stilbenoids group, which has always been regarded to have beneficial effects thanks to its manifold activity. Nevertheless, the capability to establish non-covalent cross-linking interactions with both topoisomerase II and DNA leading to cell death was described too [135]. An influence of these compounds on poisoning and/or inhibition of topoisomerases by *Alternaria* mycotoxins, also diversifying the outcomes in vivo in a mixture-dependent way, appears therefore to be possible.

On the basis of the data reported above, *Alternaria* mycotoxins and a wealth of food constituents may interfere to each other, mutually influencing their final effects. Moving further steps toward a more precise molecular-oriented understanding of the food-specific and mixture-dependent outcomes in vivo will allow mapping those categories of food might pose a higher risk for specific toxicological endpoints. In the near future, adopting such an approach will effectively pave the ground to set personalized risk/benefit assessment studies of food prone to be contaminated by *Alternaria* mycotoxins.

5. Conclusions and Future Perspectives

Alternaria mycotoxins are frequently occurring in various fresh and processed foods such as cereals, fruits, vegetables, nuts, fruit and vegetable juices, seeds and oils. In many cases, contaminated foods have been found to simultaneously contain more than one *Alternaria* mycotoxin. In addition, the co-occurrence of *Alternaria* mycotoxins along with *Fusarium*, *Penicillium* and *Aspergillus* mycotoxins is also well documented, though not routinely checked. In addition, mycotoxins co-occur with the huge number of food constituents inherently present in contaminated foods. Notably, a growing number of data pointing to significant effects of chemical mixtures of mycotoxins in combination with each other or with food components is available. On this basis, a more precise description of mycotoxin contamination in food, detailing both the co-occurrence of mycotoxins and the types of co-contaminated food categories, is urgently required to better support risk assessment studies.

In this respect, the current risk assessment of mycotoxins is mostly based on human exposure data and animal toxicity evidences of individual compounds, while the evaluation of possible effects due to chemical mixtures is only occasionally assessed. Studies on the combinatory effects of different *Alternaria* mycotoxins, also in combination with other mycotoxins, have already shown that the co-exposure may result in either additive, synergistic, or antagonistic effects, depending on the doses, time of exposure or type of combinations assessed. In addition, recent findings have shown that mycotoxins may interplay with other food constituents, with different outcomes depending on the nature of combinations tested. Taken together, these results show that the toxicity of mycotoxins may significantly change depending on the composition of chemical mixtures, whereby not only co-contaminants but also food bioactives might act as contributors. This evidence pointed out the need to carefully check the multiple co-occurrence of mycotoxins, also in combination with the other food constituents. On the other side, it is crucial to characterize the effects the various combinations with the other food constituents may cause on the toxicity of mycotoxin mixtures. However, the evaluation of combinatory effects is not easy to perform since the toxic action exerted by individual mycotoxins is often strictly dependent on the cellular model and the concentrations tested. In addition, the use of different cellular models and different tested concentrations makes the inter-laboratory comparison of results difficult. Moreover, from a practical point of view, the number of food constituents possibly co-occurring with mycotoxins and potentially able to modulate their toxicity is so huge to make the systematic assessment of any possible combination unaffordable. Therefore, the definition of a consensus to define the combinations that really deserve investigations is strongly suggested. From a toxicological point of view, the use of the Adverse-Outcome-Pathway (AOP) approach or the adoption of grouping criteria, such as read-across methodologies or other computational-based categorizing methods, might provide a convincing rational to support the early definition of combinations to be tested. Moreover, in order to improve the interpretability of the data, homogeneity in the expression of the results, as well as in the tested concentrations, used cellular models, and applied methods, should become a common objective for researchers dealing with these issues in the future.

In summary, *Alternaria* toxins in food are not yet regulated mainly as a consequence of the shortage of toxicological occurrence and exposure data. A more in-depth elucidation of their toxicity, taking into account the effects of chemical mixtures, will ensure a more precise evaluation of their effects on human health eventually resulting in a more reliable assessment of risks with an overall lower degree of uncertainty. In this framework, this review collected the main data available so far in terms of occurrence and combined actions of *Alternaria* mycotoxins and it highlighted that chemical mixture may significantly change the individual toxicity of mycotoxins. Notably, most of the combinations found naturally in food still need to be tested in terms of toxicity. Therefore, it is hard to infer with precision the actual toxicological effects due to the consumption of food contaminated by *Alternaria* mycotoxins. Nonetheless, the data presented here may serve as a ground to design further studies to deepen the knowledge about the toxicity of this class of mycotoxins and to support the assessment of risk taking into account the actual role of chemical mixtures. The proposed paradigm can be logically extended to the risk assessment of other mycotoxins, as the relevance of mixtures has been described also for other classes of mycotoxins.

Supplementary Materials: The following are available online at http://www.mdpi.com/2072-6651/11/11/640/s1, Table S1: Co-occurrence of *Alternaria* toxins in food.

Author Contributions: Conceptualization: F.C., C.D., L.D.; formal analysis: F.C.; data curation: F.C. and L.D.; writing—original draft preparation: F.C. and L.D.; writing—review and editing: G.G., G.A., E.V., D.M., C.A.; supervision: D.M., C.D.

Funding: This research received no external funding.

Acknowledgments: The study was partially supported by Fondazione Cariparma, under the TeachInParma Project. Moreover, the authors acknowledge the financial support of the Center for Studies in International and European Affairs of the University of Parma.

Conflicts of Interest: The authors declare no conflict of interest.

References

1. Berthiller, F.; Crews, C.; Dall'Asta, C.; de Saeger, S.; Haesaert, G.; Karlovsky, P.; Oswald, I.P.; Seefelder, W.; Speijers, G.; Stroka, J. Masked mycotoxins: A review. *Mol. Nutr. Food Res.* **2013**, *57*, 165–186. [CrossRef] [PubMed]
2. EFSA. Scientific Opinion on the risks for animal and public health related to the presence of Alternaria toxins in feed and food. *EFSA J.* **2011**, *9*, 2407. [CrossRef]
3. Enyiukwu, D.N.; Awurum, A.N.; Nwaneri, J.A. Mycotoxins in Stored Agricultural Products: Implications to Food Safety and Health and Prospects of Plant-derived Pesticides as Novel Approach to their Management. *Greener J. Microbiol. Antimicrob.* **2014**, *2*, 32–48. [CrossRef]
4. Eskola, M.; Kos, G.; Elliott, C.T.; Hajšlová, J.; Mayar, S.; Eskola, M.; Kos, G.; Elliott, C.T.; Hajšlová, J.; Mayar, S.; et al. Worldwide contamination of food-crops with mycotoxins: Validity of the widely cited 'FAO estimate' of 25%. *Crit. Rev. Food Sci. Nutr.* **2019**, 1–17. [CrossRef]
5. Van der Fels-Klerx, H.J.; Liu, C.; Battilani, P. Modelling climate change impacts on mycotoxin contamination. *World Mycotoxin J.* **2016**, *9*, 717–726. [CrossRef]
6. Dellafiora, L.; Dall'Asta, C. Forthcoming challenges in mycotoxins toxicology research for safer food-a need for multi-omics approach. *Toxins* **2017**, *9*, 18. [CrossRef] [PubMed]
7. Van Egmond, H.P.; Schothorst, R.C.; Jonker, M.A. Regulations relating to mycotoxins in food: Perspectives in a global and European context. *Anal. Bioanal. Chem.* **2007**, *389*, 147–157. [CrossRef]
8. Ostry, V. Alternaria mycotoxins: An overview of chemical characterization, producers, toxicity, analysis and occurrence in foodstuffs. *World Mycotoxin J.* **2008**, *1*, 175–188. [CrossRef]
9. Escrivá, L.; Oueslati, S.; Font, G.; Manyes, L. Alternaria Mycotoxins in Food and Feed: An Overview. *J. Food Qual.* **2017**, *2017*, 1569748. [CrossRef]
10. European Food Safety Authority; Arcella, D.; Eskola, M.; Gómez Ruiz, J.A. Dietary exposure assessment to Alternaria toxins in the European population. *EFSA J.* **2016**, *14*, 4654.
11. European Commission. Commission Regulation (EC) No 1881/2006 of 19 December 2006 setting maximum levels for certain contaminants in foodstuffs. *Off. J.* **2006**, 5–24.
12. Sanco, E. Summary report of the standing committee on the food chain and animal health held in brussels, 29 may 2012. *European Commission* **2012**, *2012*, 682729.
13. EFSA. *Call for Data on Alternaria Toxins in Food and Feed*; EFSA: Parma, Italy, 2016; pp. 3–4.
14. Alexander, J.; Benford, D.; Boobis, A.; Eskola, M.; Fink-Gremmels, J.; Fürst, P.; Heppner, C.; Schlatter, J.; van Leeuwen, R. Risk assessment of contaminants in food and feed. *EFSA J.* **2012**, *10*, s1004. [CrossRef]
15. Bottalico, A.; Logrieco, A. Toxigenic Alternaria species of economic importance. In *Mycotoxins in Agriculture and Food Safety*; Sinha, K.K., Bhatnagar, D., Eds.; Marcel Dekker: New York, NY, USA, 1998; pp. 65–108.
16. Scott, P.M. Analysis of Agricultural Commodities and Foods for Alternaria Mycotoxins. *J. AOAC Int.* **2001**, *84*, 1809–1817.
17. Fernández-Cruz, M.L.; Mansilla, M.L.; Tadeo, J.L. Mycotoxins in fruits and their processed products: Analysis, occurrence and health implications. *J. Adv. Res.* **2010**, *1*, 113–122. [CrossRef]

18. Fraeyman, S.; Croubels, S.; Devreese, M.; Antonissen, G. Emerging fusarium and alternaria mycotoxins: Occurrence, toxicity and toxicokinetics. *Toxins* **2017**, *9*, 228. [CrossRef] [PubMed]
19. Stinson, E.E.; Osman, S.F.; Heisler, E.G.; Siciliano, J.; Bills, D.D. Mycotoxin Production in Whole Tomatoes, Apples, Oranges, and Lemons. *J. Agric. Food Chem.* **1981**, *29*, 790–792. [CrossRef] [PubMed]
20. Puntscher, H.; Cobankovic, I.; Marko, D.; Warth, B. Quantitation of free and modified Alternaria mycotoxins in European food products by LC-MS/MS. *Food Control* **2019**, *102*, 157–165. [CrossRef]
21. Gotthardt, M.; Asam, S.; Gunkel, K.; Moghaddam, A.F.; Baumann, E.; Kietz, R.; Rychlik, M. Quantitation of Six Alternaria Toxins in Infant Foods Applying Stable Isotope Labeled Standards. *Front. Microbiol.* **2019**, *10*, 109. [CrossRef]
22. Gratz, S.W. Do plant-bound masked mycotoxins contribute to toxicity? *Toxins* **2017**, *9*, 85. [CrossRef]
23. Nathanail, A.V.; Syvähuoko, J.; Malachová, A.; Jestoi, M.; Varga, E.; Michlmayr, H.; Adam, G.; Sieviläinen, E.; Berthiller, F.; Peltonen, K. Simultaneous determination of major type A and B trichothecenes, zearalenone and certain modified metabolites in Finnish cereal grains with a novel liquid chromatography-tandem mass spectrometric method. *Anal. Bioanal. Chem.* **2015**, *407*, 4745–4755. [CrossRef] [PubMed]
24. Dellafiora, L.; Perotti, A.; Galaverna, G.; Buschini, A.; Dall'Asta, C. On the masked mycotoxin zearalenone-14-glucoside. Does the mask truly hide? *Toxicon* **2016**, *111*, 139–142. [CrossRef] [PubMed]
25. Dellafiora, L.; Galaverna, G.; Righi, F.; Cozzini, P.; Dall'Asta, C. Assessing the hydrolytic fate of the masked mycotoxin zearalenone-14-glucoside—A warning light for the need to look at the "maskedome". *Food Chem. Toxicol.* **2017**, *99*, 9–16. [CrossRef] [PubMed]
26. Puntscher, H.; Kütt, M.L.; Skrinjar, P.; Mikula, H.; Podlech, J.; Fröhlich, J.; Marko, D.; Warth, B. Tracking emerging mycotoxins in food: Development of an LC-MS/MS method for free and modified Alternaria toxins. *Anal. Bioanal. Chem.* **2018**, *410*, 4481–4494. [CrossRef]
27. Walravens, J.; Mikula, H.; Rychlik, M.; Asam, S.; Devos, T.; Ediage, E.N.; Di Mavungu, J.D.; Jacxsens, L.; Van Landschoot, A.; Vanhaecke, L.; et al. Validated UPLC-MS/MS Methods to Quantitate Free and Conjugated Alternaria Toxins in Commercially Available Tomato Products and Fruit and Vegetable Juices in Belgium. *J. Agric. Food Chem.* **2016**, *64*, 5101–5109. [CrossRef]
28. Sanzani, S.M.; Gallone, T.; Garganese, F.; Caruso, A.G.; Amenduni, M.; Ippolito, A. Contamination of fresh and dried tomato by Alternaria toxins in southern Italy. *Food Addit. Contam. Part A* **2019**, *36*, 789–799. [CrossRef]
29. Gambacorta, L.; Magistà, D.; Perrone, G.; Murgolo, S.; Logrieco, A.F.; Solfrizzo, M. Co-occurrence of toxigenic moulds, aflatoxins, ochratoxin A, Fusarium and Alternaria mycotoxins in fresh sweet peppers (Capsicum annuum) and their processed products. *World Mycotoxin J.* **2018**, *11*, 159–174. [CrossRef]
30. Ansari, A.A.; Shrivastava, A.K. Natural occurrence of Alternaria mycotoxins in sorghum and ragi from North Bihar, India. *Food Addit. Contam.* **1990**, *7*, 815–820. [CrossRef]
31. Müller, M.E.H.; Korn, U. Alternaria mycotoxins in wheat—A 10 years survey in the Northeast of Germany. *Food Control* **2013**, *34*, 191–197. [CrossRef]
32. Lou, J.; Fu, L.; Peng, Y.; Zhou, L. Metabolites from Alternaria fungi and their bioactivities. *Molecules* **2013**, *18*, 5891–5935. [CrossRef]
33. Shimshoni, J.A.; Cuneah, O.; Sulyok, M.; Krska, R.; Galon, N.; Sharir, B.; Shlosberg, A. Mycotoxins in corn and wheat silage in Israel. *Food Addit. Contam. Part A* **2013**, *30*, 1614–1625. [CrossRef] [PubMed]
34. Varga, E.; Glauner, T.; Berthiller, F.; Krska, R.; Schuhmacher, R.; Sulyok, M. Development and validation of a (semi-) quantitative UHPLC-MS/MS method for the determination of 191 mycotoxins and other fungal metabolites in almonds, hazelnuts, peanuts and pistachios. *Anal. Bioanal. Chem.* **2013**, *405*, 5087–5104. [CrossRef] [PubMed]
35. Mikušová, P.; Sulyok, M.; Šrobárová, A. Alternaria mycotoxins associated with grape berries in vitro and in situ. *Biologia* **2014**, *69*, 173–177. [CrossRef]
36. Asam, S.A.; Konitzer, K.K.; Schieberle, P.; Rychlik, M. Stable Isotope Dilution Assays of Alternariol and Alternariol Monomethyl Ether in Beverages. *J. Agric. Food Chem.* **2009**, *57*, 5152–5160. [CrossRef] [PubMed]
37. Juan, C.; Manes, J.; Font, G.; Juan-García, A. Determination of mycotoxins in fruit berry by-products using QuEChERS extraction method. *LWT Food Sci. Technol.* **2017**, *86*, 344–351. [CrossRef]
38. Zhao, K.; Shao, B.; Yang, D.; Li, F. Natural Occurrence of Four Alternaria Mycotoxins in Tomato- and Citrus-Based Foods in China. *J. Agric. Food Chem.* **2014**, *63*, 343–348. [CrossRef]

39. Scott, P.M.; Lawrence, G.A.; Lau, B.P. Analysis of wines, grape juices and cranberry juices for Alternaria toxins. *Mycotoxin Res.* **2006**, *22*, 142–147. [CrossRef]
40. Prelle, A.; Spadaro, D.; Garibaldi, A.; Gullino, L.M. A new method for detection of five alternaria toxins in food matrices based on LC—APCI-MS. *Food Chem.* **2013**, *140*, 161–167. [CrossRef]
41. López, P.; Venema, D.; de Rijk, T.; de Kok, A.; Scholten, J.M.; Mol, H.G.J.; de Nijs, M. Occurrence of Alternaria toxins in food products in The Netherlands. *Food Control* **2016**, *60*, 196–204. [CrossRef]
42. Veprikova, Z.; Zachariasova, M.; Dzuman, Z.; Zachariasova, A.; Fenclova, M.; Slavikova, P.; Vaclavikova, M.; Mastovska, K.; Hengst, D.; Hajslova, J. Mycotoxins in Plant-Based Dietary Supplements: Hidden Health Risk for Consumers. *J. Agric. Food Chem.* **2015**, *63*, 6633–6643. [CrossRef]
43. Lau, B.P.; Scott, P.M.; Lewis, D.A.; Kanhere, S.R.; Cleroux, C.; Roscoe, V.A. Liquid chromatography—Mass spectrometry and liquid chromatography—Tandem mass spectrometry of the Alternaria mycotoxins alternariol and alternariol monomethyl ether in fruit juices and beverages. *J. Chromatogr. A* **2003**, *998*, 119–131. [CrossRef]
44. Delgado, T.; Gómez-Cordovés, C. Natural occurrence of alternariol and alternariol methyl ether in Spanish apple juice concentrates. *J. Chromatogr. A* **1998**, *815*, 93–97. [CrossRef]
45. Pavón, M.Á.; Luna, A.; de la Cruz, S.; González, I.; Martín, R.; García, T. PCR-based assay for the detection of Alternaria species and correlation with HPLC determination of altenuene, alternariol and alternariol monomethyl ether production in tomato products. *Food Control* **2012**, *25*, 45–52. [CrossRef]
46. Hickert, S.; Bergmann, M.; Ersen, S.; Cramer, B.; Humpf, H. Survey of Alternaria toxin contamination in food from the German market, using a rapid HPLC-MS/MS approach. *Mycotoxin Res.* **2016**, *32*, 7–18. [CrossRef]
47. da Cruz Cabral, L.; Terminiello, L.; Pinto, V.F.; Nielsen, K.F.; Patriarca, A. Natural occurrence of mycotoxins and toxigenic capacity of Alternaria strains from mouldy peppers. *Int. J. Food Microbiol.* **2016**, *236*, 155–160. [CrossRef]
48. Oviedo, M.S.; Barros, G.G.; Chulze, S.N.; Ramirez, M.L. Natural occurrence of alternariol and alternariol monomethyl ether in soya beans. *Mycotoxin Res.* **2012**, *28*, 169–174. [CrossRef]
49. Juan, C.; Oueslati, S.; Mañes, J. Evaluation of Alternaria mycotoxins in strawberries: Quantification and storage condition. *Food Addit. Contam. Part A* **2016**, *33*, 861–868. [CrossRef]
50. Magnani, R.F.; De Souza, G.D.; Rodrigues-Filho, E. Analysis of Alternariol and Alternariol Monomethyl Ether on Flavedo and Albedo Tissues of Tangerines (Citrus reticulata) with Symptoms of Alternaria Brown Spot. *J. Agric. Food Chem.* **2007**, *55*, 4980–4986. [CrossRef]
51. Hasan, H.A.H. Alternaria mycotoxins in black rot lesion of tomato fruit: Conditions and regulation of their production. *Mycopathologia* **1995**, *130*, 171–177. [CrossRef]
52. Noser, J.; Schneider, P.; Rother, M.; Schmutz, H. Determination of six Alternaria toxins with UPLC-MS/MS and their occurrence in tomatoes and tomato products from the Swiss market. *Mycotoxin Res.* **2011**, *27*, 265–271. [CrossRef]
53. Zhao, K.; Shao, B.; Yang, D.; Li, F.; Zhu, J. Natural occurrence of Alternaria toxins in wheat-based products and their dietary exposure in China. *PLoS ONE* **2015**, *10*, e0132019. [CrossRef] [PubMed]
54. Kayode, O.F.; Sulyok, M.; Fapohunda, S.O.; Ezekiel, C.N.; Krska, R.; Oguntona, C.R.B. Surveillance Mycotoxins and fungal metabolites in groundnut- and maize-based snacks from Nigeria. *Food Addit. Contam. Part B* **2013**, *6*, 294–300. [CrossRef] [PubMed]
55. Azcarate, M.P.; Patriarca, A.; Terminiello, L.; Fernandez Pinto, V. Alternaria Toxins in Wheat during the 2004 to 2005 Argentinean Harvest. *J. Food Prot.* **2008**, *71*, 1262–1265. [CrossRef] [PubMed]
56. Li, F.; Yoshizawa, T. Alternaria Mycotoxins in Weathered Wheat from China. *J. Agric. Food Chem.* **2000**, *48*, 2920–2924. [CrossRef] [PubMed]
57. Wang, Y.; Nie, J.; Yan, Z.; Li, Z.; Cheng, Y.; Chang, W. Occurrence and co-occurrence of mycotoxins in nuts and dried fruits from China. *Food Control* **2018**, *88*, 181–189. [CrossRef]
58. Wei, D.; Wang, Y.; Jiang, D.; Feng, X.; Li, J.; Wang, M. Survey of Alternaria Toxins and Other Mycotoxins in Dried Fruits in China. *Toxins* **2017**, *9*, 200. [CrossRef]
59. Ezekiel, C.N.; Sulyok, M.; Warth, B.; Krska, R. Multi-microbial metabolites in fonio millet (acha) and sesame seeds in Plateau State, Nigeria. *Eur. Food Res. Technol.* **2012**, *235*, 285–293. [CrossRef]
60. Chulze, S.N.; Torres, A.M.; Dalcero, A.N.A.M.; Etcheverry, M.G.; Ramirez, M.L.; Farnochi, M.C. Alternaria Mycotoxins in Sunflower Seeds: Incidence and Distribution of the Toxins in Oil and Meal. *J. Food Prot.* **1995**, *58*, 1133–1135. [CrossRef]

61. Hickert, S.; Hermes, L.; Marques, L.M.M.; Focke, C.; Cramer, B.; Lopes, N.P.; Flett, B.; Humpf, H.-U. Alternaria toxins in South African sunflower seeds: Cooperative study. *Mycotoxin Res.* **2017**, *33*, 309–321. [CrossRef]
62. Bhat, R.; Rai, R.V.; Karim, A.A. Mycotoxins in Food and Feed: Present Status and Future Concerns. *Compr. Rev. Food Sci. Food Saf.* **2010**, *9*, 57–81. [CrossRef]
63. Janić Hajnal, E.; Čolović, R.; Pezo, L.; Orčić, D.; Vukmirović, D.; Mastilović, J. Possibility of Alternaria toxins reduction by extrusion processing of whole wheat flour. *Food Chem.* **2016**, *213*, 784–790. [CrossRef] [PubMed]
64. Bauer, J.I.; Gross, M.; Gottschalk, C.; Usleber, E. Investigations on the occurrence of mycotoxins in beer. *Food Control* **2016**, *63*, 135–139. [CrossRef]
65. Fanning, R.A.; Sheehan, F.; Leyden, C.; Duffy, N.; Iglesias-Martinez, L.F.; Carey, M.F.; Campion, D.P.; O'Connor, J.J. A role for adrenergic receptors in the uterotonic effects of ergometrine in isolated human term nonlaboring myometrium. *Anesth. Analg.* **2017**, *124*, 1581–1588. [CrossRef] [PubMed]
66. Müller, M.E.H.; Urban, K.; Köppen, R.; Siegel, D.; Korn, U.; Koch, M. Mycotoxins as antagonistic or supporting agents in the interaction between phytopathogenic Fusarium and Alternaria fungi. *World Mycotoxin J.* **2015**, *8*, 311–321. [CrossRef]
67. Juan, C.; Covarelli, L.; Beccari, G.; Colasante, V.; Mañes, J. Simultaneous analysis of twenty-six mycotoxins in durum wheat grain from Italy. *Food Control* **2016**, *62*, 322–329. [CrossRef]
68. Zwickel, T.; Kahl, S.M.; Rychlik, M.; Müller, M.E.H. Chemotaxonomy of mycotoxigenic small-spored Alternaria fungi—Do multitoxin mixtures act as an indicator for species differentiation? *Front. Microbiol.* **2018**, *9*, 1368. [CrossRef]
69. Pero, R.W.; Posner, H.; Blois, M.; Harvan, D.; Spalding, J.W. Toxicity of metabolites produced by the "Alternaria". *Environ. Health Perspect.* **1973**, *4*, 87–94. [CrossRef]
70. Smith, E.R.; Fredrickson, T.N.; Hadidian, Z. Toxic effects of the sodium and the *N*,*N'*-dibenzylethylenediamine salts of tenuazonic acid (NSC-525816 and NSC-82260). *Cancer Chemother. Rep.* **1968**, *52*, 579.
71. Woodey, M.A.; Chu, F.S. Toxicology of Alternaria mycotoxins. In *Alternaria Biology, Plant Diseases and Metabolites*; Elsevier: Amsterdam, The Netherlands, 1992; pp. 409–434.
72. Griffin, G.; Chu, F. Toxicity of the Alternaria Metabolites Alternariol, Alternariol Methyl Ether, Altenuene, and Tenuazonic Acid in the Chicken Embryo Assay. *Appl. Environ. Microbiol.* **1983**, *46*, 1420–1422.
73. Giambrone, J.J.; Davis, N.D.; Diener, U.L. Effect of tenuazonic acid on young chickens. *Poult. Sci.* **1978**, *57*, 1554–1558. [CrossRef]
74. Benford, D.J. Risk Assessment of Chemical Contaminants and Residues in Food. In *Persistent Organic Pollutants and Toxic Metals in Foods*; Woodhead Publishing: Cambridge, UK, 2017; pp. 3–13. ISBN 9780081006740.
75. Chou, T.-C. Theoretical Basis, Experimental Design, and Computerized Simulation of Synergism and Antagonism in Drug Combination Studies. *Pharmacol. Rev.* **2006**, *58*, 621–681. [CrossRef] [PubMed]
76. Webb, J.L. *Enzyme and Metabolic Inhibitors*; Academic Press: New York, NY, USA, 1963.
77. Chou, T.-C.; Talalayi, P. Quantitative analysis of dose-effect relationships: The combined effects of multiple drugs or enzyme inhibitors. *Adv. Enzyme Regul.* **1984**, *22*, 27–55. [CrossRef]
78. Fehr, M.; Pahlke, G.; Fritz, J.; Christensen, M.O.; Boege, F.; Altemöller, M.; Podlech, J.; Marko, D. Alternariol acts as a topoisomerase poison, preferentially affecting the IIα isoform. *Mol. Nutr. Food Res.* **2009**, *53*, 441–451. [CrossRef] [PubMed]
79. Lehmann, L.; Wagner, J.; Metzler, M. Estrogenic and clastogenic potential of the mycotoxin alternariol in cultured mammalian cells. *Food Chem. Toxicol.* **2006**, *44*, 398–408. [CrossRef]
80. Brugger, E.M.; Wagner, J.; Schumacher, D.M.; Koch, K.; Podlech, J.; Metzler, M.; Lehmann, L. Mutagenicity of the mycotoxin alternariol in cultured mammalian cells. *Toxicol. Lett.* **2006**, *164*, 221–230. [CrossRef]
81. Schuchardt, S.; Ziemann, C.; Hansen, T. Combined toxicokinetic and in vivo genotoxicity study on Alternaria toxins. *EFSA Support. Publ.* **2014**, *11*, 679E. [CrossRef]
82. Pommier, Y. Drugging Topoisomerases: Lessons and Challenges. *ACS Chem. Biol.* **2013**, *8*, 82–95. [CrossRef]
83. Fernández-Blanco, C.; Font, G.; Ruiz, M.J. Role of quercetin on Caco-2 cells against cytotoxic effects of alternariol and alternariol monomethyl ether. *Food Chem. Toxicol.* **2016**, *89*, 60–66. [CrossRef]
84. Tiessen, C.; Ellmer, D.; Mikula, H.; Pahlke, G.; Warth, B.; Gehrke, H.; Zimmermann, K.; Heiss, E.; Fröhlich, J.; Marko, D. Impact of phase I metabolism on uptake, oxidative stress and genotoxicity of the emerging mycotoxin alternariol and its monomethyl ether in esophageal cells. *Arch. Toxicol.* **2017**, *91*, 1213–1226. [CrossRef]

85. Dellafiora, L.; Dall'Asta, C.; Cruciani, G.; Galaverna, G.; Cozzini, P. Molecular modelling approach to evaluate poisoning of topoisomerase I by alternariol derivatives. *Food Chem.* **2015**, *189*, 93–101. [CrossRef]
86. Schwarz, C.; Kreutzer, M.; Marko, D. Minor contribution of alternariol, alternariol monomethyl ether and tenuazonic acid to the genotoxic properties of extracts from Alternaria alternata infested rice. *Toxicol. Lett.* **2012**, *214*, 46–52. [CrossRef] [PubMed]
87. Schwarz, C.; Tiessen, C.; Kreutzer, M.; Stark, T.; Hofmann, T.; Marko, D. Characterization of a genotoxic impact compound in alternaria alternata infested rice as altertoxin II. *Arch. Toxicol.* **2012**, *86*, 1911–1925. [CrossRef] [PubMed]
88. Fleck, S.C.; Burkhardt, B.; Pfeiffer, E.; Metzler, M. Alternaria toxins: Altertoxin II is a much stronger mutagen and DNA strand breaking mycotoxin than alternariol and its methyl ether in cultured mammalian cells. *Toxicol. Lett.* **2012**, *214*, 27–32. [CrossRef] [PubMed]
89. Fleck, S.C.; Sauter, F.; Pfeiffer, E.; Metzler, M.; Hartwig, A.; Köberle, B. DNA damage and repair kinetics of the Alternaria mycotoxins alternariol, altertoxin II and stemphyltoxin III in cultured cells. *Mutat. Res. Genet. Toxicol. Environ. Mutagen.* **2016**, *798–799*, 27–34. [CrossRef] [PubMed]
90. Aichinger, G.; Krüger, F.; Puntscher, H.; Preindl, K.; Warth, B.; Marko, D. Naturally occurring mixtures of Alternaria toxins: Anti-estrogenic and genotoxic effects in vitro. *Arch. Toxicol.* **2019**, *93*, 3021–3031. [CrossRef]
91. Vejdovszky, K.; Hahn, K.; Braun, D.; Warth, B.; Marko, D. Synergistic estrogenic effects of Fusarium and Alternaria mycotoxins in vitro. *Arch. Toxicol.* **2017**, *91*, 1447–1460. [CrossRef]
92. Dellafiora, L.; Warth, B.; Schmidt, V.; Del Favero, G.; Mikula, H.; Fröhlich, J.; Marko, D. An integrated in silico/in vitro approach to assess the xenoestrogenic potential of Alternaria mycotoxins and metabolites. *Food Chem.* **2018**, *248*, 253–261. [CrossRef]
93. Stypuła-Trębas, S.; Minta, M.; Radko, L.; Jedziniak, P.; Posyniak, A. Nonsteroidal mycotoxin alternariol is a full androgen agonist in the yeast reporter androgen bioassay. *Environ. Toxicol. Pharmacol.* **2017**, *55*, 208–211. [CrossRef]
94. Dellafiora, L.; Galaverna, G.; Cruciani, G.; Dall'Asta, C. A computational study toward the "personalized" activity of alternariol—Does it matter for safe food at individual level? *Food Chem. Toxicol.* **2019**, *130*, 199–206. [CrossRef]
95. Frizzell, C.; Ndossi, D.; Kalayou, S.; Eriksen, G.S.; Verhaegen, S.; Sørlie, M.; Elliott, C.T.; Ropstad, E.; Connolly, L. An in vitro investigation of endocrine disrupting effects of the mycotoxin alternariol. *Toxicol. Appl. Pharmacol.* **2013**, *271*, 64–71. [CrossRef]
96. Grover, S.; Lawrence, C.B. The Alternaria alternata mycotoxin alternariol suppresses lipopolysaccharide-induced inflammation. *Int. J. Mol. Sci.* **2017**, *18*, 1577. [CrossRef] [PubMed]
97. Kollarova, J.; Cenk, E.; Schmutz, C.; Marko, D. The mycotoxin alternariol suppresses lipopolysaccharide-induced inflammation in THP-1 derived macrophages targeting the NF-κB signalling pathway. *Arch. Toxicol.* **2018**, *92*, 3347–3358. [CrossRef] [PubMed]
98. Zhou, B.; Qiang, S. Environmental, genetic and cellular toxicity of tenuazonic acid isolated from Alternaria alternata. *Afr. J. Biotechnol.* **2008**, *7*, 1151–1156.
99. Bensassi, F.; Gallerne, C.; El Dein, O.S.; Hajlaoui, M.R.; Bacha, H.; Lemaire, C. Combined effects of alternariols mixture on human colon carcinoma cells. *Toxicol. Mech. Methods* **2015**, *25*, 56–62. [CrossRef] [PubMed]
100. Vejdovszky, K.; Sack, M.; Jarolim, K.; Aichinger, G.; Somoza, M.M.; Marko, D. In vitro combinatory effects of the Alternaria mycotoxins alternariol and altertoxin II and potentially involved miRNAs. *Toxicol. Lett.* **2017**, *267*, 45–52. [CrossRef] [PubMed]
101. Fernández-Blanco, C.; Font, G.; Ruiz, M.J. Interaction effects of enniatin B, deoxinivalenol and alternariol in Caco-2 cells. *Toxicol. Lett.* **2016**, *241*, 38–48. [CrossRef]
102. McKinney, J.D.; Richard, A.; Waller, C.; Newman, M.C.; Gerberick, F. The Practice of Structure Activity Relationships (SAR) in Toxicology. *Toxicol. Sci.* **2000**, *56*, 8–17. [CrossRef]
103. Juan-García, A.; Juan, C.; Manyes, L.; Ruiz, M.J. Binary and tertiary combination of alternariol, 3-acetyl-deoxynivalenol and 15-acetyl-deoxynivalenol on HepG2 cells: Toxic effects and evaluation of degradation products. *Toxicol. In Vitro* **2016**, *34*, 264–273. [CrossRef]
104. Vejdovszky, K.; Warth, B.; Sulyok, M.; Marko, D. Non-synergistic cytotoxic effects of Fusarium and Alternaria toxin combinations in Caco-2 cells. *Toxicol. Lett.* **2016**, *241*, 1–8. [CrossRef]

105. Rocha, O.; Ansari, K.; Doohan, F.M. Effects of trichothecene mycotoxins on eukaryotic cells: A review. *Food Addit. Contam.* **2005**, *22*, 369–378. [CrossRef]
106. Dellafiora, L.; Galaverna, G.; Dall'Asta, C. In silico analysis sheds light on the structural basis underlying the ribotoxicity of trichothecenes—A tool for supporting the hazard identification process. *Toxicol. Lett.* **2017**, *270*, 80–87. [CrossRef] [PubMed]
107. Solhaug, A.; Karlsøen, L.M.; Holme, J.A.; Kristoffersen, A.B.; Eriksen, G.S. Immunomodulatory effects of individual and combined mycotoxins in the THP-1 cell line. *Toxicol. In Vitro* **2016**, *36*, 120–132. [CrossRef] [PubMed]
108. Pistol, G.C.; Gras, M.A.; Marin, D.E.; Israel-Roming, F.; Stancu, M.; Taranu, I. Natural feed contaminant zearalenone decreases the expressions of important pro-and anti-inflammatory mediators and mitogen-activated protein kinase/NF-κB signalling molecules in pigs. *Br. J. Nutr.* **2014**, *111*, 452–464. [CrossRef] [PubMed]
109. Pestka, J.J. Deoxynivalenol-induced proinflammatory gene expression: Mechanisms and pathological sequelae. *Toxins* **2010**, *2*, 1300–1317. [CrossRef] [PubMed]
110. Vejdovszky, K.; Schmidt, V.; Warth, B.; Marko, D. Combinatory estrogenic effects between the isoflavone genistein and the mycotoxins zearalenone and alternariol in vitro. *Mol. Nutr. Food Res.* **2017**, *61*, 1600526. [CrossRef]
111. Dellafiora, L.; Aichinger, G.; Geib, E.; Sánchez-Barrionuevo, L.; Brock, M.; Cánovas, D.; Dall'Asta, C.; Marko, D. Hybrid in silico/in vitro target fishing to assign function to "orphan" compounds of food origin—The case of the fungal metabolite atromentin. *Food Chem.* **2019**, *270*, 61–69. [CrossRef]
112. Dellafiora, L.; Ruotolo, R.; Perotti, A.; Cirlini, M.; Galaverna, G.; Cozzini, P.; Buschini, A.; Dall'Asta, C. Molecular insights on xenoestrogenic potential of zearalenone-14-glucoside through a mixed in vitro/in silico approach. *Food Chem. Toxicol.* **2017**, *108*, 257–266. [CrossRef]
113. EFSA Panel on Contaminants in the Food Chain (CONTAM); Alexander, J.; Barregard, L.; Bignami, M.; Ceccatelli, S.; Cottrill, B.; Dinovi, M.; Edler, L.; Grasl-Kraupp, B.; Hogstrand, C.; et al. Appropriateness to set a group health-based guidance value for zearalenone and its modified forms. *EFSA J.* **2016**, *14*, 4425.
114. Aichinger, G.; Beisl, J.; Marko, D. Genistein and delphinidin antagonize the genotoxic effects of the mycotoxin alternariol in human colon carcinoma cells. *Mol. Nutr. Food Res.* **2017**, *61*, 1600462. [CrossRef]
115. Chen, W.; Lin, Y.C.; Ma, X.Y.; Jiang, Z.Y.; Lan, S.P. High concentrations of genistein exhibit pro-oxidant effects in primary muscle cells through mechanisms involving 5-lipoxygenase-mediated production of reactive oxygen species. *Food Chem. Toxicol.* **2014**, *67*, 72–79. [CrossRef]
116. Fukumoto, L.R.; Mazza, G. Assessing antioxidant and prooxidant activities of phenolic compounds. *J. Agric. Food Chem.* **2000**, *48*, 3597–3604. [CrossRef] [PubMed]
117. Braga, A.R.C.; Murador, D.C.; de Souza Mesquita, L.M.; de Rosso, V.V. Bioavailability of anthocyanins: Gaps in knowledge, challenges and future research. *J. Food Compos. Anal.* **2018**, *68*, 31–40. [CrossRef]
118. Bitsch, R.; Netzel, M.; Frank, T.; Strass, G.; Bitsch, I. Bioavailability and Biokinetics of Anthocyanins From Red Grape Juice and Red Wine. *J. Biomed. Biotechnol.* **2004**, *2004*, 293–298. [CrossRef] [PubMed]
119. Aichinger, G.; Puntscher, H.; Beisl, J.; Kütt, M.L.; Warth, B.; Marko, D. Delphinidin protects colon carcinoma cells against the genotoxic effects of the mycotoxin altertoxin II. *Toxicol. Lett.* **2018**, *284*, 136–142. [CrossRef]
120. Jan, A.T.; Kamli, M.R.; Murtaza, I.; Singh, J.B.; Ali, A.; Haq, Q.M.R. Dietary flavonoid quercetin and associated health benefits-An overview. *Food Rev. Int.* **2010**, *26*, 302–317. [CrossRef]
121. Jeong, Y.M.; Choi, Y.G.; Kim, D.S.; Park, S.H.; Yoon, J.A.; Kwon, S.B.; Park, E.S.; Park, K.C. Cytoprotective effect of green tea extract and quercetin against hydrogen peroxide-induced oxidative stress. *Arch. Pharm. Res.* **2005**, *28*, 1251–1256. [CrossRef]
122. Vila-donat, P.; Fernández-blanco, C.; Sagratini, G.; Font, G.; Ruiz, M.-J. Effects of Soyasaponin I and soyasaponins-rich extract on the Alternariol- induced cytotoxicity on Caco-2 cells. *Food Chem. Toxicol.* **2015**, *77*, 44–49. [CrossRef]
123. Rosenblum, E.R.; Stauber, R.E.; Van Thiel, D.H.; Campbell, I.M.; Gavaler, J.S. Assessment of the Estrogenic Activity of Phytoestrogens Isolated from Bourbon and Beer. *Alcohol. Clin. Exp. Res.* **1993**, *17*, 1207–1209. [CrossRef]
124. Karabín, M.; Hudcová, T.; Jelínek, L.; Dostálek, P. Biologically Active Compounds from Hops and Prospects for Their Use. *Compr. Rev. Food Sci. Food Saf.* **2016**, *15*, 542–567. [CrossRef]

125. Milligan, S.R.; Kalita, J.C.; Pocock, V.; Van De Kauter, V.; Stevens, J.F.; Deinzer, M.L.; Rong, H.; De Keukeleire, D. The Endocrine Activities of 8-Prenylnaringenin and Related Hop (*Humulus lupulus* L.) Flavonoids. *J. Clin. Endocrinol. Metab.* **2000**, *85*, 4912–4915. [CrossRef]
126. Aichinger, G.; Beisl, J.; Marko, D. The Hop Polyphenols Xanthohumol and 8-Prenyl-Naringenin Antagonize the Estrogenic Effects of Fusarium Mycotoxins in Human Endometrial Cancer Cells. *Front. Nutr.* **2018**, *5*, 85. [CrossRef] [PubMed]
127. King, R.E.; Bomser, J.A.; Min, D.B. Bioactivity of Resveratrol. *Compr. Rev. Food Sci. Food Saf.* **2006**, *5*, 65–70. [CrossRef]
128. De Waard, W.J.; Aarts, J.M.M.J.G.; Peijnenburg, A.C.M.; De Kok, T.M.C.M.; Van Schooten, F.J.; Hoogenboom, L.A.P. Ah receptor agonist activity in frequently consumed food items. *Food Addit. Contam. Part A* **2008**, *25*, 779–787. [CrossRef] [PubMed]
129. Schreck, I.; Deigendesch, U.; Burkhardt, B.; Marko, D.; Weiss, C. The Alternaria mycotoxins alternariol and alternariol methyl ether induce cytochrome P450 1A1 and apoptosis in murine hepatoma cells dependent on the aryl hydrocarbon receptor. *Arch. Toxicol.* **2012**, *86*, 625–632. [CrossRef]
130. Zhang, S.; Qin, C.; Safe, S.H. Flavonoids as aryl hydrocarbon receptor agonists/antagonists: Effects of structure and cell context. *Environ. Health Perspect.* **2003**, *111*, 1877–1882. [CrossRef]
131. Ashida, H.; Fukuda, I.; Yamashita, T.; Kanazawa, K. Flavones and flavonols at dietary levels inhibit a transformation of aryl hydrocarbon receptor induced by dioxin. *FEBS Lett.* **2000**, *476*, 213–217. [CrossRef]
132. Bandele, O.J.; Clawson, S.J.; Osheroff, N. Dietary polyphenols as topoisomerase II poisons: B ring and C ring substituents determine the mechanism of enzyme-mediated DNA cleavage enhancement. *Chem. Res. Toxicol.* **2008**, *21*, 1253–1260. [CrossRef]
133. López-Lázaro, M.; Willmore, E.; Austin, C.A. The dietary flavonoids myricetin and fisetin act as dual inhibitors of DNA topoisomerases I and II in cells. *Mutat. Res. Genet. Toxicol. Environ. Mutagen.* **2010**, *696*, 41–47. [CrossRef]
134. Bandele, O.J.; Osheroff, N. Bioflavonoids as poisons of human topoisomerase II alpha and II beta. *Biochemistry* **2007**, *46*, 6097–6108. [CrossRef]
135. Leone, S.; Basso, E.; Polticelli, F.; Cozzi, R. Resveratrol acts as a topoisomerase II poison in human glioma cells. *Int. J. Cancer* **2012**, *131*, E173–E178. [CrossRef]

MDPI
St. Alban-Anlage 66
4052 Basel
Switzerland
Tel. +41 61 683 77 34
Fax +41 61 302 89 18
www.mdpi.com

Toxins Editorial Office
E-mail: toxins@mdpi.com
www.mdpi.com/journal/toxins

www.ingramcontent.com/pod-product-compliance
Lightning Source LLC
LaVergne TN
LVHW070408100526
838202LV00014B/1413